THE PERFECT VAGINA

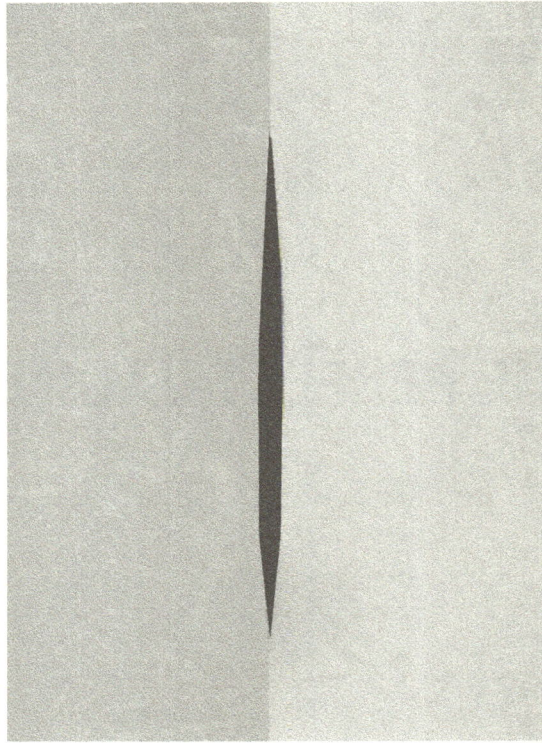

Figure 0.1. *A Clean Slit*, image by Jessica Smith, 2016.
Reproduced with permission from Jessica Smith.

I bet you're worried. *I* was worried. That's why I began this piece.
I was worried about vaginas. I was worried about what we think about
vaginas, and even more worried that we don't think about them.
I was worried about my own vagina. It needed a context of other vaginas—
a community, a culture of vaginas. There's so much darkness and
secrecy surrounding them—like the Bermuda Triangle.
Nobody ever reports back from there.

THE VAGINA MONOLOGUES (ENSLER 2001, 3)

THE PERFECT VAGINA

Cosmetic Surgery in the Twenty-First Century

—⁓—

lindy mcdougall

INDIANA UNIVERSITY PRESS

This book is a publication of

Indiana University Press
Office of Scholarly Publishing
Herman B Wells Library 350
1320 East 10th Street
Bloomington, Indiana 47405 USA

iupress.org

Manufactured in the United States of America

Cataloging information is available from the Library of Congress.

ISBN 978-0-253-05611-5 (hardback)
ISBN 978-0-253-05613-9 (paperback)
ISBN 978-0-253-05612-2 (ebook)

First Printing 2021

CONTENTS

ACKNOWLEDGMENTS

AN ACADEMIC BOOK IS ASSUMED to be the work solely of the individual researcher and writer, but this is far from an accurate description of what has been a lengthy and subsuming process. I wish to thank the institutions and individuals who supported me financially, intellectually, and emotionally as I wrote this book. I am indebted to many people, among them my informants and colleagues. Macquarie University and the Australian Anthropological Society have been particularly supportive of my project, as has Indiana University Press.

However, this book, with its focus on female genitalia, belongs to the four men in my life: my three gorgeous sons—Hunter, Lachlan, and Caleb—and even more so to Peter, who reads all I write and whose opinions I value above all others. I dedicate this book to them. For my sons, it would not have been easy growing up with a mother who researches vulvas, especially when she left illustrated books of them lying around the house, but as they have entered their own sexual and romantic lives, I believe it has been a good thing, and they have never faltered in their support of me.

Three exceptional academics from Macquarie University helped to shape this manuscript: Lisa Wynn, Greg Downey, and Victoria Loblay. They liberally provided their insights into my research and writing. Lisa Wynn was endlessly generous with her time, intellectual stimulation, and directions (and we share a love of nature, children, and issues outside the academy). Greg Downey helped me situate my writing anthropologically and provided the scaffolding for this book. In earlier drafts of this work, Victoria Loblay was indispensable, assisting with editing and pointing out where my arguments wandered off track. Many thanks also to Kirsten Bell and Alexander Edmonds, who inspired me to pursue this enquiry many years ago.

Being part of Macquarie University over many years has been enriching for me, and there are many fellow staff members and students I would like to acknowledge, but they are too numerous to mention. I have enjoyed the collegiate nature of our encounters. Particular thanks, however, go to Michaela Stockey-Bridge and Sumant Badami for making even the worst days sunny as we shared ideas, coffees, and laughs. Payel Ray, the anthropology administrator, was endlessly helpful and has become a firm friend. Many thanks, also, to Wendy Monaghan for her meticulous editing services and Frances D'Arcy-Tehan for sharing resources with me.

Most importantly, I wish to acknowledge my extremely generous informants. I shared some especially intimate moments with women, and I was amazed that so many physicians were happy to discuss the topic with me. Without the participation of my informants, there would be no book.

PROLOGUE

Mandy's Story

MANDY WAS ONE OF THE first women I spoke with in my endeavor to gain a further understanding of why female genital cosmetic surgery, particularly labiaplasty, has increased in popularity in Australia (and globally). I wanted to know how women discover that this surgery is available, where it is promoted and for what reasons, why more women are anxious about the form and function of their genitalia today, and why they consequently seek cosmetic surgery. Also, I wanted to explore the role of the medical profession in the rise of female genital cosmetic surgery.

When I asked Mandy why she was considering having genital surgery, she replied, "I'm interested in vaginal tightening to repair and restore my bits after naturally delivering my children. This is for a combination of sexual enhancement, for myself and my husband, as well as to restore my weakened pelvic floor. I'm also interested in labiaplasty as I have always been extremely self-conscious about how I look, so much so that I hardly ever let my husband see me naked—we have been together eight years and married for five—and I never, *ever*, let anyone go down on me."

As I listened to Mandy's reasoning, I endeavored to hide my astonishment at her extreme self-consciousness within a marriage. When explaining how she became ashamed and embarrassed about her genital appearance, Mandy pinpointed one encounter as the root of her genital anxiety: "I had a bad experience with a boy when I was eighteen, which was probably the beginning of my body image issues. He made negative comments about my protruding labia minora, and I have never been able to get past it, even after ten years with a loving partner. During sex ed at school, it was very well explained that some girls are innies and some are outies.[1] After the incident when I was eighteen, though, I thought I was wrong, that I was ugly and abnormal for being an outie. I think it certainly has had an impact on my confidence. I mean, I think I was twenty-five or twenty-six before I had my first Pap smear. I just couldn't bring myself to do that, to have someone look at me."

Discovering that surgery was available to "correct" her condition confirmed Mandy's feelings about herself. "It's only recently that I've realized most women are probably more like me, but that doesn't change the way I feel about myself," she said. "If done for the right reasons, which I believe mine are, cosmetic surgery can enhance and improve a person's sexual activities and self-esteem. It should not be done to please someone else, although I know this is probably the case for many women."

"Have you only thought of surgery since you've had your children?" I asked.

Mandy replied, "Um, well I think a few years ago, I heard it mentioned on a TV program. That was the first time I had heard of there being this type of surgery, labiaplasty. Um, and I thought, 'I'd like to have that, but I probably never will,' because at that stage I don't think I had even met my husband, and I couldn't bring myself to be naked—it was not me at all. But it has hung in the back of my mind, and there has been a lot more about it on the internet and on those TV programs, definitely.

"I can't even remember what I looked like as a child, but from what I have read, a girl's labia minora get bigger during puberty, so I don't know if that happened to me or not because I don't remember what I looked like before. I knew what I looked like by the time I was fourteen or fifteen, and I was told that I was normal, and I accepted it. But later I felt, given the issue that I had [with the comments from the boy—she gave me no more details of the incident] and other people's opinions, possibly even media, magazines and stuff—but I don't remember looking at any porn and things, I don't think I saw much even at university—but I think those things probably compounded it as well as my thinking that, 'Oh, they [her labia] are wrong; I am abnormal.'"

I asked Mandy if anyone else had ever commented on her labia. She said, "My husband commented to me once. I don't know how much of it is inexperience on his part, because both of us had been with very few people before we met each other. We have only been with a handful of people each, and he didn't comment, like, he was just . . . can I be um, um, candid?"

"Yes, of course," I replied.

"I had knickers on, and he was just brushing my leg and then moved his hand up, and he said, 'Oh, what's that?' [*giggles*], feeling it through my knickers, and I thought, 'Oh!' It wasn't even that long ago, probably a couple of years into the relationship. It might have been something he had noticed but hadn't had the guts to really ask me about up till then. I don't know."

Like the rest of the women whose stories are featured in this book, Mandy researched female genital cosmetic surgery on the internet, contacted surgeons, and watched clips on YouTube and television programs such as *The Perfect Vagina* (2008), a British documentary exploring labiaplasty.

"You wouldn't want to go in blind," she said. "After the kids go to bed at seven o'clock, I guess I can either watch TV, play on my computer, or read a book. My husband is often not here three or four nights a week as he also does shift work. With the kids, I can't go anywhere, so I have time to explore what I am interested in. I am just making sure that I am doing it [genital surgery] for me, not for anyone else. I think that I am, but I am a bit concerned about where my feelings come from."

"Because you had that experience when you were eighteen?" I asked.

"Yeah, yep." Mandy laughed softly. "It is the same thing, even with simple things like haircuts and waxing. Yes, we do it for ourselves, but who are we really trying to impress?"

"How would you convince yourself that you are doing it for the right reasons?"

"I think that [in] the last couple of months my motivations have changed slightly. What I am more interested in now is vaginoplasty rather than labiaplasty because of having my kids. Having them so close together—I don't know whether that makes me any different to people who have them far apart—but I am certainly not in any way, shape, or form anything like I was before childbirth and, you know, that was always going to be the case. I didn't expect to have children and stay the same. What I am looking at putting myself through is not necessary—it is not really medical—it is for my own sort of satisfaction and for my husband as well."

Mandy has had numerous noncosmetic surgical procedures. She comes from a medical family; her father is a doctor. "I am not shy of the needle or the knife," she remarked.

I mentioned to Mandy that leading medical bodies, such as the Royal Australian and New Zealand College of Obstetricians and Gynaecologists, caution against female genital cosmetic surgery unless it is for what are purportedly medical reasons.

Mandy retorted, "You can make anything into a medical problem even if the motivations are entirely separate. I can say it is all to do with incontinence or problems with sex, and that would be perfectly acceptable, and then I could say, 'While you are down there can you please tidy up my labia?'" She laughed.

When I asked about her husband's opinion, Mandy said, "He says, you know, he says he has no problem with me, and if it would make . . . It's a joint decision. He says he loves me however I look but feels at a loss to help me with my body issues. He would do anything to make me happy. I think he thinks the thing that would make it better for him is if my confidence improved. If I feel that I look good, and I feel good, then I am likely to be less inhibited and more confident and make the first move."

"Sexually?"

"Yep."

Mandy and I chatted about what is normal for vulval morphology. "Normal isn't the right word," she said emphatically. "There is no normal. The word I would like to use is *aesthetically pleasing*. After I watched *The Perfect Vagina* and saw the plaster casts [of a wide variety of vulvas], that certainly changed my opinion a lot. The majority of women are so different to the ideal, and everyone is in the same boat—we are all different to the ideal, so what is normal? You know, there are women who accept much more difference than I do, and they aren't worried. And then—I can't say that it is what your partner thinks—and, well, my partner doesn't worry about it, and yet I still do. So, I suppose, if he did worry about it, I would be more inclined to be saying, 'OK, you can pay for it!'" She giggled.

I asked Mandy if she thought vulval aesthetics were important for relationships and notions of desirability and femininity. "On the whole, yes, like from the point of view of the man going out to catch a hot woman, but when it comes to selecting a partner to settle down with, I don't think it has a whole lot to do with it. It then becomes more about values and personality—getting along with a person rather than trying to appear desirable. But then, on the other hand, I don't want to be physically undesirable to my husband. Just because we get along, and we have the same values, and we raise our children well—I still want to feel desired by him. Like dyeing your hair or buying a new dress, being attractive to your partner is important. I think, going back to what we were saying before, feeling attractive makes men more attracted to you because you have got that confidence and that air of feeling good."

Mandy spoke of having body issues and low self-esteem. We chatted about her three pregnancies over three years. Mandy had wanted a family and had chosen to have her children in rapid succession so that she could then move on with her life. "I want my body back. I think that if my body issues are taken care of, my inhibitions will go away. In addition, I will have more confidence and be more adventurous and be more willing to explore whatever else there is to explore."

"You mean sexually?"

"Yes, absolutely. I don't know if how I feel is entirely the reason for our sex life being the way it is [somewhat unsatisfactory], or if it would be that way even if I were comfortable and confident. I don't want all of a sudden for everything to change, but I wouldn't mind if I *do* gain more confidence and get rid of my inhibitions and my self-esteem problems. Um, slowly introducing more of those—I don't know—different things, different positions, um, times of the day—I don't know, having the lights on would be—I am still uncomfortable with oral sex."

"Does your husband find this difficult?"

"I think he has accepted it by now. Towards the beginning, he made sure that it was my decision, not his. I was very explicit. I said, 'I do not want that. I cannot handle that.' He said, 'I am happy to do it if you want me to do it.' But . . .'"

I gently suggested that it's possible that her husband is not worried about the look of her vulva.

Mandy agreed. "I don't blame him for anything."

"But he doesn't blame you for anything either, does he?"

"Probably not, but I still blame myself. As women, we feel we should be servicing our husband's needs. There is this feeling that if we are not there for them, they will stray, sort of thing."

Incredulous, I said, "You are a working mother of two young people and pregnant!"

Mandy said her husband is supportive and a wonderful father. He has agreed to have a vasectomy once the new baby arrives. Mandy wants a more than satisfactory relationship with her husband, "to keep it alive and not just go down the path of, you know, we have been married for fifteen or twenty years. We love each other, but we are not 'in love.' I want to keep the spark and keep things rolling along and exciting."

We were coming to the end of our conversation. "I don't think I have spoken to anyone like I have talked to you tonight," she said. "It's nice to be able to talk about things that I can't with other people.

"Like I was saying before, my husband doesn't have an incredibly high libido. I lean towards thinking that if I were more attractive, or I were better, or if I were more . . . [*pauses for a long time*] he would be more interested."

"Because you want more sex or because you want to be loved more?"

"Probably because I think that if he desired me more, then that would make me feel more attractive. Because if we just climb into bed and go to sleep, I sort of think, 'Oh, but he works a lot. He works long hours, and he has a very early start and probably has a zillion other things on his mind.' You know? I try and remind myself of those things so as not to get depressed, and I have Googled 'guy's issues' and things to see if there is any relevance there, but I don't think there is. I just think he is simply not that kind of guy. And it [sex] is great sometimes—really, really great sometimes." She laughed. "But the number of times I have had to say no is a handful."

"I am barely thirty, and I don't want to be worrying about stupid little things when I can have something done to fix it. I have made a lot of sacrifices, and now I want to get my body back to its pre-baby state to some degree."

—⚏—

As a twenty-nine-year-old married woman with children, Mandy is not necessarily typical of women contemplating or choosing to undergo genital surgery: some are younger, some are childless, some are considerably older. I include Mandy's account here because her poignant story demonstrates the manner in which some women express their anxiety about their bodies and their genitalia. Some women want to be perfect, others have low self-esteem, some have received negative comments from lovers, and others think their genitalia are not normal. Highly specific and individual accounts such as Mandy's are of value to anthropological research. Mandy's story demonstrates how aesthetic concerns can intersect with relationships, body-image issues, self-esteem, and experiences of sexuality in the current milieu in which biomedical opportunities are increasingly available, media images of the "desirable body" (and the "desirable vulva") abound, and expectations to work on the self are relentlessly promoted. Mandy's narrative echoes some of the recurring themes that emerge throughout this book, such as the vulnerability of women to culturally defined bodily, aesthetic, and functional expectations and their willingness to address these perceived shortcomings through surgery.

NOTE

1. An "outie" is when the labia minora, or inner lips of the vulva, protrude past the labia majora, or outer lips.

THE PERFECT VAGINA

INTRODUCTION

Vulnerable Vulvas

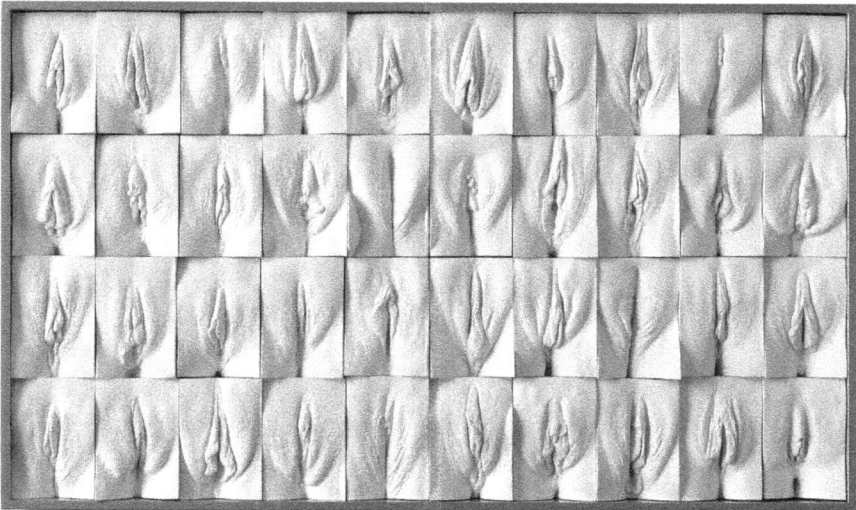

Figure i.1. *The Great Wall of Vagina* (panel 5 of 10), image of an artwork by Jamie McCartney, 2014. Reproduced with permission from Jamie McCartney.

Big C	Labiaplasty 1992 (rough draft)
When I passed her yesterday in the street I was reminded I've been trying to write aesthetically about hers for a long time	First World version Of Genital Mutilation. Performed by surgeons in sterile operating room with the best medications. Anesthesia.
you see she's an erotic dancer and I happen to have been offered a peek at hers twice at least	Everything to make you comfortable. But you will never be comfortable. Never again. Unconscious.
and it's pearly perfect kind of pure	Physical societal norm achieved With severed meat.
she's about fifty still with the niftiest in half the nation	A little stitch in the clit. Death
she's worked at it obviously been cosmeticised?	For the little death. But what a beautiful flower
doesn't matter it's to die for . . .	it will be.
(Penelope Grace, 2010)	(Quill Shiv, 2011)

THE JUXTAPOSITION OF THE TWO poems above encapsulates the contrasting ways in which labiaplasty is typically represented—beautification and awe on the one hand and physical subjugation on the other. The results are the same either way. Opinions differ about the legitimacy of surgically altering women's genitalia, but the lure of "a beautiful flower" or a look "to die for" is increasingly persuasive. Such aspirations are no longer confined to erotic dancers; concern about genital aesthetics now pervades the thoughts of many women. As such, female genital cosmetic surgery is a growing, complex, provocative, and polyvalent practice worthy of examination. There is no one definitive answer to why female genital cosmetic surgery is gaining in popularity—rather, the reasons for its increase are multifaceted.

According to medical opinion, female genitalia vary in appearance as much as snowflakes: they are all different. They come in a wide range of shapes and sizes. However, the acceptability of this diversity is narrowing for women today as a new desexualized genital aesthetic ideal—the clean slit—gains currency.[1] This aesthetic is one lacking hair, with the labia minora (or inner lips) contained within the labia majora (or outer lips) of the vulva. All skin folds and protrusions are neatly tucked away. Increasingly in the West,[2] women are choosing to alter their genital appearance through hair removal, piercing, bleaching, and vajazzling (a form of decoration of the female pubic area with crystals or glitter) and, more invasively, through female genital cosmetic surgery in their quest for a supposedly more appealing "designer vagina." The incidence of female genital cosmetic surgery as a form of body modification has escalated globally in recent years, and in this book, I seek to understand this phenomenon by listening to women's stories and doctors' accounts while also examining the cultural milieu in which the practice of female genital cosmetic surgery has arisen.

Working as a pharmacist in Australia and abroad, I never questioned the appropriateness of medical intervention into everyday lives or the massive influence of the pharmaceutical and medical industries. During my time living in the Middle East, Africa, and Indonesia, I became aware of and interested in the practice of female genital cutting (FGC), or female circumcision. When in Kenya, I was initially pleasantly surprised at the efforts of Australian aid agencies to curtail the practice. As I became more familiar with African culture, however, I began to see that the issue of FGC, and Western efforts to eradicate the practice, was extremely complex. On my return to Australia, I was therefore surprised to discover that women in the country of my birth were choosing to undergo genital cosmetic surgery and that their numbers were rising dramatically. Certainly, there are significant differences between female genital cosmetic surgery and FGC in terms of age, consent, numbers, and the conditions under which these operations are performed. However, are they radically different?

I am curious about female genital cosmetic surgery. I respect the decisions women make when choosing to undergo these procedures, and I acknowledge that some doctors may feel they are genuinely helping women. However, questions remain: Why are more women in the West altering their genitalia today? Why do some women suffer genital anxiety? Is genital surgery used to alleviate genital anxiety or enhance femininity, or both? What is the role of biomedicine in this endeavor? What are the opinions of surgeons who perform female genital cosmetic surgery? When I began my exploration of female genital cosmetic surgery, I had these questions in mind but no firm idea of where my investigations might take me. They brought me here.

In this book, I describe the environment in which certain women in Australia choose genital cosmetic surgery. I offer individual snapshots by way of their narratives, but these are contextualized, positioned within the broader discourse on cosmetic surgery. The women whose stories inform this ethnography have rationalized their motives for undergoing surgery given the social and cultural pressures and the medical opportunities available, and this is reflected in the way they narrate their experiences. Women find meaning in their experiences by telling their stories. The meanings of female genital cosmetic surgery and vulval aesthetics are thus recreated through narration and subsequent interpretation. While it is imperative to take women's stories of surgery seriously, they must be understood as filtered through individual logics of meaning-making, and these logics can be elucidated by examining the complex cultural milieu in which women make the choices they do about their bodies.

Although there are many (often strident) opinions critical of the powerful set of discourses and practices that surround cosmetic surgery, such positioning can result in the demonization of women who choose these procedures. Therefore, it is more fruitful to examine the environment in which the clean-slit genital ideal has arisen. Meredith Jones (2008, 29) argues that such an approach "does not mean condescendingly offering 'understanding' to cosmetic surgery recipients (implying that they are dupes of the beauty myth) but instead accepting that cosmetic surgery is now a meaningful part of our world." Because we are all makeover citizens (in that we are persuaded to constantly improve ourselves), it is imperative that we "find ways to constructively understand, examine, and live with this fact" (Jones 2008, 29). In this ethnography, I have applied Jones's sensibility by balancing an examination of the social space (one I share) in which surgery is offered as a solution to genital anxiety with a careful listening to women's narratives.

My position in this research requires some clarification. As Virginia Braun (2012) suggests, everyone has an opinion about female genital cosmetic surgery. There are ethical concerns, human rights concerns, and sociopolitical concerns, but there are also the concerns that individual women have about their bodies, and these cannot be discounted. Although I set out to understand more about genital cosmetic surgeries, I came to the project carrying a certain amount of baggage. I am a feminist, an older woman to whom certain cosmetic procedures have been offered unsolicited; some I have rejected, but other nonsurgical procedures, I have embraced. I am not against cosmetic procedures. However, I am critical of the perceived need to engage with what I can only describe as a form of *competitive* embodiment.

By way of a vignette, I recently met the (then) chief pharmacist from Great Ormond Street Hospital, London, where I worked more than thirty years ago—we had not seen each other in the interim. She told me she imagines all her previous staff as twenty-five-year-olds, the age most of us were at the time. If she was shocked by my aged appearance, she managed to disguise it well. We sat there, me with my short, dyed-blond hair and she, comfortably in her late seventies, a single woman with gray hair and a perfect English complexion, discussing vulvas, body image, and pharmacy. As we conversed animatedly about my research, she said, "Do you think we should just ban mirrors, Lindy?" How ironic that the vulva, the part of a woman's body least subject to the mirror's reflection, has not escaped its scrutiny—it is the invisible intimate, the mark of a woman.

I have attempted to be reflexive in my account of female genital cosmetic surgery and realize that my own experience and gender cloud my ability to be objective. Perhaps this has resulted in me empathizing more with the women who choose surgery and less with the medical profession. This could be because "studying up" (Nader 1969, 284) is more difficult than is studying your peers, or it could be related to issues of gender. Laura Nader challenged anthropologists to "study up," by which she meant study the middle and upper end of the social power structure, a category into which biomedicine falls. By doing so, connections between groups in society and links between groups and individuals are revealed and workings of power are exposed. By interviewing surgeons and attending medical conferences, I experienced these workings of power firsthand. I had to deal with gatekeeping (from surgeons' receptionists and nurses) along with other issues of access and ethics that revealed the attitudes of surgeons to their patients, often in quite revelatory ways. Although I spent time in surgeons' clinics and hospitals, where I could make observations of the interactions between surgeons, patients, nurses, and receptionists as well as examine items such as before and after photograph albums and testimonials neatly piled on coffee tables, the professional nature of the discipline of medicine meant that my interactions with doctors were primarily limited to interviews. In contrast, I found it easier to build a personal relationship with women, something forged over time in an equal and relaxed environment, one where female empathy (and solidarity) often allowed us to share intimate truths.[3]

I am also a "native" anthropologist, studying my own (mostly white, middle-class) society, which may make some of the nuances of observation on issues such as body image, imperatives for self-enhancement, and the desire to seek medical intervention for cosmetic purposes more difficult to detect. However, as Kirin Narayan (1993) suggests, it is more useful to abandon the distinction between dichotomies such as insider or outsider, native or nonnative, because the fixity of these is false. In my research, my identification shifted depending on which group I was observing—women or surgeons—as power relations varied within these interpenetrating communities. This interconnectedness reflects the rhizomatic nature of cosmetic surgery itself, in which there are myriad intersecting positions, realities, and discourses. Drawing on Gilles Deleuze and Félix Guattari's (1987) notion of the rhizome as a multidirectional and asymmetrical network of lines and connections enables a better understanding of female genital cosmetic surgery. From this perspective, cosmetic surgery appears not to be solely the result of medicalization, commercialization, or the media. Rather, the practice appears "as a complex network of relationships and issues," as opposed to a phenomenon that can be described in terms of "a simple linear causality running from, for example, patriarchy to woman-as-victim" (Fraser 2003, 25). Similarly, this book embodies a rhizomatic perspective. Throughout the chapters, many points overlap and intersect, thus mimicking and echoing—both in structure and style—the key argument of this book; that is, a multitude of causal factors intersect to make female genital cosmetic surgery a productive choice for certain women. There is no one answer to why female genital cosmetic surgery is increasing in popularity in the West, and as such, the perhaps convoluted nature of the text that follows mimics the "problem" of female genital cosmetic surgery itself.

My research approach followed the method advocated by Cheryl Mattingly (2010, 29): a "narrative phenomenology of practice" involving person-centered, event-centered, and discursive-centered ethnography. Women convey their experiences of genital cosmetic surgery through storytelling, beginning with a desire for surgery, then the procedure itself, and finally the transformation. Their narratives describe events, their experiences with their surgeons, and the outcomes of the surgery. These narratives are constructed within a certain discursive terrain, one that is informed by the media, particularly the internet and social media, an arena where surgeons, patients, academics, feminists, and the public discuss female genital cosmetic surgery, illuminating the structural and discursive environment in which women make choices about their personal lives. Mattingly (2010, 44) suggests that social theorists have been reluctant to "*theoretically* privilege experience" over structure—that is, to treat social life in explicitly phenomenological terms. I believe both are essential to understanding cosmetic surgery. Although it is imperative to examine the structural environment in which women choose genital cosmetic surgery, women's stories and experiences must be equally valued. In addition, language is important when endeavoring to understand the circumstances in which surgeons and women come together. Language manipulates events, turning surgery into a meaningful experience, as language itself is simultaneously manipulated to persuade women that surgery may be beneficial to them.

I have included comments from social media sources, such as weblogs, message boards, and other online communities. Since the internet is a key source of information and action regarding female genital cosmetic surgery, comments on social media sites were important data sources for my research. As Tom Boellstorff (2008, 61) states about virtual worlds, "To demand that ethnographic research always incorporate meeting residents in the actual world for 'context' presumes that virtual worlds are not contexts in themselves; it renders ethnographically inaccessible the fact that most residents of virtual worlds do not meet their fellow residents offline." Similarly, most women discussing genital cosmetic surgery online do not expect to meet in "real life" the others who post there. Female genital cosmetic surgery cannot usefully be understood without examining social media as a source, not only of information but also of legitimate social interaction for individuals. As Debra Spitulnik (1993, 307) prophetically wrote before social media blossomed, "Many of these new developments supplant the 'mass' of mass media, making them more individual and interpersonal." Online social media offer places where individuals can go for advice and information, and the sharing of bodily concerns.

In this book, I illuminate some of the complexities and contingencies that surround female genital cosmetic surgery as an emergent biomedical practice, a practice garnering considerable attention in the popular media, in the medical field (particularly women's health), and in academic and feminist discourse. I examine contemporary femaleness and the attempts to attain this through medicine—the biomagical—and to thereby display a femininity that is considered not only appropriate but also desirable.[4] This book is primarily about labiaplasty and Australian women, but it is also about surgeons and emerging medical markets, and about how biomedicine can take on magical qualities. The neologism *biomagical* conveys the transformative nature of biomedicine when it is harnessed for cosmetic purposes. By juxtaposing biology (the scientific) with magic (the transformative), the boundaries of medicine are reconfigured, allowing it to enter new spaces. When biomedicine becomes biomagical, there is an imperative to constantly improve the (female) body. Magic implies transformation, and although cosmetic surgery involves risk, pain, and recovery, it is both marketed and imagined as a permanent solution to aesthetic or functional concerns. Today, magic and the aesthetic are bound up with both consumption *and* technology (biomedicine). As Michael Taussig (2012, 6) notes, "Not only is the inseparability of the aesthetic and the magic of the economy now *back* in the saddle but, under the rubric of the postmodern, new worlds of aesthetic intensification and libidinal gratification bound to a new body have taken center stage," a stage on which the medical profession can capitalize. New technologies and social practices (such as female genital cosmetic surgery) provide "emotional value" and "magical status" for consumers (de Waal Malefyt 2017, 1) who are lured by not-impartial information and advertising. Aesthetics (as always) are important and attainable, and the aura that surrounds cosmetic surgery—its magic—is more powerful than the procedures themselves.

I did not set out to determine whether women who undergo female genital cosmetic surgery are making sound liberating choices or uninformed culturally coerced ones, although such arguments underpin much of the discourse surrounding cosmetic surgery. Rather, I was interested in the experiences of women who engage with these procedures, how the medical profession (without which there would be no such thing as female genital cosmetic surgery) sees its role, and how this coming together is interpellated through the media and consumption, where cosmetic surgery is presented as a permanent, viable solution to bodily concerns. The units of analysis that inform this book are the creation of a particular vulval ideal for women, the complex relationship between norms and ideals, and female genital cosmetic surgery as an example of an enhancement technology—a ritual of sorts—employed in the pursuit of

bodily perfection. Through these units of analysis run two threads: biomedicine (represented by doctors and medical discourse) and the media, particularly the internet and social media.

WOMEN, DOCTORS, AND THE MEDIA: FIELDS OF ENQUIRY

The core of my research in Australia involved interviewing women who had
had or were contemplating genital cosmetic surgery, and interviewing plastic
and cosmetic surgeons and gynecologists who perform female genital cosmetic
surgery. All surgeons and women completed a consent form approved by the
Macquarie University Ethics Committee. Approval was contingent on using
pseudonyms for all the women and surgeons I spoke with in Australia. Also,
I attended several conferences and presentations where female genital cosmetic
surgery was the sole topic or an included matter. In particular, I attended a
medical congress held in Las Vegas that specifically promoted and taught female genital cosmetic surgery, or what their society terms *cosmetogynecology*.
At this event, surgeons shared their knowledge and expertise about these procedures: it was a significant event for knowledge production. However, it also
served a political purpose, with notions of brotherhood and boundary erection
invoked to counter opposition to female genital cosmetic surgery. As I was a
member of the public attending this congress, I have not used pseudonyms
when referring to those who spoke there. Most proceedings were recorded on
a compact disc, which I purchased. Similar congresses are held annually in
the United States.

The fieldwork was multisited and conducted over a four-year period between 2009 and 2013. The analysis of the media and the medical literature
continued until the writing of this book. Because my research involved medical practice, women, and an analysis of the discourse surrounding female
genital cosmetic surgery, my methods of data collection varied according to
context. Overwhelmingly, my research methods involved following female
genital cosmetic surgery around and across these different sites in order to
build an understanding of the practice: how it is defined, imagined, represented, described, and spoken about by various players. Female genital cosmetic surgery has only grown in popularity since this research was conducted,
and its promotion and defense by some physicians has become more strident.
Simultaneously, these practices have drawn increasing criticism from certain
professional medical bodies.

All the Australian surgeons I interviewed were recruited through the internet, by word of mouth, or from their advertisements in cosmetic surgery

magazines—the same method used by women seeking surgery. I spoke with more than forty surgeons; I visited most of them in their private or hospital office. Some I interviewed on several occasions. Five of the cosmetic or plastic surgeons were female, as were three of the gynecologists. All other doctors were male. Most of the surgeons who participated in the research resided in major cities in the eastern states of Australia, from Cairns in the far north to Melbourne in the south. The majority of Australians live on the coastal fringes of the continent, and several surgeons suggested that the beach culture that pervades these spaces contributes to the popularity of labiaplasty.

To recruit women for my research, I posted an anonymous questionnaire on Survey Monkey. Not all women whose stories inform this book completed the questionnaire. Some I interviewed directly. The questionnaire itself provided limited information, but it was my most successful form of recruitment. I received more than forty responses. I also asked doctors to distribute cards explaining the research and asking women to participate. A link to the questionnaire was posted on weblogs and online health discussion boards in Australia when the topic of genital surgery arose. Overall, twenty-two women gave me their contact details, and it is these women whose narratives contribute to this book. A list of the women, indicating their age, marital status, and parity, appears in table 1 in appendix 1. Table 2 in appendix 1 gives a summary of women by age, marital status, parity, and occupation. Nine women were students, five were psychologists, and the remainder were from a breadth of professions. Two were retired, and two were homemakers. Most women were middle-class white Anglo-Australians with an educational level of secondary school or higher. Just over half were single and childless, and most lived on the eastern seaboard of Australia. Appendix 2 includes the original interview questions for women who had either had or were contemplating having female genital cosmetic surgery.

I also interviewed ten beauticians who were offering Brazilian waxing in Sydney. Although this procedure is less invasive than genital surgery, its prevalence indicates a change in genital aesthetics, one that may help explain what triggers genital anxiety in women, given that it exposes labia previously obscured by pubic hair. Laser pubic hair removal is also growing in popularity in Australia because it shares with female genital cosmetic surgery some of the magical promise of permanency.

I carried out an extensive internet search during the period of the research, mostly using the Google search engine. This led me to online health discussion boards, newspaper articles, weblogs, and television stories. Other media sources included women's magazines—both online and offline—soft-core pornography, and social networking sites. I also extensively reviewed surgeons' websites and subscribed to several cosmetic surgery magazines. The internet plays a major role in supporting and publicizing cosmetic surgery through both advertising and the provision of easy access to texts and images online. These influence the decisions women make about their bodies and fuel the perception of appearance as a medical problem. I examined medical literature concerned with female genital cosmetic surgery, including medical journals, textbooks, conference proceedings, and material generated by medical institutions for the public. This text and image-based analysis allowed me to compare the different perspectives of female genital cosmetic surgery portrayed in the media.

FEMALE GENITAL ALTERATIONS: AN OVERVIEW

Female genital alterations have a long history. They encompass traditional FGC, also referred to as circumcision or female genital mutilation, an ancient practice that predates the Abrahamic religions; surgeries that were performed on women in the West to "cure" so-called deviant sexual behavior; operations on those with ambiguous genitalia; sex reassignment surgery; and, most recently, female genital cosmetic surgery. This list is not exhaustive. Some alterations are performed without the consent of the girl or woman; others are "freely" chosen. As Braun (2008, par. 1) notes, "What unites all these procedures is an understanding of the way women's genitalia should be, if girls and women are to be appropriately gendered and sexually desirable." In different cultures and different eras, how women's genitalia should look and function has been prescriptive.

Terminology is both important and contested. What I refer to as FGC, for instance, is frequently called female genital mutilation. World bodies that censure these operations (such as the World Health Organization and the United Nations Children's Fund) adopt the latter term for rhetorical effect in their critique of these practices typically performed on non-Western girls and women, and this has drawn the ire of some in practicing communities. The term *mutilation* implies judgment; it connotes barbarism and cruelty, and ontologically separates FGC from other female genital operations (Whitcomb 2011). This book is about female genital cosmetic surgery; other practices are referred to only obliquely. However, the fact that FGC is illegal in Australia (as in many countries) while female genital cosmetic surgery is growing in popularity cannot be ignored. Female genital cosmetic surgery has ethical and political implications. These two procedures are presented very differently in medical discourse, although, in the transcultural context, they cannot be so easily separated. The World Health Organization (2014) describes FGC as any procedure that involves partial or total removal of the external female genitalia or other injury to the female genital organs for nonmedical reasons. Clearly, female genital cosmetic surgery falls under this purview given that it involves altering female genitalia for cosmetic—not medical—purposes and labiaplasty involves the removal of external female genitalia. Although Western medical institutions recognize a woman's right to choose lawful medical and surgical treatments, tension arises when some women's desires are considered legitimate while others' desires are not, particularly if such decisions are based on cultural preferences rather than medical expertise and resources.

Western medicine has a long history of gynecological intervention after childbirth, including procedures to correct fistulas, tears, prolapses, and incontinence (Adams 1997; Braun 2010). After childbirth, it was not unusual for doctors to insert an extra stitch into a woman's vagina for the subsequent satisfaction of her husband, and even today, "midwives and obstetricians are trained to sew up tears and episiotomies firmly to avoid 'gaping'" (Manderson 2004, 297). Until recently, episiotomies were routinely performed on women to prevent tearing during childbirth. Current research has shown, however, that this results in more complications than allowing the perineum to tear naturally (Lappen and Gossett 2010).

Female genital surgical operations without a medical indication are commonly attributed to non-Western societies and the practice of FGC, but in England and North America during the Victorian era, surgeons performed clitoridectomies to prevent masturbation and other socially defined "unfeminine" behaviors, such as hysteria, lesbianism, and promiscuity—conditions thought to compromise women's primary roles in society, that of marriage and reproduction (Green 2005; Manderson 2004). Isaac Baker Brown, an eminent British obstetrician-gynecologist, was an outspoken advocate of clitoridectomy, and although his reputation was tarnished after the publication of his 1866 book *On the Curability of Certain Forms of Insanity, Epilepsy, Catalepsy, and Hysteria in Females*, medical texts continued to recommend clitoridectomy into the mid-twentieth century (Baker Brown 1866). With the improved surgical techniques of the 1950s, genital operations became routine for those with ambiguous genitalia. Frequently, the size of the clitoris of people of indeterminate sex was reduced and, despite criticism of the practice, feminizing surgeries (clitoroplasties) continue today (Coventry 2000; Fausto-Sterling 2000; Kessler 1998). Another example is that of Dr. James Burt, an American gynecologist, who began performing his "love surgery" in the 1960s. This surgery involved, at a minimum, realigning the vagina and reducing the clitoral hood (Adams 1997). Dr. Burt believed that women were anatomically inadequate for intercourse given that they often failed to achieve orgasm, a condition he considered pathological. Consent for genital operations was not always obtained or deemed necessary. Often, the women were in the hospital to give birth or for other gynecological procedures (Adams 1997), and sometimes patients were not even informed that they had been subjected to these procedures (Braun 2010).

Clearly, the surgical alteration of female genitalia is not new. Female genitalia in their natural state have historically been seen as troublesome, both to women and to society (Braun 2012). Female sexuality has been regarded as a challenge that requires management, and "given this context, FGCS [female genital cosmetic surgery] has been framed as 'the latest chapter in the surgical victimization of women in our culture.' The alternative account, promoted by some surgeons and sections of the media, is that, finally, women's genitalia and sexual problems are getting the attention they deserve" (Braun 2010, 1393). Genital surgery today, particularly labiaplasty, is performed primarily for aesthetic, not functional, reasons (despite protestations to the contrary). Women's genitalia are being altered to more closely approximate the culturally generated aesthetic ideal that defines female genitalia as contained, neat, and tidy—the opposite of protuberant male genitalia.

LABIAPLASTY AND OTHER FEMALE GENITAL COSMETIC SURGERIES

While an array of female genital cosmetic surgeries is available, labiaplasty is the most prevalent procedure in Australia. According to one cosmetic surgery website:

> Labiaplasty is a surgical procedure that will reduce and/or reshape the labia minora—the skin that covers the female clitoris and vaginal opening. In some instances, women with large labia can experience pain during intercourse, or feel discomfort during everyday activities or when wearing tight-fitting clothing. Others may feel unattractive or wish to enhance their sexual experiences by removing some of the skin that covers the clitoris. The purpose of a labiaplasty is to better define the inner labia. During this procedure, the urethral opening can be redefined, and if necessary improvements to the vagina may be made. The problem can be caused by genetics, sexual intercourse or difficulties in childbirth. (Esteem Cosmetic Studio 2013)

Here, labiaplasty is presented as a solution to a woman's genital shortcomings. The definition mixes lay and anatomical terms in a confusing and unscientific manner. What is involved in "redefining the urethral opening" and "improving the vagina" is left vague, but the wording suggests these anatomical features are likely to be lacking in their natural state. While the quality of the information on surgeons' websites varies, procedures are uniformly portrayed as rational and simple, and it is to these websites that women frequently turn for information about surgery.

In contrast to the encouraging tone of surgeons' websites, some rather skeptical reports present female genital cosmetic surgery as both scary and ridiculous. Headlines such as "Designer Vagina Surgery: Snip, Stitch, Kerching! Demand for Cosmetic Gynecology Has Never Been Higher. And for Plastic Surgeons, Business Is Booming" (Lee 2011) and "Popular Cosmetic Procedure Called the 'Barbie' Hacks Off Women's Labia so She's Smooth Like a Doll" (Baker 2013) regularly appear in the press and on feminist weblogs. Regardless of its portrayal, female genital cosmetic surgery has entered the everyday, not because numerous women are undergoing these procedures but because it has become part of popular discourse along with other sensationalized reports of cosmetic surgery, often involving celebrities. Surgeons' websites and women's magazines regularly frame genital cosmetic surgery as a rational and empowering choice for women, whereas other sources are more circumspect. An increasing number of doctors in Australia and elsewhere are offering female genital cosmetic surgery, which has given rise to concern, particularly within the women's health sector and feminist networks, as well as among medical regulatory bodies.

While body modification, both historically and currently, is a universal phenomenon, its medicalization in the West has allowed the cosmetic surgery industry to flourish, and the notion of what constitutes health has expanded to include beauty and sexuality. This trend generates new opportunities for action while constricting the range of acceptable difference. With its power to render unacceptable not only disease but also a less-than-perfect body, biomedicine appears to possess near-magical properties. Within the media and Western medicine, there are elements driving an increase in female genital cosmetic surgery by promoting the belief that normal biological variation in women is pathological and that surgery can cure this. This results in a more clearly demarcated gendered body becoming the acceptable norm. Cosmetic surgery is not routinely portrayed as constraining or detrimental to women (unlike FGC) because women are portrayed as individuals who freely choose surgery, and choice is presumed to lie outside culture rather than being firmly embedded within it.

One of the first reports of cosmetic labiaplasty appeared in 1984 in the article "Aesthetic Vaginal Labiaplasty" published in the journal *Plastic and Reconstructive Surgery* (Hodgkinson and Hait 1984), although as early as 1976, labiaplasty for "marked hypertrophy" was described by H. Melvin Radman (1976), who considered enlarged labia a congenital condition. In the late 1990s, clinical reports began appearing in academic journals along with articles in the popular press, particularly glossy women's magazines, where the result of surgery to beautify or improve the function of female genitalia was frequently referred to as a "designer vagina" (Braun 2010). While female genital cosmetic surgery may have emerged in the West, specifically in the United States, it is increasingly being offered globally and is garnering worldwide attention (Ashong and Batta 2013; Dorneles de Andrade 2010). According to a 2016 report published by the International Society of Aesthetic Plastic Surgery (ISAPS 2016), labiaplasty is the world's fastest-growing cosmetic surgery procedure, with a 45 percent increase in procedures performed in 2016. The countries performing the most labiaplasties in 2016 were the United States, Brazil, Russia, Spain, Germany, Turkey, Colombia, France, Italy, and Mexico (ISAPS 2016). However, labiaplasty is also practiced in the Middle East, Africa, Australia, New Zealand, South America, Asia, and many other parts of Europe. Female cosmetic genital surgery has also entered the sphere of medical tourism, and procedures are promoted on the internet and at exhibitions such as Sexpo, an Australian adult lifestyle and sexuality trade fair. In an article in the *British Medical Journal*, Ronán Conroy (2006, 16) asserts that the "practice of female genital mutilation is on the increase nowhere in the world except in our so called developed societies," thereby drawing a strong link between female genital cosmetic surgery and FGC.

Female genital cosmetic surgery involves a range of interventions, from the purely cosmetic to those that profess to enhance sexual pleasure. Procedures include, but are not limited to, labia minora reduction (labiaplasty), labia majora augmentation, liposuction of the mons pubis or labia majora, vaginal tightening ("rejuvenation"), clitoral hood reduction, clitoral repositioning, G-spot amplification, perineum rejuvenation, genital whitening, and hymen reconstruction (Braun 2010; Women's Health Queensland Wide Inc. 2007). Labiaplasty of the labia minora is the most frequently performed procedure in Australia and is done primarily for aesthetic reasons, either to stop the labia minora protruding below the labia majora or to correct asymmetry. Some women request labiaplasty because they experience discomfort during physical activities, such as cycling, horse-riding, and walking, or during sexual intercourse (Women's Health Queensland Wide Inc. 2007). Others report having issues with hygiene. Labiaplasty is sometimes accompanied by clitoral hood reduction, which involves paring back the skin folds around the clitoris.

Although no reliable statistics are recorded in Australia, 1,129 "medically" indicated labiaplasties were funded by Medicare between July 2014 and June 2015. However, there are no definitive criteria defining medically indicated labiaplasties in Australia—rather the decision is left to the treating physician. Medicare is the Australian federal health-care system providing primary health care to all Australian citizens and permanent residents, similar to the National Health Service in the United Kingdom. It is partly funded by a tax called the Medicare levy. This is very different from Medicare in the United States, which is a federal health insurance program applicable only to people sixty-five years or older or to those with certain disabilities or end-stage renal disease. During the ten-year period to 2013, the number of labiaplasties claimed through Medicare in Australia increased by 457 percent (Belt 2013), which led to closer scrutiny of such procedures by the Medicare Claims Review Panel. However, these Medicare figures are not indicative of the number of labiaplasties performed in Australia, given that most procedures are performed in private practice and not claimable through Medicare or private health insurance and are therefore not audited.[5] One of the cosmetic surgeons I interviewed said she performs around two hundred labiaplasties each year and submits none of these through Medicare; others said they performed fifty to one hundred operations annually. Some surgeons said they are wary of being investigated by Medicare, a potential outcome of submitting multiple claims. Over the ten years prior to 2011, there was a fivefold increase in the number of labiaplasties performed under the National Health Service in the United Kingdom (Crouch et al. 2011). However, statistics such as these are merely indicative, because surgery is performed by a wide variety of players, and numbers are not routinely captured.

The popularity of cosmetic surgery in general has increased exponentially over the past few decades. In the United States in 2016, more than thirteen million cosmetic surgical and nonsurgical procedures were performed by board-certified doctors. Of these, over 1.9 million were surgical procedures. Americans spent more than US$15 billion on cosmetic procedures in 2016, and surgery accounted for 56 percent of that expenditure. Women are the main consumers of cosmetic surgery (91 percent). Labiaplasty procedures increased by 23.2 percent in 2016 (ASAPS 2016). More than ten thousand labiaplasties were performed in the United States in 2016, with 36 percent of all plastic surgeons now offering the procedure in their practices (ASAPS 2016). Several of the surgeons I interviewed speculated that female genital cosmetic surgery is as popular today as breast augmentation was several decades ago.

The age of women seeking labiaplasty appears to vary widely, but women in their twenties and thirties predominate. Some of the surgeons I spoke with said younger women are now requesting surgery; others do so after having their children or before embarking on a new relationship. The women I interviewed who had had labiaplasty ranged in age from eighteen to fifty-nine. The Medicare data for labiaplasty in Australia show that most women undergoing surgery fall into the fifteen to fifty-five age bracket (Malone 2013). A seventy-nine-year-old woman I interviewed had the procedure suggested to her by her gynecologist because she suffered vulval discomfort. One plastic surgeon told me she had operated on a twelve-year-old girl with labial asymmetry. This wide age range has been documented by other researchers.

When performing labiaplasty, surgeons employ a range of surgical techniques from simple amputation to more complicated procedures, such as the wedge resection, z-plasty, w-shaped resection, de-epithelialization, laser labiaplasty, composite reduction, fenestration, and flask labiaplasty. Amputation removes the (often darker) free edge of the labia. It was the original technique, and it is still used. The various resection techniques, however, involve cutting shaped wedges or sections out of the labia, and the incised edges are then sewn together, leaving the natural edge intact. With de-epithelialization, sections of the labia are excised or thinned out. Composite reduction entails labial tissue reduction as well as reduction of tissue closer to the clitoris. Fenestration allows for a reduction in both the height and length of the labia minora. Flask labiaplasty is purported to be a customized procedure that assures symmetry and the preservation of nerve and vascular supply (Oranges, Sisti, and Sisti 2015). All these techniques give slightly different results and have been developed and refined by various surgeons. New ways of performing labiaplasty—sometimes employing novel instruments, sometimes using different incisions—appear regularly in the medical literature, demonstrating that techniques are continually being tweaked and developed. Which technique provides the "more perfect" or "more natural" result is hotly contested. One cosmetic surgeon, for example, describes her recently added Dove technique as producing "a very delicate result with little evidence that the labia have been altered. The technique takes longer than other labiaplasty techniques because of the delicate, painstaking work involved. However, the results justify the additional time taken" (Konrat 2014)—and, presumably, the extra cost.

No surgery comes without risks, from both the anesthesia and the surgery itself. The main risks are bleeding, infection, and local swelling. There can be problems with healing, such as incision dehiscence (wound breakdown), under- or overcorrection, scarring, and pain. The possibility of altered sensation is glossed over by surgeons, even though genital surgery performed on people with ambiguous genitalia and women with vulval cancer has resulted in reduced sexual function (Braun 2010). In addition, no studies have been done to determine whether these surgeries will cause problems during subsequent childbirth. According to some surgeons, requests for the revision of "botched jobs" performed by other practitioners are quite common. Despite this, few women I spoke with seemed overly concerned about the risks of nerve damage and subsequent issues with diminished sensation. The American College of Obstetricians and Gynecologists and its Australian equivalent, the Royal Australian and New Zealand College of Obstetricians and Gynaecologists (RANZCOG), have issued public position statements cautioning against genital cosmetic procedures, as has the Australian Federation of Medical Women. The RANZCOG statement reads, in part:

> Gynaecological conditions that merit surgery include genital prolapse, reconstructive surgery following female genital mutilation and labioplasties to repair obstetric trauma. Medical practitioners performing any vaginal surgery should be appropriately trained.
>
> Obstetricians and gynaecologists should have a role in educating women that there are a large number of variations in the appearance of normal female external genitalia and that there are normal physiological changes over time, especially following childbirth and menopause. Patients requesting procedures other than for gynaecological conditions should be assessed thoroughly and the reasons for such a request assessed carefully. . . .
>
> The College strongly discourages the performance of any surgical or laser procedure that lacks current peer reviewed scientific evidence other than in the context of an appropriately constructed clinical trial. . . .
>
> At present, there is little high quality evidence that these procedures are effective, enhance sexual satisfaction or improve self-image. The risks of potential complications such as scarring, adhesions, permanent disfigurement, infection, dyspareunia and altered sexual sensations should be discussed in detail with women seeking such treatments. (RANZCOG 2016, 2)

This nonbinding position statement for obstetricians and gynecologists does not apply to cosmetic and plastic surgeons. The 2015 RANZCOG statement referred to "labioplasties with clinical indications," but this vague statement has since been replaced with "labioplasties to repair obstetric trauma," thereby tightening the recommendations. Although some bodies, such as Women's Health Victoria in Australia and the Royal College of Obstetricians and Gynaecologists in the United Kingdom, have issued position statements recommending further research and the imposition of regulations, female genital cosmetic surgery remains an unregulated area globally. Medical experts have called for well-designed prospective studies to evaluate the long-term satisfaction, benefits, and risks of female genital cosmetic surgery, but very little information is currently available.

Regarding long-term satisfaction with female genital cosmetic surgery, only anecdotal evidence is available. Doctors report high satisfaction rates for labiaplasty, typically over 90 percent (Braun 2010; Likes et al. 2008), but it should be borne in mind that studies of patient satisfaction do not typically undergo scientific validation and rely on "usually satisfied" patients voluntarily responding to surgeons' questionnaires. As Braun (2010, 1394–98) attests, "Psychometrically robust psychological measurement is needed for FGCS [female genital cosmetic surgery], with long-term follow-up, alongside appropriate clinical outcome studies that assess sexual and psychosocial outcomes; ideally assessment should not be conducted by those with fiscal interest in the outcome." Lih-Mei Liao, Lina Michala, and Sarah Creighton (2010, 22) point out that "consumer satisfaction should not be confused with clinical effectiveness." Cosmetic surgery, however, is not subject to the same principles as other medical intervention. Although some changes are afoot, most cosmetic surgery is not evidence based (Eaves III, Rohrich, and Sykes 2013; Goodman 2011). In Australia, there is fierce competition between plastic and cosmetic surgeons, with the former highly disparaging of cosmetic surgeons, who do not undergo the same rigorous training as plastic surgeons.[6] Gynecologists, general surgeons, and general practitioners also perform these procedures. However, general practitioners who pose as cosmetic surgeons do not have recognized surgical training, and in one Australian state, Queensland, they are forbidden from referring to themselves as "surgeons."

THE SETTING

Current concepts of the body and notions of choice are articulated in an increasingly medicalized world. The body has become central to identity, a corporeal indicator of a willingness to take care of the self, which has emerged contemporarily as an almost obligatory endeavor, making cosmetic procedures more difficult to resist. As one cosmetic surgeon who specializes in labiaplasty explained to me:

> There is not a correlation between a physical feature and how you feel about it. It's not a one-to-one sort of thing. You can't say that if it was half the

size, you would be twice as happy, or if the size was doubled, you'd be half as happy—there is no correlation. People are still going to look at the big billboard outside and say, "I want to look like that because that is what our society is built around." You know, our society is built for us to desire to look and be a particular way, to buy a particular sort of house, eat a particular sort of food. It is obviously very complex, but I think this [female genital cosmetic surgery] sort of gets mixed up with that. The women who are looking for a partner, they want to look like the billboard. They want to look desirable.

When you are young, and you are trying to form a particular image for yourself in the world, you are trying to project yourself into the world in a particular way. You look at what you are least happy with, and you address that. If you don't like your hair, you get it done in a way that you like. If unhappiness remains, you look at something else. You might be a bit overweight. You have your basic level of happiness. I think human nature is . . . We are removing obstacles from our path, but we are still looking for obstacles to remove. There is always something we can improve.

In his comment, this surgeon captures some of the key elements that persuade women to undergo genital cosmetic surgery, including the power of the media—the "billboard"—to drive consumption in a culture where happiness is portrayed as achievable through constant self-improvement. While we have been "looking for obstacles to remove"—in this case, parts of the external genitalia—new biomedical technologies and skills have been emerging as a panacea for genital anxiety.

Choice, agency, and desire have been much discussed in academia in relation to cosmetic surgery, but these debates are not the focus here. Rather, I concentrate on female genital cosmetic surgery as a phenomenon, which is much more radically embedded in cultural strategies than debates about choice and agency can elucidate. Feminist scholars have highlighted that the rhetoric of choice underpins discussions about cosmetic surgery and that this rhetoric disguises any cultural coercion that may lead to physical conformity (Moran and Lee 2013). However, as Rosemary Gillespie (1997, 82) argues, although "conformity to social and cultural norms may on the one hand represent collusion by women in dominant constructions of femininity, nevertheless at the individual level it may also be rational and empowering for them." Whether or not they appear to be, women are vulnerable to the technological beauty imperative because many of its messages are absorbed subliminally. Cosmetic surgery has become normalized, and as Virginia Blum (2003, 44) writes, "The bodies of women in a postsurgical culture are all compromised regardless of whether we choose or refuse surgical intervention. . . . We are inevitably in a relationship to surgery regardless of whether we actually become surgical." As more women undergo cosmetic surgery to emulate the vulval depictions found in the media, the ideal gains currency.

There is a complex relationship between aesthetic ideals and understandings of normality. Many women are unconvinced that normal genitalia are adequate for happiness and social inclusion. Cosmetic surgery is offered as a tool that "rational" women can freely choose in their search for self-esteem and happiness. Exploring these themes allows us to reflect on the influence of the media and medical science in a consumer-driven makeover culture and highlights how the production of ideals and their association with notions of normality are increasingly impinging on bodily integrity. In *Skintight: An Anatomy of Cosmetic Surgery*, Meredith Jones develops the concept of makeover culture (Jones 2008). She describes how, in the West, we are expected to improve ourselves constantly, often through technological means. Makeover culture values and rewards processes of working on the self. Individuals are increasingly expected to take responsibility for their health and well-being, and since the health and beauty industries have become increasingly entwined, taking care of oneself is an ongoing and complex project.

Although cosmetic surgery in general has become normalized and less stigmatized, female genital cosmetic surgery is proving to be a testing ground for the extent to which vanity and self-care should become part of the surgical domain. Perhaps this is because of the private nature of genitalia and their centrality to sexuality, or perhaps it is because of the comparison between genital cosmetic surgery and FGC (a comparison stridently denounced by doctors). As both Kirsten Bell (2005) and Lenore Manderson (2004) point out, women's sexuality is imagined as easily upset and more vulnerable to culture than men's, as demonstrated by debates about male and female circumcision. Despite this assumed susceptibility of female sexuality to outside incursions, genital cosmetic surgery can be considered a form of self-care ("care of the self" in Foucault's terms), particularly when it is undertaken to alleviate genital anxiety, which has arisen in the current cultural milieu where standards of sexual attractiveness now include the invisible, intimate genitalia. These aesthetic standards are increasingly precise for the vulval region. For the women whose stories inform this book, genital cosmetic surgery has relieved their genital anxiety and afforded them greater sexual confidence. "While the psychological underpinnings of genital anxiety as well as its origins as a cultural production and social construction must not be ignored, it is similarly problematic to universally admonish as disingenuous a woman's newfound sexual and personal self-confidence and experience of pleasure as a result of FGCS [female genital cosmetic surgery]" (Rodrigues 2012, 790).

Because it is considered taboo for women's genitalia to be on public display, increased importance is placed on them. They constitute what I term the *invisible intimate*. Although the invisible intimate is profoundly shaped by cultural expectations, this dimension of body image is particularly susceptible to critique. Consequently, a new body-image vulnerability has emerged. For some women I interviewed (such as Mandy from the prologue), a negative comment from a partner or the negative portrayal of protruding labia minora in the media led to their genital anxiety and propelled them to seek surgical solutions. In conditions of intimate invisibility, genital anxiety is amplified because it cannot be discussed in the same way as other anxieties. In addition, women who suffer genital anxiety display a receptivity bias; despite being reassured that they are normal, they remain concerned about their vulval appearance.

THE BODY

Female genital cosmetic surgery cannot be understood without looking more broadly at the role of the body in lived experience. Rather than being determined by nature, the body is increasingly understood as a social and cultural construct and therefore capable of constant transformation. "The body is a metaphor of the social world (Sontag 1978), but the social world, its structures and institutions, leaves physical imprints on the body, mnemonics of global and local moral, social and political relationships" (Manderson 2011, 29). Markers of cultural distinction, or preference, can be written on the body, ensuring that our anatomy reflects our culture. The body then becomes a site of human expression and agency (Mason 2013), and in a biomagical milieu, "body maintenance, renewal and embellishment builds on the constant rewards of scientific discovery, technical advance and fantastic possibility" (Manderson 2011, 31). Whereas genital cosmetic surgery may be one of "fantastic possibility" for sufferers of genital anxiety in that it provides relief from feelings of inadequacy, it produces a certain form of constrained femininity. Female genital cosmetic surgery, therefore, marks the female form with the values of our moral and social world.

Common threads run through the discourse surrounding cosmetic surgery. On both sides of the debate, it is portrayed as acting on a presurgical natural body untouched by culture—a blank canvas—rather than a body already imprinted by culture (Jones 2008). While there may be no natural precultural body, cosmetic surgery does focus on what Alexander Edmonds (2010, 32) refers to as "biologized selves," and this corporeal body becomes the object of transformation. Cosmetic surgery acts on the "bare" physiological organism (Edmonds 2010, 241). Body parts are often isolated and fragmented, drawn out of the symbolic and cultural realm, "quantified in clinical measurements" (Edmonds 2013b, 77), manipulated, and then reincorporated into the social. The cosmetic surgery body is therefore both "a cultural phenomenon and biological entity" (Braun and Wilkinson 2001, 18).

With female genital cosmetic surgery, sexuality is framed visually through biology, and what is considered attractive is determined by the supposedly objective terms and parameters of medicine materializing a "biological body" (Edmonds 2013b, 65). However, as Edmonds (74) makes clear, despite some women (and their surgeons) believing that cosmetic surgery liberates them from biological constraints, the possibility of medical intervention may "paradoxically heighten consciousness of a flawed, though malleable, biological body." Edmonds goes on to explain that, "Plastic surgery not only inscribes culturally variable aesthetic norms, but also clinically describes a biologically ageing, reproductive and sexual body. It reduces sexuality and beauty to physiological structures and processes, and has the potential to create biologically self-aware subjects who select medical technologies to calibrate the feedback relationships between body image, sexual health and psychological well-being" (79).

Mandy, whose story opens this book, is a mother of three young children with a demanding job. She blames her lackluster sex life not on her busy schedule but on her bodily changes and imperfections (in this case, attributed to pregnancy and childbirth). Mandy has projected her dissatisfaction onto her body, which she views as an entity that can be "fixed" surgically. For Mandy, surgery offers a simple solution to her complex social problems. Women who choose genital cosmetic surgery have a heightened biological awareness, which manifests in genital anxiety. The biological body, even the invisible, intimate vulva, is not absent but present, felt, and experienced, and surgery may be employed to disappear its unwanted presence (Manderson 2011). Whereas body modification usually works against nature by marking the natural body with culture (Edmonds 2010), cosmetic surgery presents the aesthetic and erotic body as the natural, desirable object, a hyperreal image (Baudrillard 1994) that is displayed and normalized in the media, thus persuading some women to act. Not only bodies are malleable, but so too are desires. These desires are fueled by consumerism, ensuring that bodies are "molded and disposed by history and culture" (Manderson and Jolly 1997, 1), a milieu in which biomedicine plays a vital role.

Although, as Christopher Lasch (1979) suggests, it could be argued that a narcissistic preoccupation with the self exists today, there is also an imperative to care for the self. This form of individual policing has arisen within a particular set of circumstances: a consumer culture in which the body and its appearance, fitness, and health are foregrounded. The body is an ongoing personal project, which we refashion according to the "dictates created in the market but felt individually" (Orbach 1999, 2). In late modernity, the body has become a source of individual identity, a self-reflexive project (Giddens 1991). "In a context where there no longer exist shared systems of meaning [such as religion or ideologies] which construct and sustain existential and ontological certainties residing outside of the self, individuals have turned towards the body as a foundation on which to reconstruct a reliable sense of self. . . . Paradoxically, however, as our capacity to re-fashion our bodies increases with the advances in surgical procedures and other bio-technologies, our sense of who we are becomes less and less certain" (Negrin 2002, 37).

Here, Llewellyn Negrin highlights how our expanding ability to refashion our bodies is accompanied by a sense of public uncertainty. The biomagical has given us the power to transform our bodies, and yet, as with other emergent medical technologies, there is an excitable imagination surrounding female genital cosmetic surgery. As Gary Downey and Joseph Dumit (1997, 7) posit, medical technologies "routinely contribute to the fashioning of selves." Their proliferation ensures that we live "liminal lives," a term that Susan Squier (2004) adopts to describe the workings of biomedicine on contemporary personhood. Human life is no longer tethered (Turkle 2008) to biology, because biomedical interventions ensure that the "form and the trajectory of our lives can be reshaped at will" (Squier 2004, 9). Ironically, this freedom to continually fashion our bodies is enacted at the biological level. Consumption, the media, and the biomedical imaginary coalesce within an environment of constant becoming and self-transformation, ensuring that female genital cosmetic surgery appears to be a viable option for some women (Tanner, Maher, and Fraser 2013).

Anthony Elliott (2008, 46) describes contemporary society as one of advanced globalization where "disposability has been elevated over durability, plasticity over permanence." This creates a milieu in which "fundamental anxieties and insecurities are increasingly resolved by individuals at the level of the body" (46), allowing "considerable scope for personal opportunities" but also ensuring that these come at an emotional, and often financial, cost (47). In an environment where personal makeovers are valued, many women have a free-floating anxiety about their bodies, as evidenced in the women's narratives that inform this book. Bodies are routinely portrayed as deficient and subject to control and embellishment. Bodily anxiety may be projected onto certain body parts and functions, thereby somatizing a sense of deficiency or inadequacy, one that is disseminated in the media and confirmed by the availability of cosmetic procedures to correct perceived defects. Fears about unattractiveness, imperfection, or sexual undesirability can be projected onto a fragmented part of the body (such as the vulva), and when that body part is excised or altered, so too are feelings of inadequacy (at least temporarily). Cosmetic surgery then becomes a powerful transformative ritual.

RITUAL AND SACRIFICE

Victor Turner (1967, 19) defines ritual as "prescribed formal behavior for occasions not given over to technological routine, having reference to beliefs in mystical beings and powers." With our contemporary faith in biomedicine, it is not difficult to envisage biomedical intervention as a ritual imbued with magic. Robbie Davis-Floyd (1994, 2) describes ritual as "patterned, repetitive, and symbolic enactment of a cultural belief or value; its primary purpose is alignment of the belief system of the individual with that of society," and a rite of passage "is a series of rituals that move individuals from one social state or status to another." Ronald Grimes (2000) points out that in Davis-Floyd's definition, almost any routine behavior could be termed "ritual." However, cosmetic surgery has a more transformative aspect than other, more pedestrian daily rituals, such as hair care and makeup. The change is more permanent, the transformation more promising and more complete, thus ensuring that it is more than "masochistic submission" to the coercive forces of consumer and beauty culture (Blum 2003, 59). Cosmetic surgery has a powerful ritualistic component. Surgical interventions adhere to strict procedural guidelines dictated by biomedicine, and although surgery is a technological routine, biomedicine has symbolic qualities because we increasingly place our faith in its power to transform our lives.

Cosmetic surgery is also a rite of passage. Women often undergo genital cosmetic surgery at a significant stage in their life. They may be entering the sexual realm (referred to as the "sexual market" by some surgeons) as young women, beginning a new relationship, or coming to terms with their bodies after childbirth. Mandy wants to return to her prematernal body. An older woman, Jane (whose story appears in more detail in chap. 2), described her vulva as "old," "uncomfortable," and with "a couple of tongues sticking out." She desired a younger-looking vulva in keeping with her sexual aspirations. Female genital cosmetic surgery can offer passage to "normality," "perfection," comfort, and heightened sexuality. As with a rite of passage, surgery works sequentially, with the liminal stage (Turner 1967) being the surgery and with the recovery period—although hardly a period of antistructure—being perhaps a stage of withdrawal, renewal, and contemplation.

Female genital cosmetic surgery also involves sacrifice; there are risks of a poor result, pain, and uncertainty. This is evidenced in some of the women's narratives about the postsurgical period: "The first few weeks, I felt so mutilated and mortified that I was thinking, 'Oh God, what has gone on with you, woman?' [and] that I won't be able to have sex anymore, and I felt all different and that I would be too small and that I've got funny bits here" (Jane, single, fifty-nine years, labiaplasty patient).

Jane not only suffered an extended recovery period but also found herself in a powerless position due to her lack of knowledge about the intricacies of the surgery itself and what to expect. Another woman I spoke with underwent genital cosmetic surgery three times before achieving a "perfect" result. She said, "Since May, I've constantly been sick and cried myself to sleep, taken time off work, honestly fearing I was going to be (in my eyes) 'deformed.' And now, I am so utterly grateful for what my last doctor has done for me. She has given me so much more confidence than I ever could have imagined. I feel truly blessed" (Kylie, single, thirty-one years, labiaplasty and clitoral dehooding patient).

Mirroring more traditional ritual events, for these two women, female genital cosmetic surgery was clearly a traumatizing experience. Yet apart from these statements, neither woman dwelt on the negative aspects of surgery. Rather, they moved on to what they consider a more satisfactory state, where they are no longer troubled by the appearance of their genitalia. As women seeking new sexual partners, they feel transformed and less self-conscious. Female genital cosmetic surgery is a ritual enacted at the individual level, one that promises reintegration through a newfound feeling of social inclusion and so-called normality. Cosmetic surgery has an inherent narrative quality. The stages of ritual are reflected in women's narratives of surgery—the before, the process, and the after—a subject I return to in chapter 3.

MEDICALIZATION

The biomagical is a transformative aspect of medicalization, one that brings the biomedical and beauty industries closer together through the medium of cosmetic surgery, thereby affirming its ritualizing potential. Leonore Tiefer (1996, 253) defines medicalization as "a major social and intellectual trend whereby medicine, with its distinctive ways of thinking, its models, metaphors, values, agents, and institutions, comes to exercise practical and theoretical authority over particular areas of life." Since the early nineteenth century, medicine has become a medium through which bodily experience gains meaning (Lock and

Nguyen 2010; Rose 2007). Biomedicine sets parameters for bodily deviation from a statistical norm—that of the healthy or average body. The abnormal or pathological is associated with disease, which requires treatment to facilitate a return to normality (Lock and Nguyen 2010). However, medicine not only cures disease but also, through the process of medicalization, transforms the social and subjectivity into the biological. Medical definitions and treatments are offered for what were previously considered social or psychological problems or, in the case of cosmetic surgery, no problem at all (Braun and Tiefer 2010; Conrad 2005). Medicalization works not only to alleviate stigma and shame (by medicalizing conditions otherwise portrayed as individual failings, such as alcoholism and obesity) but also to foster anxiety when new arenas are co-opted into discourses of normality or optimization (Lock and Nguyen 2010; Tiefer 1996).

Women's bodies have been particular targets for medicalization and normalization—psychologically, hormonally, reproductively, and as they age (Braun and Tiefer 2010; Conrad 2005; Gillespie 1997; Parker 2010). Reproductive function continues to be the focus of much medicalization of women's bodies, although there has been a noted shift to include sexuality more broadly, thereby providing a new scope for intervention. The emergence of female genital cosmetic surgery and the frenzied search for pharmaceutical and medical treatments for female sexual dysfunction (Moynihan 2003) are examples of this increased medicalization of female sexuality.

Biomedicine is usually presented as objective "value-free and ahistorical" knowledge (Healy 2006, 79). As such, rational behavior is presumed to respond to it (Good 1994). However, as Emily Martin (2001) suggests, medical science is also a hegemonic and often uncontested system, which has resulted in invasive procedures and treatments appearing natural and acceptable. Medicine can be employed to optimize and enhance subjectivity, leading to new ways of envisioning and achieving personhood (Rose 2007). It is usually assumed that medicalization is a recent phenomenon, inextricably associated with modernization in the West. For many commentators, its origins lie in the professionalization of medicine and the emergence of medical specialties. Practicing surgeons are intent on establishing genital cosmetic surgery as a legitimate subspecialty and founding vulval aesthetics and female sexual pleasure as worthy of medical attention. However, when medicine expands into consumer services, as is the case with cosmetic surgery, "physicians have a vested economic interest in the medicalization of appearance and shape" (Gillespie 1997, 74). The result is a shifting, unstable divide between rational, scientific medicine and commerce-oriented consumer medical services, made apparent by my labiaplasty informants, who frequently emphasized functional rather than aesthetic concerns when seeking surgery.

The fragmentation of the body that medical science perpetuates is employed to particular effect in cosmetic surgery, where body parts are isolated for aesthetic critique, fetishized, and subjected to market forces and the possibility of being serially upgraded (Frank 2002). "Fragmentation distorts because it renders bodies like other merchandised commodities: collections of 'features' that can be added and upgraded, enhancing value" (Frank 2002, 24). Although perfected body parts have no intrinsic value, they can have a derivative value (Frank 2002), as Edmonds (2007) reveals with regard to women who choose to have cosmetic surgery through the public health system in Brazil. Edmonds (2007, 363) refers to a "neoliberal libidinal economy" that describes the nexus between beauty, sexuality, and medical consumerism, one that affords the marginalized an opportunity to improve their position through cosmetic surgery. In Australia, women seeking surgery (or indeed Brazilian waxing) are often on the sexual market, looking for a partner. Here, medical technology is aimed at personal optimization, "securing the best possible future" for individuals (Rose 2007, 6).

Medicalization is an interactive, rather than a one-way, process. Medicalizing a condition makes intervention more likely. Women desire surgery and doctors provide it, but power relationships are uneven. The medical profession is in a privileged position in relation to those it treats because it has the necessary scientific knowledge and skills, and therefore authority, to transform women's bodies. The print and electronic media, along with personal interactions and current fashions, define appropriate femininity and attractiveness for patients and their surgeons. How women experience their bodies, their embodiment, is individual to them, but doctors must interpret women's desires and decide what they want from cosmetic surgery (Parker 2010). As Sander Gilman (1999, 334) says, "When we turn to the physician, we demonstrate our autonomy and abdicate it simultaneously." Surgeons work within the boundaries of technology, but they also have their own notions of aesthetics (see chap. 4). The genital aesthetic and functional ideals of doctors, both male and female, are influenced by the same cultural forces to which their patients are subjected. It is therefore inevitable that doctors' personal tastes will be physically imprinted onto the bodies of their patients.

—m—

Vulvas have a long history of vulnerability globally, but the rise of female genital cosmetic surgery, particularly labiaplasty, in recent decades has brought new attention to female genital aesthetics in the West. Consequently, similarities between genital cosmetic surgery and FGC, wherein some women's desires are considered legitimate and others' are not, cannot be summarily dismissed, despite differences regarding matters of age and consent. The Western medical-ization of cosmetic surgery gives it a legitimacy that is not afforded to FGC even if medicalized. Cosmetic surgery is a multibillion-dollar industry, and its popu-larity shows no signs of abating. In a makeover culture, self-transformation is valorized, and individuals are increasingly being persuaded to improve them-selves, often employing medical technologies. Female genital cosmetic surgery is not an isolated biomedical trend but part of a complex web of cultural forces and discourses centered on the body.

The neologism *biomagical* conveys the transformative properties of biomedi-cine, with its assertion that cosmetic surgery can magically alter the body and thus facilitate happiness, boost self-esteem, and increase feelings of social in-clusion. Biomagical imaginaries act on the body, including the vulva, in an en-vironment in which the health and beauty industries are increasingly entangled and images of eroticized, and therefore desirable, female genitalia abound in the media. Female genital cosmetic surgery is a beauty ritual focused on a previously less visible body part, the vulva, which is now fetishized and subject to aesthetic judgment and novel market forces in the contemporary medical-ized and media-driven milieu. As the poems that preface this introduction suggest and as current medical opinion affirms, the lure of "a beautiful flower" or a look "to die for" has resulted in an increased demand for, and practice of, female genital cosmetic surgery.

Like all social events, female genital cosmetic surgery involves a multitude of players, and in this field, power operates unevenly. By interweaving women's narratives with the supposed rationality of medical science, this book elucidates the complexity of these structures, highlighting the convoluted and changing cultural and social field in which concepts of gender, the body, ideals, normality, and biomedicine coalesce in the first decades of the twenty-first century.

This book comprises five chapters. Two of the chapters contain exten-sive narrative elements where I quote women's stories of their experiences at length to highlight that the way in which they recount their experiences of surgery or genital anxiety works to constitute that experience.

Chapter 1 focuses on the production of ideals and reveals that the current genital ideal for women is one of absence, a clean slit comprising a smooth vulval exterior with no flesh protruding. This ideal has historical underpin-nings, but it also allows the trafficking of images of female genitalia in the popular press in Australia, particularly in soft-core pornography, where female genitalia are minimalist, hairless, and frequently digitally altered to comply with censorship classification standards. Women's genitalia are thus rendered asexual and safe for general viewing, and the clean-slit ideal is particularly potent because it reaches a wide audience. Ironically, the second-wave feminist movement, which encouraged women to embrace their genitalia and become aware of their genital appearance and function, has led women to compare their genital morphology with others', but frequently, the genitalia with which they compare their own (mostly in the media) have been altered. Apart from in hard-core pornography, medical texts, and rare vulval art, vulval diversity is not shown. The medical profession is also complicit in generating the clean-slit ideal via their websites, where, through a particular use of language as well as before and after photographic images, they validate women's concerns about their genital appearance.

Chapter 2 discusses normativity and the contradictory nature of the term *normal*. Norms are created in the media and reinforced through medical science in a way that often persuades women that they are not normal. What is considered normal in the pubic area is changing. Although a wide variation of normal is acknowledged both in the popular press and by physicians, this variation is not desirable, because overtly visible genitalia, for women, are considered unattractive and a sign of inappropriate femininity. Therefore, although most genital variation is normal, only a limited range of "normal" (i.e., acceptable) is shown, and this fuels genital anxiety in some women. Normality as a concept is ambiguous. To be normal is desirable but also mediocre, not ideal. In medical terms, one should be normal (i.e., healthy), but in aesthetic terms, women desire to be better than average.

Chapter 3 reveals that some women who undergo female genital cosmetic surgery are aiming for perfection rather than normality. Cosmetic surgery uses the biomagical power of medicine to transform bodies, and by association minds, in a society that values technology itself (its salvational and magical properties) and "technologies of the self"—attributes that in a makeover culture are central tenets to living. Our bodies, including our vulvas, tell a story of who we are. A tension therefore exists between "care of the self" and excess (a perhaps inappropriate use of biomedicine). This tension is mediated through consumption, making the biomagical promise of cosmetic surgery difficult to resist in a milieu where working on the self is expected and enhancement technologies are available.

Chapter 4 is an ethnography of a conference I attended in Las Vegas that was hosted by the International Society of Cosmetogynecology. At the conference, female genital cosmetic surgery was taught and its practice defended. Following

Lawrence Cohen (1995, 320), I describe the conference as an "epistemological carnival," a site of knowledge production and contestation—a celebration of knowledge, to an extent—but one that hides as much as it reveals. Although most doctors ostensibly attend medical conferences to gain further knowledge and skills in what is a rapidly changing scientific field, there is frequently more at stake. The conference was strategic and as much about professional politics as it was about knowledge sharing. A strong sense of brotherhood was invoked, one that involved the establishment of boundaries in order to found and protect this new area of expertise, which is coming under criticism from medical bodies and feminist scholars for being unscientific and possibly dangerous to women.

Chapter 5 brings the threads of my observations together as I reflect on bodily autonomy, risk, desire, and magic. I utilize a particular personal experience with injury and medical care in an endeavor to draw some parallels between the risks and choices attributed to cosmetic surgery and other forms of risk so as to contextualize the subject of this book. I discuss the clean-slit ideal as a simulacrum, which has its original version or prototype in prepubescent girls only, and I discuss how vulval ideals are generated as much through what is *not* represented in the media as by what *is* represented. In this chapter, notions of ritual and sacrifice are examined in more detail, and using this frame, the idea that female circumcision and female genital cosmetic surgery are radically different is interrogated. The role of biomedicine—the biomagical—in producing what is considered desirable femininity is examined through the lens of female genital cosmetic surgery.

NOTES

1. I use the term *clean slit* to refer to a particular minimalist vulval aesthetic. I credit the term to Simone Weil Davis (2002) but cannot confirm its origins as a descriptor for female genitalia.

2. I use the expression *the West* as a gloss to refer to the two countries where I carried out my research—Australia and the United States—while signaling that these practices are found in other European and Anglo-Pacific contexts, including, for instance, the United Kingdom, France, Greece, Germany, Italy, Scandinavia, Canada, and New Zealand.

3. When I refer to "women" throughout the text, I am referring to my female informants who had undergone or were considering undergoing genital cosmetic surgery, not female doctors.

4. I credit Lisa Wynn for the neologism *biomagical*.

5. Medicare funding for labiaplasty in Australia (under Item 35534) is available only if the surgery is deemed necessary for a woman's health and

performed in a hospital. If surgery is covered by Medicare, a rebate may also be available through private health insurance. Labiaplasty in Australia costs between AUD$4,000 and AUD$8,100 (Malone 2013). The average cost of labiaplasty in the United States is US$2,924, according to 2018 statistics from the American Society of Plastic Surgeons. However, this average cost is only part of the total price; it does not include anesthesia, operating room facilities, or other related expenses (American Society of Plastic Surgeons, 2020).

6. Any qualified doctor can perform cosmetic surgery in Australia; however, plastic surgery is a medical specialty requiring at least an additional five years of training. Specialist plastic surgeons are accredited by the Australian Government through the Australian Medical Council. Despite that, female genital cosmetic surgery is not always taught during plastic surgery training.

ONE

—ᗯ—

MELTING SNOWFLAKES
Toward a Clean Slit

FEMALE GENITAL AESTHETICS HAS ARISEN as a topic of discussion in the media, as the following excerpt from an article that appeared in *Sirens* magazine attests.

> Even enviably beautiful women are totally freaked out by their vaginas. Maybe that means labia are the great equalizer. Or maybe it means we all need some serious help.
>
> The problem with this variety of anxiety, though, is that it's tough to assuage. Guys have grappled with genital insecurity since penises were invented, but at least there's a yardstick by which they can measure their adequacy—literally, a yardstick. Bigger is better, the end. . . . With this dilemma, I don't know where I stand: What is the ideal here?
>
> It's tough to find a standard, realistically speaking, not only because we don't spend a lot of time staring into other women's vaginas, but also because labia vary about as much as snowflakes. (Armstrong 2008, par. 6–8.)

Sirens magazine (now titled *Sexy Feminist*) claims to be an alternative online women's magazine that intellectualizes the topics found in standard women's magazines in fresh ways. According to the article, both female and male genitalia vary substantially, but some female genitalia are increasingly considered more aesthetically pleasing than others. Traditionally, it has been assumed that men are more concerned than women about the appearance of their genitalia; aesthetically, or at least functionally, bigger is presumed to be better. Conversely, for women, modesty and cleanliness have been the genital ideal. The physicality of women's genitalia has not been exposed to public scrutiny. However, some women are now more anxious about the appearance of their genitalia, and contrary to Jennifer Armstrong's (2008) words quoted above, they are now more likely to see other female genitalia because of the mainstreaming of the sex industry and increased exposure to nudity in magazines, in movies, and on the internet. This has occurred at the same time as fashions and a gym and beach culture (where female genitalia are expected to be out of sight while encased in tight fabric) are driving a certain aesthetic ideal.

The increasingly specific and visible female genital ideal is that of the clean slit (Weil Davis 2002) or *single crease*, a term used in the Australian pornographic magazine industry (Drysdale 2010). Although many women may not aspire to this ideal, it is the aesthetic most frequently encountered in the media. In *Being and Nothingness*, published in 1943, Sartre commented, "The obscenity of the female sex is that of everything that gapes open" (quoted in Greer 2000, 39). The clean-slit ideal seeks to rectify this image of female genitalia. The ideal is one of absence, a smooth exterior with no flesh protruding and with skin folds completely contained: this can be attained through the removal of pubic hair and, increasingly, through surgery. The clean-slit ideal has been largely created by the media, which generates contradictory messages for women. The popular press, backed by medical opinion, acknowledge that a wide range of variation is normal, but by showing only altered, minimalist vulvas, the implicit message is that women should be worried if their genitalia do not match up to this exacting ideal. The clean-slit aesthetic represents desirable femininity as it is portrayed in the visual media, and genital cosmetic surgery allows the women who choose it to assuage their genital anxiety and increase their self-esteem. The tidy minimalist look is also endorsed as desirable by practicing doctors who profess to understand women's genital anxieties and why they seek surgery. In an environment where bodies are generally seen as malleable and perfectible, striving to achieve a more perfect body is normalized, even valorized. Whether this acceptance extends to female genital cosmetic surgery is more uncertain.

THE CLEAN SLIT

In *I'll Show You Mine*, a photo study of women's vulvas, compiled by Wrenna Robertson, a Canadian editor, one participant wrote:

> A few years ago, I looked up labiaplasty on the web. I'd become very self-conscious about the size of my labia minora after being with female sex partners and seeing their vulvas up close and personal. Like the porn actors I had seen, their labia minora were nicely tucked into a centerfold and hidden between their labia majora, like a letter perfectly folded and slipped into an

envelope. My labia minora most certainly were not folded perfectly; they were crumpled and protruding obnoxiously from between my legs. What was the point of an envelope being held, licked, and sealed if it couldn't contain a letter? (Robertson 2011, 39)

Robertson's aim in this publication is to relieve women of genital anxiety by showing genital diversity. Accompanying each image is text written by the woman whose vulva is shown, explaining her relationship with her genitalia. A number of similar books exist, but the women participating in my study were more likely to obtain information on vulval morphology from the internet.[1]

As the above quotation from Robertson demonstrates, the genital ideal for women is minimalistic; the labia minora should be symmetrical and not protrude past the labia majora (Weil Davis 2002). Using Robertson's analogy, the letter fits neatly within the envelope. There must be no gaping; the vulva should be flat and closed tight. A slit is a long, straight, narrow opening or cut, an aperture. It is also an obscene term for female genitalia (Princeton University 2013b). When it comes to contemporary genital appearance in the West, however, the term *slit* takes on a more positive resonance. The ideal echoes that of the model female body, which is represented as tall, straight, and slender, voluptuous only in the "right" places.

Before and after photographs of genitalia found on cosmetic surgery websites confirm this aesthetic ideal. One surgeon in the United States, Dr. Red Alinsod (who has trained several Australian surgeons), has labeled his most minimalist vulval look the "Barbie," which results in "a 'clamshell' aesthetic: a smooth genital area with the outer labia appearing 'sealed' together with no labia minora protrusion at all" (O'Regan 2013, 3), reflecting the iconic American doll's lack of genital detail. According to Alinsod, "I had been doing more conservative labiaplasties but I kept getting patients who wanted almost all of it off. They would come in and say, I want a 'Barbie.' So I developed a procedure that would give them this comfortable, athletic, petite look, safely" (O'Regan 2013, 3).

How a vulva can look "comfortable" and "athletic" is perplexing, although the Barbie look certainly appears to be a prepubescent, smooth, and plastic aesthetic. This surgeon's website describes three vulval looks: the Rim, the most conservative choice, which Alinsod suggests is the look most commonly achieved with labiaplasty worldwide; the Barbie, which is complete excision of any protruding labia minora and the aesthetic most frequently requested by Dr. Alinsod's patients, particularly those on the West Coast of the United States; and the Hybrid, a recent addition to this aesthetic selection, which is a combination of the Rim and the Barbie, giving "a very fine, petite, natural looking hint of a rim around the vaginal opening" (Alinsod 2013). Just a few years ago, the options were the Rim and the Barbie, and this third choice reflects current trends to continually "improve" labiaplasty techniques to produce a particular aesthetic result. However, although aesthetic choices may vary marginally, the overall aim is for minimization of skin folds, and Alinsod is obviously proud of his ability to offer alternatives to the Rim.

All surgery has risks, and given that the labia minora serve a purpose, excising them may alter sensation and function. The labia minora are rich in nerve endings, blood vessels, and estrogen receptors and therefore add to pleasure and sensation during sexual arousal. They also keep the entrance to the vagina moist, and they direct the urine stream (Battaglia et al. 2013; Dobbeleir, van Landuyt, and Monstrey 2011; Puppo 2013; Schober et al. 2010; Yang et al. 2005). According to Justine Schober et al. (2010), labia minora become engorged during sexual arousal, making them important for sexual response. Labiaplasty, therefore, removes tissue that makes an important contribution to sensory sexual arousal.

Despite the body of medical literature describing the physiology of the labia minora, a gynecologist who specializes in female genital cosmetic surgery and who has been trained by a leading proponent of the practice in the United States responded with conviction when I asked him about the function of the labia minora, "Oh no, there are no pleasure receptors in the labia, none at all." In contrast, when I questioned plastic surgeons about labia minora, they routinely assured me that they did indeed contain nerve endings that function for both pleasure and pain and that these may be compromised in the search for the "comfortable, athletic, petite look" of the Barbie aesthetic. However, because of their surgical skills, doctors performing female genital cosmetic surgery believe they can minimize risk.

Barbie

Referring to images of vulvas in *Playboy* magazine, Carlin Ross, who with Betty Dodson runs a sex-positive educational website, observes, "Here's the formula: not one woman has pubic hair, not one woman has visible labia. Their sex organ is just a slit and they all look alike. Even their outer lips are tight and barely visible. It's like they took a Barbie doll and drew a line down the middle of her crotch and, voila, it's a vulva. They don't look anything like the vulvas I see in the Bodysex groups" (Ross 2012, par. 2).

Ross's critique of the clean slit is understood through her use of a Barbie-doll analogy. It comes as no surprise that ideal female genitalia are often described in terms of a Barbie-doll aesthetic given that Barbie is modeled on the supposed pinnacle of (hyperreal) Western femininity (Baudrillard 1994).

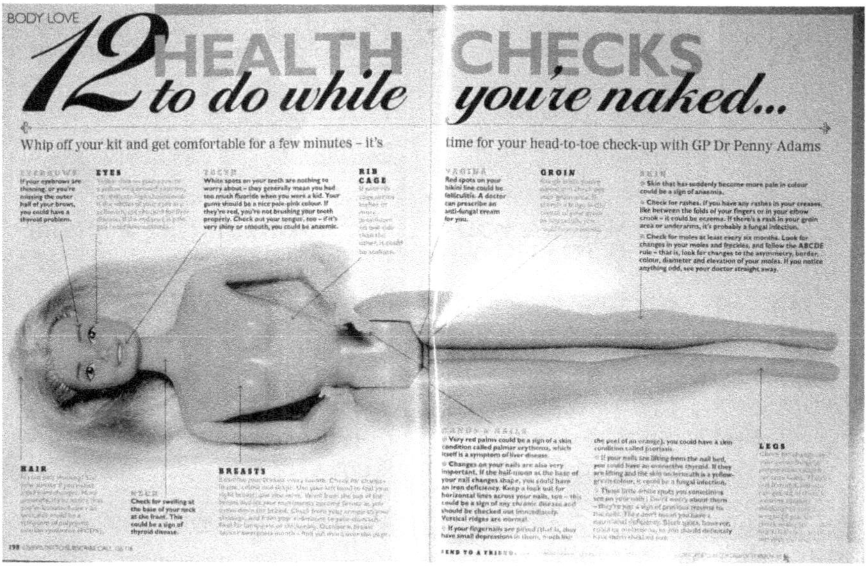

Figure 1.1. "12 Health Checks to Do While You're Naked," published in Issue 447 of the Australian edition of *Cosmopolitan*, Bauer Media Pty Ltd, October 2010, pp. 198–99. Reproduced with permission from Bauer Media Pty Ltd.

Unlike the original doll, Barbie often now comes with molded underpants, so she has become more modest and, although her vulva is flat and lacks detail, her (lack of) genitalia are now more difficult to critique as a result. Photographs of Barbie dolls are sometimes used as educational tools in women's and teenagers' magazines in Australia, such as *Cosmopolitan* and *Dolly*, where articles have appeared with body parts labeled as requiring health checks or as sites for cosmetic surgical intervention.

The use of Barbie as an educational tool in a section titled "Body Love" (see fig. 1.1) is provocative; any parallel drawn between Barbie's physique and real bodies carries the assumption that women should compare their bodies with this plastic, extremely unrealistic ideal. While Barbie is bereft of much anatomical detail, including the vulva (labeled in fig. 1.1 as "Vagina"), Barbie-related anxieties tend to cluster around specific markers of idealized femininity—breast size, waist-to-hip ratio, slenderness, and smooth genitalia. As Jacqueline Urla and Jennifer Terry (1995, 13) suggest, "Because Barbie's body is statistically deviant compared to most women, the doll has functioned to underscore the predicament of femininity: no female body is ever appropriate" without intervention. Indeed, "the female body has increasingly become, like Barbie herself, a form of cultural plastic," and the vulva has now succumbed to this plasticity (Urla and Terry 1995, 13).

Cleanliness

When associated with the notion of a clean slit, the word *clean* primarily refers to a visual aesthetic of neatness and tidiness. However, given the historical construction of female genitalia as smelly, dirty, and leaky, the ideal for women also extends to keeping their genitalia as clean and sweet-smelling as possible. Cleanliness, particularly female bodily cleanliness, is valued. Women, predominantly young women, frequently ask in women's magazines and on the internet about feminine hygiene. "Do I smell and can people tell?" is a major topic (Teens Health 2008). As most women's health sites attest, the smell of vaginas can vary significantly. However, this is not always reassuring for women, as the following illustrates.

> My vagina stinks!?!!??!?!?!?
> Yeah. My vagina stinks. I don't know why. I talked to my doc on the phone and I have an appointment in 4 days. BUT I have a date TOMORROW with this really awesome guy, and I've tried shaving, putting lotion or baby powder. NOTHING HELPS. I even tried Vagisil. Doesn't work either. I can't postpone the date. I already did that last week. Ugghh I'm so embarrassed! Please make my vagina not stink. (Abbie K 2009)

While a malodorous vagina may indicate an infection requiring treatment, the number of young women asking these questions coincides with a resurgence of feminine hygiene products in pharmacies and supermarkets, supported by advertisements in magazines and on television. Chemist Direct, an Australian online retailer, listed thirty-four feminine hygiene products on a particular day in 2013, including washes, sprays, and a recently introduced product, wipes. The advertisements suggest that women's genitalia are naturally offensive, despite the vagina being a self-cleaning organ requiring nothing but water for upkeep (Herbenick and Schick 2011). A market exists for feminine hygiene products because of culturally mediated female genital insecurity. One 2013 advertisement for feminine wipes, published in Issue 47 of the Australian *Cosmopolitan* (2013, 99), declared, "Hooray for a fresh Hoo-ha. With Libra Get Fresh Wipes. They're not only compact and super discreet, they're also gentle enough to use all over. Slip some in your handbag so you don't get caught out." The implication here is that women should not only be vigilant about policing their feminine odor but also discreet in doing so. By implying that women need this product, Libra is perpetuating the notion that female genitalia are dirty, shameful, and in need of management.

Older women are also concerned about hygiene. One fifty-two-year-old woman I interviewed said that having a labiaplasty has solved her concerns with hygiene:

> Ann: I like to smell nice and fresh as much as I possibly can. Before, by the end of the day, I would always find I was very fastidious. I always carried little wipes, little feminine hygiene wipey things. I don't want to smell. I don't want to be talking to someone—well, to be honest, it's offensive. I don't like to smell fishy or yucky or have any sort of odor. But I must say since I've had this done—like, you know, I sort of go for a wee or something late in the afternoon and I go, "Oh! I don't have that pungent smell." Whether that is because my labia were trapping extra bits that I never actually got to properly or not, I don't know.

Hygiene issues such as toilet paper sticking to the labia after micturition or difficulties maintaining personal cleanliness during menstruation are reasons some women give for considering labiaplasty. However, most surgeons I spoke with dismissed the suggestion that surgery could resolve hygiene issues or reduce the incidence of recurrent yeast infections (candidiasis); rather, they emphasized discomfort, aesthetics, and self-esteem as reasons for surgery. Beauticians, on the other hand, do emphasize the importance of cleanliness and neatness as a major advantage of Brazilian waxing. "Girls just prefer it without hair. It is a hygiene thing," one commented. Neatness is linked to cleanliness, control of one's environment, and, increasingly, one's body. Historically grounded negative portrayals of female genitalia are thus perpetuated in the media and in society more widely, and the anxiety they generate in women sells products and services (such as waxing, depilatory products, vaginal deodorants, and wipes).

Liminality, Containment, and Absence

The ideal of the clean slit extends beyond aesthetics to include cleanliness and bodily control, a form of containment of marginal zones (Douglas 1966). The "mysterious" liminal nature of female genitalia threatens order. Unlike male bodies, "the vagina sports moist, textured tissues like bodily insides while it is accessible from the outside without an incision" (Kapsalis 1997, 19). Women's bodies are always in need of control to ensure there is no leakage of menstrual fluid, no secretions, and no odors—signs of this liminality and abjection (Kristeva 1982). To these leaky feminine attributes has been added the more material labia. Unruly, large, and protruding labia minora are abject, despite their (until now, in the West) permanence on the body.

> To the dangers and allures of what's hidden about the vagina, now is added the "too muchness" of labial tissue. In their heterogeneous dappling and their moist curves, labia mark the lack of tidy differentiation between inside and outside and that's just *too much*. One effect of this procedure is to reduce this sense of a "marginal" site between exterior and interior corporeality. . . . This indeterminacy, actually a function of the labia's protective role, may be part of their association with excess. (Weil Davis 2002, 15)

Female genital cosmetic surgery addresses genital excess. For many women seeking cosmetic surgery, excess is desirable for breasts but not for labia. The clean slit, as an ideal, renders the genital area less problematic (visually) by demarcating the boundary between the "fetishized gloss of the outer dermis and the wet, mushy darkness of the inside" (Weil Davis 2002, 15) through the removal of excess tissue (and hair), thus making this marginal zone more distinct. Elizabeth Grosz asks, "Can it be that in the West, in our time, the female body has been constructed not only as lack or absence but with more complexity, as a leaking, uncontrollable, seeping liquid; as formless flow; as viscosity, entrapping, secreting; as lacking not so much or simply the phallus but self-containment" (Grosz 1994, 203). Grosz suggests that this lack of self-containment, this "seepage," defines women's corporeality. So, let seepage be contained. Leaking menstrual fluid is considered socially unacceptable, making the tampon—although a liberating technology for women—the quintessential "plug." It puts the vagina in its place by sealing it up. Similarly, labiaplasty does this visually by removing any "gateway" tissue, thereby giving a sealed appearance to the vulva (Weil Davis 2002, 15).

Leaky, protruding representations of the female body echo the grotesque, which for Mikhail Bakhtin (1984) is celebratory and inclusive, and a central theme of the carnivalesque. However, the body of which Bakhtin speaks is not the individual body but the social body. With the grotesque body, "Stress is laid on those parts of the body that are open to the outside world, that is, the parts through which the world enters the body or emerges from it, or through which the body itself goes out to meet the world. This means that the emphasis is on the apertures or the convexities, or on various ramifications and offshoots: the open mouth, the genital organs, the breasts, the phallus, the potbelly, the nose" (Bakhtin 1984, 26).

Bakhtin's emphasis on the "apertures" and "convexities" through which the body goes out to meet the social world is pertinent, because it is these parts of the body that are particularly targeted by cosmetic dentistry and surgery. When the grotesque is applied to the individual female body, it requires management, not celebration. "The images of the grotesque body are precisely those which are abjected from the bodily canons of classical aesthetics. The classical body is transcendent and monumental, closed, static, self-contained, symmetrical, and sleek" (Russo 1994, 8), as represented by the clean slit itself. Conversely, "the grotesque body is open, protruding, irregular, secreting, multiple, and changing" (Russo 1994, 8), descriptions frequently attributed to female genitalia— the "everything that gapes open" to which Sartre refers.

Unclad female genitalia, particularly in magazines, in articles about female genital cosmetic surgery, and on websites, are routinely depicted as a V or, if including the legs held together, a Y; they end in a perfect point of *nothingness*. This minimalist look implies that female genitalia are thoroughly internal, the opposite of male genitalia. The sexual opening is disguised, rendering a closed appearance that, while obscuring where the vaginal opening is and what else is there, simplifies female sexuality for safe consumption. This ideal makes the slit the dominant anatomical feature of the genitalia, when it is, in fact, merely the gateway to a set of structures. Except in hard-core pornography, in medical texts that typically show stylized drawings, and in rare vulval art (such as drawings, photography, and plaster casts), the complexity and fascination of female genitalia are hidden. There is no melding of the external and internal genitalia. Female genitalia are reduced to a single, smooth, and desexualized assemblage, an obstacle-free opening readily accessible for male penetration, affording direct access without effort or complications. "The sanitized, deodorized, sterilized, always accessible vagina and womb," says Germaine Greer (2000, 43) in *The Whole Woman*, "are more, not less, passive than they ever were."

According to the surgeons I interviewed, an absent and smooth aesthetic is the look that patients request. "My patients uniformly want their genitals to have nothing hanging down or protruding below the labia majora," said one male doctor. Another said, "Some people want their mons pubis reduced. It's just fat. We liposuck that bit, so it doesn't stick out." This language suggests that bumps and protrusions need to be reduced and made smooth. The flat, absent look, which also extends to clad genitalia, is largely dictated by current fashions. Fashions have become progressively skimpier and tighter, particularly lingerie, jeans, leggings, and swimwear, and nothing is hidden—hair or labia. A study conducted by Ros Bramwell (2002) of photographs in glossy women's magazines in the United Kingdom concluded that the ideal clad female genital area is presented as a flat, smooth curve.

The antithesis of this is *camel toe*, a colloquial term referring to the outline of the vulval cleft showing through tight fabric, a look ridiculed in the popular press. Nonsurgical solutions to camel toe have emerged on the market. These include supportive underwear, such as the aptly named Camelflage, and even a shoehorn-like device called SmoothGroove, which ensures no vulval "seam" or bulge appears underneath clothing. The possibility that camel toe may be more obvious as a result of pubic hair removal is unaddressed, because having bushy hair is, for many, as unthinkable as camel toe itself. As one woman explained to me, "It wasn't just in the bedroom that my labia were a problem—wearing jeans was painful because they'd dig into my labia, and I couldn't wear tight shorts or even a swimsuit because you could see a bump." Bumps and genital structures "hanging down" or "sticking out" need to be reduced and made flat. This ideal of absence for female genitalia is "consistent with a social norm that considers women's genitalia should be invisible" (Bramwell 2002, 190).

Appropriate Femininity

The ideal of genital absence is inextricably linked to female sexuality. The clean-slit aesthetic allows the trafficking of images of women's genitalia in the media that would otherwise not be possible, because it renders them safe for public viewing, not too sexually loaded. Desirable, eroticized (censored and airbrushed) but appropriate femininity involves large breasts and minimal genitalia. This ideal is a strange paradox in which a woman's body has every other marker of female sexuality enhanced and exaggerated (breasts, curves, lips, and flowing locks, yet no body hair) but with the primary markers of her sexuality (labia and clitoris) reduced to absence. Men, but especially women, are sold this desexualized image as an erotic version of the body, a nonassertive but acceptable form of femininity. In this paradigm, the erasure of sexuality allows absence and invisibility to play a role in the erotic imagination. While many models are androgynous rather than curvy (perhaps representing a nulliparous body shape), pornography and cosmetic surgery websites often display a more traditionally feminized body.

Female sexualization is everywhere; it is used to sell products and services and to create desire, yet only one form of sexuality is presented as publicly acceptable. Women who seek the perfect vulva reflect the dominant order of female sexuality, which idealizes a flawless body, a body disciplined through dieting and fitness regimes and, at times, enhanced by cosmetic surgery. We live in an era of sexual self-marketing in which (healthy and beautiful) bodies are increasingly used to express identity and to garner social status.

The clean slit defines femaleness as opposite to maleness in a clear, uncomplicated manner, an aesthetic of heteronormative complementarity. The gaping hole that resists closure, the liminal field, is rendered more visually closed through female genital cosmetic surgery, making the area less problematic, less leaky. It is snapped closed like a clam formed by the labia majora, which in some instances are made to appear more obvious and "useful" through the injection of fillers.

One female plastic surgeon, Dr. Marcos, told me that she plumps up the labia majora in approximately 50 percent of her genital cosmetic surgery patients. Dr. Marcos has a busy practice in a regional city in Australia. Her surgery, an unpretentious two-story wooden house, is some distance from the town center. On visiting one afternoon, I found the small waiting room full. A kind man gave up his chair for me and went to sit on the step. The sofas were squidgy, their homely character too intimate for a waiting room. A number of women were present but also several older men whom I (perhaps incorrectly) assumed were there for reconstructive surgery. The staff members were friendly, but the atmosphere was rather chaotic. After a long wait, I was ushered upstairs into a small treatment room furnished with only a bed and stool. I was told that a patient who was feeling faint had been put in Dr. Marcos's office downstairs.

I had begun to feel somewhat uncomfortable when in bounced Dr. Marcos, a short woman wearing a tight-waisted cotton dress that showed off her rounded figure. She was perfectly groomed, with bright lipstick and a beaming smile. I was instantly at ease. "So you want to talk about fannies?"[2] Dr. Marcos gushed as she sat on the stool. "You have to look at the patient standing up. That is how they look at themselves. They don't want to see anything. No one wants a granny fanny." Describing labia majora augmentation, she said, "It is a good procedure and it only takes ten minutes. I tell my patients that I can't make them look like some 'Fluffy Galore' in a porn picture. I stress the unpredictability of surgery. I have learnt my technique by trial and error."

Dr. Marcos was proud of her handiwork. As she showed me a PowerPoint presentation she had delivered at a recent plastic surgery conference, she said, "Look at a pretty fanny as compared to a scraggy, rather limp one. I must confess, as far as shaven fannies go, there is definitely a new neatness and plumpness to the altered one. The crescent shape of filler placement gives a natural look. You mustn't overdo it, as when standing it will then be too bulky. It would be a disaster to have it protruding too far." The labia majora need to be plumped up to hide the labia minora but not to the extent that they themselves protrude, thereby spoiling the flat, absent look.

Genital ideals vary over time and place. In the West, longer labia have historically been associated with racial stereotyping, sexual promiscuity, or lesbianism (Bramwell, Morland, and Garden 2007; Dickinson 1949; Nurka and Jones 2013). However, long labia now appear to be associated with inadequate and undesirable femininity. This contrasts with other cultures. For example, in Japan, the term *winged butterfly* is used to describe protruding labia minora, and this aesthetic is considered a sexual delicacy rather than unattractive or unfeminine (Sager 1999). As part of a feminine beautification ritual, the women of the Buganda people of Uganda stretch and massage their labia and clitoris from childhood in order to extend them (Weil Davis 2002), as do women from other areas of central, eastern, and southern Africa, where "long lips" are deemed "a source of pleasure and beauty" (Manderson 2012, 7). Hellen Venganai (2016) explains how Shona-speaking women in Harare, Zimbabwe, associate the practice of labia elongation with modernity rather than rural tradition. These women emphasize discourses of fashion and self-improvement, thus affirming their modern, middle-class identities. Clearly, genital ideals are strongly shaped by cultural preferences and meanings. The clean-slit ideal is therefore a natural desire to alter one's body so as to adhere to aesthetic preferences.

Some male surgeons I spoke with drew an analogy between protruding labia minora and inappropriate femininity. One plastic surgeon, Dr. Hoffman, specifically asked me to visit his clinic when a woman from a rural region was consulting him about labiaplasty. I am uncertain why he suggested this. I always felt uncomfortable when waiting in surgeons' offices if women were there for an appointment or surgery. This was not because I was embarrassed that someone might think I was there to enquire about genital (or other) cosmetic surgery for myself; rather, I felt I was intruding on other women's medical choices. I met Dr. Hoffman in his office before the patient arrived, and he told me how prevalent female genital cosmetic surgery was in Europe, Asia, and South America, and that women in Australia had a poor understanding and awareness of surgical possibilities for "improving" their sexual functioning and genital aesthetics. When the woman, an attractive forty-four-year-old, went in to see Dr. Hoffman, I sat outside reading a tome he had given me on genital surgeries and sexual disorders in Korea. There were no other patients in the waiting room and I began to feel uneasy while also absorbing the myriad surgical possibilities put forward in the text I was perusing. Finally, the woman emerged, and I was ushered into the surgeon's office once more to finish our conversation. There he showed me before and after photographs of some of his patients' vulvas. Pointing to one photograph of protruding labia, Dr. Hoffman said, "It looks like a penis, doesn't it? It's a disability." On a different occasion, another surgeon commented, "They see it as a problem, too bulky, you know. It looks like they have got testicles." By describing these women's genitalia in terms of male genitalia, these surgeons are insinuating that longer labia are not just aesthetically displeasing but also masculine in nature and therefore inappropriate for a heterosexual woman. Similar notions are echoed in circumcising societies, as Janice Boddy elucidates in her book *Wombs and Alien Spirits*.

Wombs and Alien Spirits

In *Wombs and Alien Spirits*, Janice Boddy describes what constitutes appropriate femininity for the Hofriyati of Northern Sudan. The Hofriyati practice pharaonic circumcision, or infibulation, a procedure that involves the excision of most of the external female genitalia and the stitching or narrowing of the vaginal opening. For the Hofriyate, particularly women, bodily orifices make people vulnerable and are therefore "considered most appropriate when closed or, failing that, when minimized" (Boddy 1989, 52) in a manner echoed by the clean-slit aesthetic. The essential attributes of a circumcised woman are those of purity, cleanliness, smoothness, and enclosure. Boddy (1989, 55) explains that "by removing their external genitalia, female Hofriyati seek not to diminish their own sexual pleasure—though this is an obvious effect—so much as to enhance their femininity." For Hofriyati women, infibulation is a symbolic act that deemphasizes their sexuality, thereby allowing them to assert their social indispensability as mothers of men (Boddy 1989). Their principal concern is fertility, and sensation is sacrificed in order to achieve socially approved reproduction. By enclosing the womb through infibulation, uterine blood—the source of fertility—is "contained and safeguarded," thus ensuring the well-being of the village (Boddy 2016, 50). The principle concern of women who choose labiaplasty, however, is not fertility. Rather, they risk diminishing sensation to gain a certain (more feminine) aesthetic, thereby facilitating feelings of attractiveness and social inclusion. As with the Hofriyati, women undergoing female genital cosmetic surgery endeavor to display what is currently accepted as desirable femininity. Visually, the results of infibulation and the more radical forms of labiaplasty and clitoral hood reduction are not dissimilar.

As Boddy (2007) explains, infibulation for Hofriyati girls strengthens and symbolizes their social roles. "A girl's body is feminized, enclosed both by infibulation and the courtyard walls behind which she should now remain; a boy's body is masculinized, opened to confront the world" (Boddy 2007, 63). Female genital cutting (FGC), then, has a representational meaning that extends beyond the physical. Boddy argues that "in Western thought, the sexed body is primary and gender is derived, whereas in Northern Sudan, gender is primary and the conventionally sexed body is derivative" (61). In other words, in infibulating societies, genitalia are altered to fit a specific feminine identity ideal. Now that more women in the West are altering their genitalia in order to display appropriate femininity, Boddy's distinction appears less emphatic. In the West, the desire for female genitalia to appear absent is at this stage mostly a visual ideal, which can be attained by editing images of female bodies in the media rather than the widespread surgical alteration of women's genitalia. However, the aesthetic ideals of smoothness and invisibility for female genitalia do converge across cultures, and in the West, there is an increasing acceptance of the malleability of female genitalia, something that has long been attributed to those in circumcising societies.

The Problem of Pubic Hair

The clean-slit ideal is also an anti-hair ideal. A lack of pubic hair, or its minimization, particularly on the labia majora (if hair is left on the genitalia, it is typically on the mons pubis, above the labia), exposes the desirable slit. As one surgeon explained, "You often get to see that area—very few women these days have hair that grows bushy." Another surgeon commented, "Having hair in those areas is very natural, but it is not very nice." The hairless ideal is complex. It extends beyond a female ritual (which, for many, it has become) or the desire for a prepubescent appearance. Rather, there is a desire for smoothness, which is associated with cleanliness and sexiness. "Single women worry all the time [about the state of their pubic hair] in case they meet Mr. Right. They think once they have a Brazilian, it will please the man more," said one beautician. This concept of smoothness and cleanliness is shared by the Hofriyati, whose brides remove all body hair prior to marriage and after marriage when the woman "wants to attract the attentions of her husband" (Boddy 1989, 65). However, some stories of hairlessness are more disturbing. One labiaplasty recipient with whom I spoke had been sexually abused as an adolescent, and she divulged, "One day I heard a young guy on a bus comment on how awful this girl's vagina was because it had hair on it. I also know about pubic hair because I had chemotherapy and my husband loved my hairless, emaciated, prepubescent-looking body. I discovered he was a pedophile and divorced him."

While depilation may produce a prepubescent look, it is more accurately, according to the women in this study, an extension of grooming and bodily maintenance, echoing the myriad other technologies with which women engage to enhance their bodies. Not all the women I interviewed who had undergone labiaplasty removed or trimmed their pubic hair, although pubic hair removal was more prevalent among the younger participants. Some women said that prior to surgery, they had been too embarrassed to have a Brazilian wax or a Pap smear but had subsequently taken up these practices.

A study of pubic hair removal practices in the United States found that sexually active younger women are more likely to engage in pubic hair removal than older women and that total hair removal is less common than retaining at least some pubic hair (Herbenick et al. 2010), thus refuting the notion that a prepubescent ideal is favored. A 2008 Australian study of pubic grooming among 235 undergraduate students found that 60 percent of respondents removed at least some of their hair, with 48 percent removing most or all of it. Reasons given for adopting pubic grooming practices included sexual attractiveness and self-enhancement (Tiggemann and Hodgson 2008). The authors of the study suggest that "the removal of pubic hair, in particular, is associated with glamour and sexiness to a much greater extent than the more 'mundane' removal of underarm or leg hair" (Tiggemann and Hodgson 2008, 895). The study showed that hair removal practices also appear to be linked to reading fashion magazines and watching television programs such as *Sex and the City* and *Big Brother*. In a 2012 edition of the Australian magazine *Cosmopolitan* (2012a, 66) under the title "What Do You Like to Find When You Head Down There?" 50 percent of the male respondents said "completely bare," 44 percent "a well-groomed lady garden," and only 6 percent "all natural." None of the women I interviewed drew a direct link between pubic hair removal and their desire to have surgery.

Mandy, whose narrative appears in the prologue, was anxious about her genital appearance and contemplating surgery. She explained that she now regularly removes her pubic hair.

Mandy: Now I go all the time [to the beautician], once every six weeks.
Lindy: Does your husband prefer it like that, does he comment?
Mandy: Um, it is interesting because, well, I only have one girl [beautician] that I go to. I can't bring myself to go to anyone else. I had my first session, and when I got home my husband said, "How did it go?" Because I had not been able to let the [waxing] lady do everything because I wasn't comfortable with her looking at me—I still have that shy factor—so as much as I like the girl who waxed me, I still have to wear the little plastic G-string . . . I just remember when I got home and he said, "How did you go?" Um [*sighs deeply*], and I explained to him that I took off as much as I had been able to get done. He was surprised because it was basically everything down to the labia. I couldn't go any lower than that. I certainly couldn't let her see me. He was surprised because I took the whole of the front off, and he said, "Aren't you going to leave a strip?" I said "No"

> [*laughs*], and he said, "Oh, why not?" So, he expected that I would leave
> something there, but I had every intention of taking everything off.
> We haven't discussed it any further—we probably should.
> Lindy: Since you have an issue with your labia, don't you think having no hair
> makes it more obvious?
> Mandy: No, because I don't think the hair covers things up. It is part of the
> problem.

At this point, Mandy became lost for words, so I interjected that perhaps she felt that way because hair is also one of her body issues, and we went on to discuss other things. With the beautician, Mandy cannot expose her labia for fear of embarrassment. However, despite her acute genital anxiety, she engages in depilation. Mandy finds both pubic hair and protruding labia minora unattractive and unhygienic. She desires a clean slit but does not perceive a causal link between hair removal and her dislike of her protruding labia.

HOW THE CLEAN-SLIT IDEAL EVOLVED

A complex web of history, art, and language has combined with the medical profession, the media, and feminist understandings of the body to create the clean slit as an aesthetic ideal for women. A corollary of this ideal is female genital anxiety.

History

Vulvas were frequently depicted in the Paleolithic era, and images appeared as Venus figurines and etched or painted on rock surfaces at various Stone Age sites in France, Spain, and Russia. The size and shape of the vulvas differ widely (Blackledge 2003). What these representations meant (and whether they were created by women or men) is unclear; they may have been associated with childbirth or fertility, or used in rituals or as a source of male erotica (Blackledge 2003; Nesbitt 2001; Wolf 2012). Vulval depictions have been interpreted by many scholars as early signs that female sexuality and fertility were considered sacred, and that such prehistoric images represent humankind's first use of symbolism (Blackledge 2003; Wolf 2012). In Australia, the Aboriginal people etched vulvas into sandstone walls. At one particular site, Carnarvon Gorge in Queensland, vulvas are a common motif. Dated as being thirty-five hundred years old, they were most probably a symbol of fertility (Kirtley 1996).

However, more recently in many Western cultures, women's genitalia have been imbued with negative sociocultural meanings, and the manner in which the vagina moved from the scared to the profane—particularly with the advent of Christianity—is well documented by scholars such as Catherine Blackledge (2003) and Naomi Wolf (2012). Female genitalia increasingly became problematic—an area for concern, a source of shame—and therefore hidden and veiled rather than celebrated and revealed: "Perceived as powerful yet vulnerable, a source of pleasure yet smelly and ugly, passive yet hungry, the vagina and its surroundings get more disrespect than honor" (Tiefer 2008, 475). Female genitalia are depicted as problematic (Braun and Wilkinson 2001) and polluting in ways suggested by Mary Douglas (1966) in her seminal work *Purity and Danger*. Bodily margins, particularly female genitalia, are invested with power and danger; therefore, they can be manipulated in order to establish social control and define appropriate sexuality. "By taking up less space, the female genitalia are further controlled and made absent in the world" (Priddy and Croissant 2009, 183). At this point in history, in which "the embodiment of space often denotes power, this reduction can also represent a reduction of power for the female body" (Priddy and Croissant 2009, 183). Genital absence, therefore, is not only a signifier of appropriate femininity; it also reinforces gender hierarchies by determining not only how a woman should look but also how she should act—she should be modest.

In the West, in the late eighteenth and early nineteenth centuries, an earlier acceptable notion of women's natural lustiness was transformed into the myth of feminine modesty (Weil Davis 2002). Appropriate modest decorum, although appearing innate, has been a huge and ongoing project for women. The same social world that saw (and perhaps, less convincingly, continues to see) the ideal woman as a spectacle for male pleasure, aesthetically pleasing, unchallenging, and devoid of rampant sexuality has also "spawned and recycled dirty jokes about 'vagina dentata,' fatal odors and other horror story imagery of female genitalia" (Weil Davis 2002, 9). Vagina dentata, the vagina with teeth, is an ancient and enduring motif that existed individually in North and South America, across Africa and the South Pacific, and in India and Europe before global communication arose. The myth varies from location to location, but there is a common narrative of the vagina as something to be feared (Blackledge 2003; Rees 2013; Wolf 2012). Sexual folklore abounds with stories of "snapping vaginal teeth" and a male fear of castration (Blackledge 2003, 165). Many dentata stories are found in creation myths, and perhaps not surprisingly, they often involve brave male heroes removing the vaginal teeth. The reasons for the ubiquitousness of the myth of vagina dentata are not clear; do men fear what lies within the mysterious interior of the vagina, which is likened to a mouth, or do they fear what Blackledge (2003, 165) refers

to as the "insatiable vortex of female sexual energy"? Wolf (2012, 129) believes
that vagina dentata imagery is not about aversion to the vagina but a "necessary balance to the reverence for women's life-giving powers." Although the
myth of vagina dentata has largely receded, Emma Rees (2013) argues that
its symbolism continues in horror films and artwork. A history of negative
female genital imagery has resulted in many women internalizing a fear of
being associated with these unfavorable connotations. Disgust and desire
have long been conflated when describing female genitalia, and this paradox
is one that women constantly and individually negotiate.

Images are instrumental in creating ideals. Whereas medical science has
defined the pathological, art has defined the grotesque. Representations of
female genitalia in contemporary mainstream media are in stark contrast to
the (presumed) rampant sexuality of figures such as Saartjie Baartman—
the Hottentot Venus—whose labial folds were ogled and sketched by early
nineteenth-century scientists, who saw African female sexuality as animal-like
and pathological (Blackledge 2003; Gilman 1999; Nurka and Jones 2013; Weil
Davis 2002). Saartjie Baartman was a Khoi Khoi (Hottentot) woman born in
southern Africa around 1790. In 1810, she was taken to Europe, where she spent
time in both London and Paris. In London, she was exhibited as a circus at-
traction because of her elongated labia minora and prominent buttocks. While
longer labia were admired in her home country, they represented sexual and
racial difference (and inferiority) to Western society and became the subject
of scientific investigation when she went to Paris, where her labia came under
the scrutiny of the anatomist Cuvier (Blackledge 2003; Nurka and Jones 2013).
Georges Cuvier was fascinated by Baartman, particularly her labia, which he
dissected and described in great detail after her premature death in 1815 at the
age of twenty-six. Her labia were then preserved and put on display in the Musée
de l'Homme in Paris until 2002, when they were returned to South Africa. These
"scientific" studies of Baartman sought to establish white superiority, thereby
justifying the colonial project by suggesting that what colonialists termed at the
time as "the Negro race" were the lowest form of human, something akin to apes
(Nurka and Jones 2013). "The white, colonial understanding of the female 'Hottentot' genitals was that they were both animal and anomalous; the labia functioned as the primary signifier for deviance from not only civilized humanity, but
also femininity" (Nurka and Jones 2013, 422). Camille Nurka and Bethany Jones
(2013) theorize that the present-day dislike of protruding labia minora stems
from the colonial past and a desire to distinguish white ("civilized") femininity from black ("uncivilized") femininity. By the twentieth century, however,
"the scientific obsession with the measurement of the labia had moved away

from race to concentrate more firmly on sexuality" (Nurka and Jones 2013, 419). The turn to concerns about so-called deviant sexuality (lesbianism, prostitution, and masturbation) and its link to vulval morphology are reflected in the works of Robert Latou Dickinson (1949) and Havelock Ellis (1900).

During the colonial period, white women's genitalia were shown in art as hairless and absent, safe for the male voyeuristic gaze (Berger 1972). One icon of female beauty, the nude odalisque, was heralded as the epitome of femininity—the naked harem woman. Orientalism (Said 1978) in art therefore represented the aesthetic branch of European colonialism, a form of Western social propaganda, while medical science, by defining the pathological, was used to justify colonization. However, tracing the historical construction of women in the arts as merely a show for the male gaze presents an incomplete picture of women today, because they are increasingly producers and consumers of their own image. Historically, as now, the white female nude and her genitalia were aesthetically altered to make them suitable for public consumption. Nudes have long been a classic art form, even in periods when public (particularly female) nudity was anathema, but these nudes were not meant to be erotic, as many are today. "While the invisible white vulva of the eighteenth and nineteenth centuries represented desexualized purity, the contemporary post-surgical vulva allows for sexual availability, and replaces sexual shame with confidence" (Nurka and Jones 2013, 429), thus demonstrating that genital ideals can connote different meanings over time.

Language

The clean-slit ideal is also generated through language. The word *vagina* is often used colloquially to describe the entire female genital region, despite this term actually referring only to the canal that leads from the vulva to the cervix. The term *vulva* refers to the external genitalia (labia majora, labia minora, clitoris, mons pubis, perineum, introitus, and hymen), although what is in fact included under this label is unclear (Barnes and Lumsden 2010). How we name female genitalia is important. The American feminist and psychologist Harriet Lerner (1994, 31) believes that neglecting the word *vulva* has serious consequences and calls the practice a "psychic genital mutilation. . . . Language can be as powerful and swift as the surgeon's knife. . . . What is not named does not exist." Some health professionals and sex educators believe that the public should adopt anatomical terms. They feel such a practice is more appropriate than using nicknames that fail to represent the genitalia accurately (Buni 2013). The use of the word *vagina* to include all the anatomical features of female genitalia is reflected in the popular term *designer vagina*, which refers to genitalia that have been surgically modified. However, naming individual structures anatomically, although appearing rational, may not be a neutral practice. For instance, Debby Herbenick and Vanessa Schick (2011) point out that the term *labia minora* may itself be misleading because it infers these lips should be small. They suggest adopting the term *inner labia* or *inner lips* instead.

The words *vulva* and *vagina* remain largely taboo except in medical situations. This is hardly surprising in a culture where a recent television advertisement for a feminine hygiene product drew criticism from Australian audiences for mentioning the words *vagina* and *discharge* instead of resorting to the usual visual euphemisms—allusions to flowers, sunsets, and women in white bikinis (Rosewarne 2012). Very few of the women I interviewed employed these terms to describe their genitalia, which is not unusual. In their study of the language of sexual health, Lisa Wynn, Angel Foster, and James Trussell (2010) found that language reflects people's thinking about sexuality and the body, and what is deemed culturally appropriate, and this informs both their experience and their actions. According to Virginia Braun and Celia Kitzinger (2001b), women's genitalia are often considered unmentionable. They refer to one study in which only 7 percent of respondents felt it was acceptable to use the term *vagina* freely. Another study found that 53 percent of women "felt some discomfort using the word *vagina*" (Braun and Kitzinger 2001b, 146). Since many women, and men, are unable to identify all the components of the female genitalia using medical terms, they resort to using epithets. One reason for this linguistic trend may be that female genitalia have been associated with pudendal disgust. The word *pudenda* (plural of *pudendum*) has its roots in the Latin word *pudēre*, meaning "to be ashamed" (Dictionary.com 2014). The term *pudenda* refers specifically to the external genital organs of women. Genital shame is not shared; quite the reverse: "There is an enormous societal cache for shame when it comes to publicly exposing female genitalia, verbally, visually, or metaphorically" (Ramos 2011, 36). Naming erogenous body parts is more than superficial. Societal notions about the female body are reflected in naming—through either the adoption of euphemisms, positive or negative, or the use of nonspecific language about the constitutive parts of female genitalia.

Frequently, derogatory terms are used to refer to female genitalia (as they are to male), and this reinforces women's insecurity about their genitals' appearance and odor. The terms *cunt, batwing, beef curtain, meat seat, stench trench*, and *wizard sleeve*, to name but a few, are in stark contrast to the more euphemistic monikers such as *down there, bits, vajayjay*, and *yoni*, which are favored by many women when referring to their genitalia (Braun and Kitzinger 2001b;

Herbenick and Schick 2011). The use of negative epithets for female genitalia disallows women a positive or enabling view of their genitalia. In *The Female Eunuch*, first published in 1970, Greer argued, "Part of the modesty about female genitalia stems from actual distaste. The worst name anyone can be called is cunt. The best thing a cunt can be is small and unobtrusive: the anxiety about the bigness of the penis is only equalled by anxiety about the smallness of the cunt. No woman wants to find she has a twat like a horse-collar: she hopes she is not sloppy or smelly" (Greer 2006, 44–45). While Greer is implying here that the extended use of the word *cunt* as an insult stems directly from a dislike for what it denotes, the same logic could be applied to male genitalia. No one wants to be called a *dick* or a *prick*, because these terms are equally offensive.

When men use negative terms for female genitalia, it can affect how some women experience their genitalia, even if men have not commented to them directly.

> Janice: I've heard men say at barbecues, "Oh, she's got a crotch bigger than Gene Autry's saddlebag." I don't know who that is, must be a cowboy or something.
> Lindy: Sounds big, anyway.
> Janice: It does. And I heard, I heard [*laughs slightly*], and this person is still with his partner. He said that about his partner, not in front of her, but in front of a lot of other men, and I heard that and thought—well, then I heard other women commenting on how they had heard other men commenting on, you know, the size of the labia, and I just thought, "Oh, that's an issue. People don't like it, it can't be right. It must be wrong to have this." So, I started, I started developing this very self-conscious image.

In this extract, Janice, a labiaplasty recipient, describes how she evolved her own sense of genital self-consciousness based on discussions she overheard. Greer's insight that "the best thing a cunt can be is small and unobtrusive" is evidenced here too, particularly in the loaded—and clearly negative—phrase "a crotch bigger than Gene Autry's saddlebag." Gene Autry was an actor who played the role of a cowboy, and indeed, his saddlebags were large. The use of derogatory terms to describe female genitalia helps inform an ideal that is, as closely as possible, the opposite of that alluded to in these referents. As such, aesthetic ideals are produced through language.

In the British Channel 4 documentary *The Perfect Vagina* (2008), Lisa Rogers, the presenter, asks her male painters and decorators what they would say is the "perfect vagina."

Painter 1: Ah, a shaven one.

Painter 2: No, I do like a bit of hair.

Painter 1: I prefer them tucked in. I don't like a squashed hedgehog . . .
some women have flaps they could tuck in their socks, beef curtains.
I do like oral sex, you know, giving and receiving, and it is like having a
presentation with your meal; if it is all slapped on the plate and it is all
mushy peas everywhere, it puts you off a bit, you know. You have to have
something that looks nice before you taste it—if she's got an ugly fanny,
sorry mate, if you are having sex for the first time with a woman, if she has
an ugly fanny, sorry mate. (*The Perfect Vagina* 2008)

Although this comment may well have been made especially for the cam-
eras, such sentiments are echoed in the concerns of some women, particularly
of young women, who ask about genital attractiveness on the internet. These
women are worried about what their sexual partners might think about their
vulvas. In a hurt and damaged voice, one woman disclosed to me that she had
been ridiculed and humiliated by men about her labia on multiple occasions:
"Men are cruel if women are different. I would not have had a labiaplasty otherwise. More than one person was rude about it and used offensive language.
What would men feel like if we criticized their penises?" Because of these comments, she had not had sexual intercourse for twelve years. To blame men,
however, is to fail to recognize that vulval ideals are created and propagated
in the media (and increasingly fashioned by beauticians and surgeons). Men
and women aspire to ideals that are not necessarily innate but generated in a
particular time and space. The ideal becomes so familiar, however, that it is
perceived as natural.

Feminism

The second-wave feminist movement had a major impact on women's knowledge of their bodies, allowing women to wrest back control of their corporeal
selves to some extent from the authority of the postwar male-dominated medical profession (Kline 2010). Before second-wave feminism, genitalia were often
a source of shame and embarrassment for women, a part of their body that
they rarely examined themselves. Over the years, feminist voices have sought
to address this negative representation of female genitalia and the derogatory
language frequently used to describe them. Publications such as *Our Bodies,
Ourselves*, first published in 1971 by the Boston Women's Health Book Collective, and *A New View of a Woman's Body*, published in 1981 by the Federation

of Feminist Women's Health Centers, sought to bring accurate anatomical information to women while acknowledging vulval (and clitoral) diversity.

Our Bodies, Ourselves "promoted the concept that experiential knowledge based on personal stories is a crucial component of women's health" (Kline 2010, 5), allowing a "reconceptualization of biology that privileged women's experiences over clinical research" (Kline 2010, 11). Second-wave feminists challenged Sigmund Freud's (1905) championing of the vaginal orgasm, and William Masters and Virginia Johnson (1966) affirmed the role of the clitoris in sexual response (although Masters and Johnson's emphasis on orgasm suggests that it is central to sex rather than recognizing that sex can be pleasurable even if orgasm does not eventuate). These were emancipatory steps. Because of the feminist movement, attitudes toward women's role in sex and the appropriateness of self-touching changed. Dodson (1974), a prominent American feminist, wrote *Sex for One: The Joy of Self-Loving*, affirming the appropriateness of masturbation. With the advent of the contraceptive pill and the women's liberation movement, there was a change in Western sexual mores, with women having a higher number of sexual partners and more sexual freedom. In this sense, feminism has undoubtedly been liberating for women and has encouraged them to be more comfortable with their bodies and their sexuality. However, there have been unexpected consequences, not because of feminism per se but because of the intersection between the body awareness that feminism promotes, the influence of the media, and the resurgence of medical authority with regard to genital aesthetics.

One male cosmetic surgeon I interviewed drew a direct connection between feminism encouraging women to familiarize themselves with their own genitalia and increased demand for genital cosmetic surgery. He noted, "Traditionally, in Western society, women have not been encouraged to explore their genitals, although this has changed since second-wave feminism. Now we are freer to talk about these things. Now we talk about penis, vagina, and menarche. When a woman reads something, she says, 'Let me examine my genitals.' She knew it was there but didn't want to see it. Now women are more open and want to see themselves—see what is so important."

Women, from both a medical and a feminist perspective, have been encouraged to embrace their genitalia and are freer to talk about and view them. However, these movements, which were intended to be liberating for women, have been somewhat of a double-edged sword. Being aware of your genital appearance allows you to compare it with others. Unfortunately, the female genitalia with which women compare their own are not likely to be in the flesh but in altered images in the media. Consequently, women have not become liberated about their genital appearance, but anxious. As Faith Wilding (2001) explains, "The jouissance and libidinal excess pursued by many feminists as a path to autonomy and power, is being replaced in public discourse by the full-scale consumer spectacle of the cyborg porn babe, whose predatory surface is adorned by every well-worn sign of coded sexuality that the market will bear" (Wilding 2001, 6). This "coded sexuality" in Western makeover culture has extended beyond breasts and buttocks to the genital region. Female sexual characteristics are being accentuated as the opposite of their male equivalents—scarcely a feminist or liberating goal. The "cyborg porn babe" image, so readily found in the media, deems some zones in need of augmentation, while others must be stripped away in an effort to approximate this hyperfeminine ideal.

While second-wave feminism centered on collective empowerment for women, identity today is more likely to focus not on collective female power but on power gained through self-control, with "an intensive and critical focus on controlling one's body" (Kline 2010, 160). Wendy Kline concludes, and I concur, that second-wave feminism has failed the female body to some extent: "Rather than expand and enhance knowledge and power, and create a collective consciousness, it [the body] continues to restrict and contain women" (160). If feminine power comes from individual bodily control rather than collective knowledge and action, women are subject to manipulation—by the media, the medical profession, and societal expectations. Women today are concerned about their individual bodies and selves, not the communal "our bodies, ourselves," and this puts enormous pressure on them to comply with strict aesthetic and functional standards.

Pornography

Debates about whether the pornography industry is detrimental or emancipating abound in academia, feminist circles, and the popular press. With the pervasiveness of the internet, pornography has become mainstream and, as such, more popular with women. According to a survey of internet pornography consumption in Australia, a third of pornography consumers are now female (Horin 2007), and *The Porn Report* (Albury, Lumby, and McKee 2008) found that women consume 20 percent of soft-core pornography. Other international studies have estimated pornography consumption rates to be between 86 and 98 percent for men and 54 and 85 percent for women (Hald 2006). I asked women about the influence they thought pornography had on establishing

genital ideals. Most were aware that images in unrestricted material, particularly in magazines, might be digitally altered.[3] Although their opinions varied
about how they personally were influenced by pornography, they spoke of it in
a normalized fashion and considered pornography an accepted part of everyday
experience. Only two of the twenty-two women I interviewed said they did not
access pornography at all.

The normalization of pornography, along with the proliferation of "crotch
shots" in music clips and other visual material, has contributed to women's genitalia being less hidden than in the past. Their increasingly visible yet contained
nature confirms the vulval ideal. One of the most accessible sources of images
of female genitalia is soft-core pornography, where contained genitalia represent
a safe, nonthreatening version of female sexuality. The women's genitalia shown
in unrestricted magazines such as *Playboy*, *People* (a men's magazine in Australia,
not the American *People* magazine), *Picture*, and *Penthouse* have no or very little
hair. They are neat, symmetrical, and, in most images, digitally altered, often
resulting in vulvas that have the appearance of weirdly fuzzy, indeterminate
triangles. As an editor of one soft-core pornography magazine explained on the
television program *Hungry Beast*, "It's not because they've chosen to only photograph women with 'innies.' Many of the models actually have 'outies' in real life,
which have been 'healed to a single crease' with the aid of image editing software.
Think of it as 'digital labiaplasty'" (Drysdale 2010). Even in restricted material,
labia have no dark edges, and anuses are usually bleached (Drysdale 2010).

In Australia, the censorship classification system insists that unrestricted
pornographic magazines and women's magazines are subject to the Guidelines for the Classification of Publications, which state, "Realistic depictions
of sexualized nudity should not be high in impact. Realistic depictions may
contain discreet genital detail but there should be no genital emphasis. Prominent and/or frequent realistic depictions of sexualised nudity containing genitalia will not be permitted" (Attorney-General's Department 2005).

This ruling also affects women's magazines, as Mia Freedman, former editor
of Australian magazines *Cosmopolitan*, *Cleo*, and *Dolly*, describes: "To this day,
any magazine showing any 'genital detail' must be sold in a sealed plastic bag.
Like [restricted] pornography. And I'm not talking about explicit legs akimbo
shots, just shots of a normal girl standing up with her legs closed. She must
look like Barbie or the airbrush will be deployed to make the censors happy
and protect our sensitive eyes from OFFENSIVE VISIBLE LADY PARTS"
(Freedman 2009).

However, what exactly constitutes "discreet genital detail" is not clear, and
the basis for industry decisions about this lacks transparency. In *Hungry Beast*,

which aired on the ABC in Australia in 2010, an ABC board member responded as follows when asked about "discreet genital detail": "Yeah, well, I guess genital detail is that we can have discreet genital detail in unrestricted and I guess that means genital, well, detail is pretty straightforward, so discreet means little or no, or very little, detail or not prominent, so it's sort of quite clear, if that makes sense" (quoted in Drysdale 2010). There is nothing clear about this comment other than that women should not have anything "prominent," or obviously protuberant, about their genitalia. So, why are labia minora considered to have "high genital impact"? Why should they not protrude?

The "problem" of female genitalia was highlighted in 2013, when the student newspaper of the University of Sydney, *Honi Soit*, attempted to promote acceptance of female genital diversity by publishing on its cover eighteen photographs of students' vulvas depicting the normal range (see fig. 1.2). The editors of *Honi Soit* had originally intended the photographs to be uncensored, but the Student Representative Council, which publishes the newspaper, requested the vulvas be covered by black bars; otherwise it would be illegal, too pornographic. However, within hours of distribution, the publication was withdrawn despite the censorship—the black tabs were apparently too translucent. A flaccid penis was shown on a *Honi Soit* cover in 1993 without incident. It seems vulvas are still too scary or too offensive for public viewing, even when presented for a positive cause—body acceptance—at what one would assume is a liberal institution. Although the uncovered vulvas did show genital detail, which is against classification specifications, it is unclear why their use for educational purposes as opposed to erotica was deemed unsuitable. Anyone can log on to the internet and view doctors' websites or the Labia Library (2017), an educational website about vulval diversity, and see similar images.

One woman I interviewed, Hilda, a forty-one-year-old labiaplasty recipient, was extremely angry about the need for women's labia to be out of view in pornographic magazines. She said, "Growing up in a society that 'doctors' women's genitalia in magazines like *Playboy* results in people being conditioned to think of different types of vaginas as horrible. No wonder many women have a complex about their most private parts. No partner has made me feel uncomfortable, but it is generally my own insecurity about it that prompted me to do something. I am horrified that in this day and age, it is still OK for magazines to 'remove' part of a woman's body because it's considered offensive, while men don't have any of their bits removed." Magazines routinely airbrush photographs of models and celebrities to conform to perceived aesthetic ideals. Many younger women were ambivalent about this practice. However, this form of enhancement is optional, whereas when

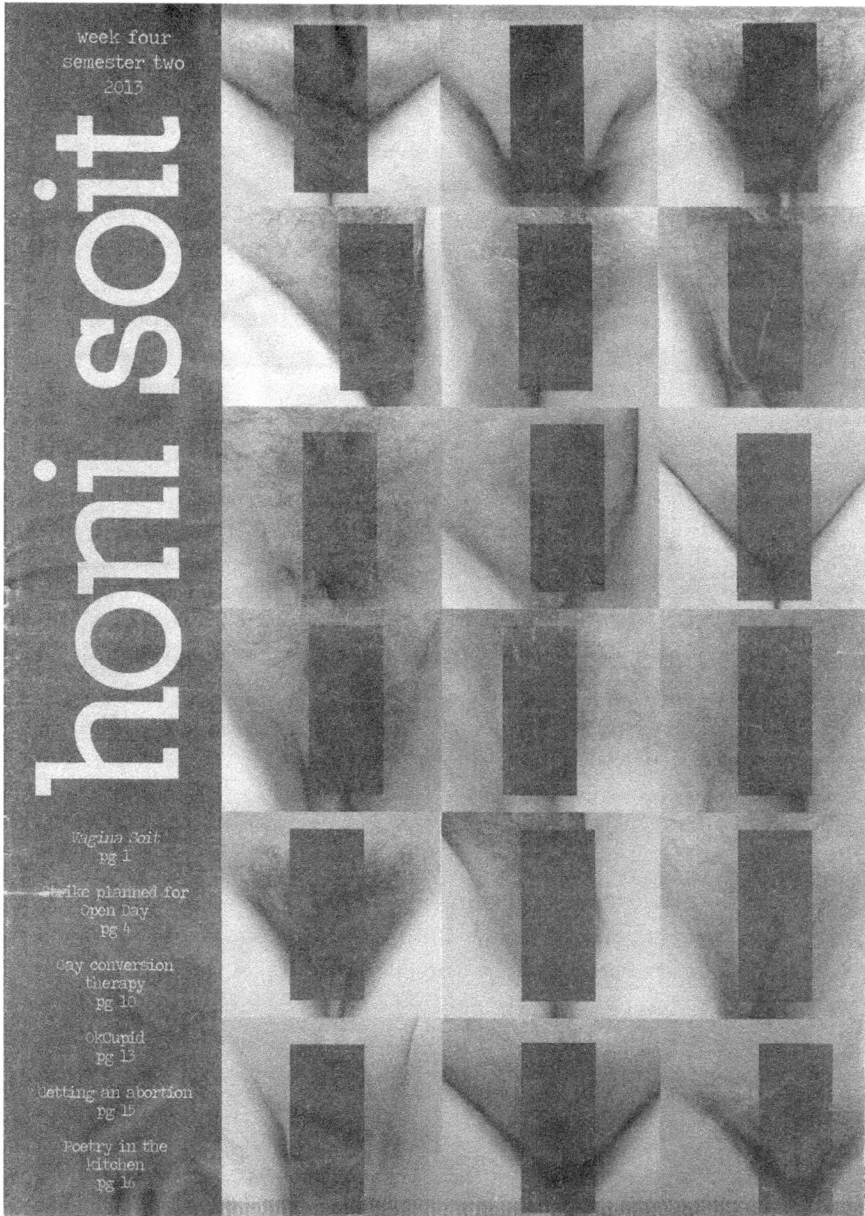

Figure 1.2. "Are you seriously offended by a body part half the population has?" (Honi Soit 2013). Reproduced with permission from the Students' Representative Council, University of Sydney. (The Students' Representative Council never published the uncensored image, which can be found on the internet.)

images of naked women are to appear in unrestricted media, the airbrushing of protruding labia is compulsory and regulated.

Some women spoke freely about their desire to emulate the aesthetic of the neat, tidy vulvas that they see in pornography. Kylie, a thirty-year-old labiaplasty and clitoral dehooding recipient, said, "Women want to be perfect, and if we see trim and tidy vaginas in pornographic material, magazines, movies, and adult videos, we start comparing our own and it doesn't look as good as theirs. Then of course we're going to want to change ourselves." Others were adamant that their decision to have surgery was unrelated to pornography and claimed they are not as gullible as some women. Bella, a twenty-six-year-old labiaplasty recipient, said, "I don't doubt for one second that some women are made to feel insecure by the seemingly perfect genitals and bodies of women in porn. However, due to my research into labiaplasty and personal interest in all the details of the procedure, I know that every woman's vagina is different, and there really is no 'normal' or 'perfect' type of vagina. But I don't doubt that not all women understand that." Despite their awareness of genital diversity, all the labiaplasty recipients I interviewed aspired to the same aesthetic displayed in pornography without necessarily acknowledging the source of the ideal. Like slenderness, the minimalist closed look is the ideal to which some women aspire.

Pornography, particularly soft-core pornography, normalizes a certain aesthetic, and this can affect the lives of ordinary women. This occurs despite the fact that a wider variety of female forms are now easily accessible on the internet. In the same way that women's fashion magazines, the movie industry, and television generate a collection of images that reflect and determine what is considered a beautiful or perfect body in Western society, the proliferation of soft-core pornography has created an assemblage of images that define the perfect vulva. These images are increasingly consumed by women, who—more than their male counterparts—prefer to see idealized body types. According to *The Porn Report* (Albury, Lumby, and McKee 2008), women are drawn to "fantasy or plastic porn" with a strong visual aesthetic appeal. Male consumers prefer to view hard-core pornography, where it is more likely that "real" women will be depicted (Albury, Lumby, and McKee 2008; Hald 2006). The fantasy porn star ideal suggests a single form of acceptable sexuality for women, one driven largely by women themselves. As one surgeon said, there seems to be a disjuncture between the sexes. Ideals are being generated (and mandated) in the media and adopted by women without any conversation with men. Despite this, some women are concerned about what men think of their vulvas and, as one woman told me, they feel that men "assume our lady bits all look like the ones they see in pornography."

Idealized female genitalia are rated G (for general viewing) so they can be consumed by a wider range of viewers and therefore generate more income. Restricted magazines, XXX-rated websites, and the increasingly popular amateur, or gonzo, internet pornography sites show a less romanticized, more realistic female form, in sharp contrast to the sleek, smooth bodies shown in *Penthouse, People, Picture,* and *Playboy* magazines. While a diluted (and less erotic) ideal of female genitalia has been pursued in the mainstream media, hard-core pornography has become a multibillion-dollar industry (Dines 2010). However, hard-core pornography is primarily consumed by men and has little effect on the choices women make about their genital appearance (Albury, Lumby, and McKee 2008). In addition, more-explicit imagery usually shows women with their legs spread wide, their inviting vulvas glistening like oysters, and in these positions, it is expected that the labia minora would be on display. Conversely, in unrestricted material, whether women are standing or posing in more-suggestive positions, their labia are out of sight. This hampers an understanding that it is normal for the labia minora to be visible in the more modest positions permissible in soft-core material (Drysdale 2010). Consequently, cultural mores demand two versions of female genitalia in pornography: the real and the ideal. It is ironic that the real—the full range of normal genitalia—is more likely to be found in hard-core pornography, an industry that many argue demeans women. Presumably, the safe clean slit does not threaten cultural stability or offend the viewer, because it represents contained and accessible female sexuality. Actual female sex organs are considered too dangerous for public viewing. Women's real sexuality is censored and erased and replaced with the desexualized clean slit, which itself is eroticized to create aspirational desire and, by association, consumer desire in men and women.

Pornography functions by selling libidinal desire, both as a form of entertainment and as a form of ideal creation—that is, ideals about what is considered desirable in the human form and in the sexual act itself. However, Bethany Jones and Camille Nurka (2015) suggest that the relationship between pornography and female genital cosmetic surgery is not linear, as is often suggested—rather, a more complex model is required to understand motivations for surgery. Emphasizing the role of pornography in driving genital ideals is political because it diverts attention from other drivers, such as the medical profession and the commercialization of medical practice, particularly cosmetic surgery. The existence of an ideal and its attendant genital anxiety is financially advantageous for surgeons. It would be simplistic to blame pornography alone for the rise in genital cosmetic surgery. However, after the publication of the article "Clinical Characteristics of Well Women

Seeking Labial Reduction Surgery: A Prospective Study" by Naomi Crouch et al. (2011) in the *British Journal of Obstetrics and Gynaecology* in 2011, articles appeared in the digital media discussing the study, with titles such as "Is Porn Pushing Popularity of 'Designer Vaginas'?" "Porn Blamed for 'Designer Vagina' Epidemic," and "Pornography Linked to Huge Rise in Plastic Surgery for Women." This was despite the fact that in the Crouch et al. (2011) study of thirty-three women, only four (12 percent) reported having viewed pornography, while eleven (33 percent) said they had seen surgeons' advertisements for genital cosmetic surgery. Pornography, although a pervasive influence, is often employed as a scapegoat when discussing female genital cosmetic surgery. Pornography and Brazilian waxing are routinely blamed for the rise in these procedures. However, as Laura Kipnis (1993, 7) argues, images do not "simply and immediately lead directly to actions," as antipornography activists claim. Pornography is merely one element that creates desire for genital cosmetic surgery. The divisive potential of pornography sells media and diverts attention from the aestheticization and medicalization of women's genitalia by the surgeons whose income depends on generating genital dissatisfaction and driving demand for surgical solutions.

The Mainstream Media

Today's media speaks directly to women and their wayward genitalia, but it is a reciprocal conversation. In addition to pornography, the mainstream media (of which pornography is now a part) is a key producer of aesthetic ideals and information, and the media has never been more invasive and all-consuming than it is today. However, the distribution of knowledge and ideals is complex, and the media reflects the interests and concerns of the society and culture in which it is situated—in this case, sociocultural unease with female genitalia. Makeover culture (see chap. 3), the biomagical, and the media go hand in hand.

As a form of mass communication, the media includes women's and men's magazines, newspapers, radio and television, movies, and the internet. The internet serves differing purposes for women. Information can be accessed through message boards or online forums, which are driven by women seeking others' opinions of ideals and experiences. Articles about female genital cosmetic surgery are frequently posted on weblogs and online magazines, and surgeons' websites contain information and before and after photographs of altered genitalia at the same time as the visual media reaffirm genital ideals. As one prominent provider of genital cosmetic surgery in Australia comments on its website, "Labiaplasty and vaginal rejuvenation are becoming more popular, mostly due to the internet. While it may not be the most well-known of cosmetic medical procedures, labiaplasty is fast becoming a popular treatment for women who are unhappy with the overall shape of their vagina. Why is this? The access and immediacy of the internet has been an invaluable source of information for a lot of women. Their initial concerns can be researched and answered very discreetly within the privacy of their computer, iPhone or tablet" (Aesthetica 2012).

Surgeons suggest the internet is beneficial to women as a site of information (even though the information is about procedures that may not be warranted and for which there is little scientific evidence of long-term efficacy or safety), and the information provided normalizes the need for these procedures.

Women see unrealistic images of other women in the media, aspire to wear the up-to-date, revealing fashions on display there, and frequently embrace a gym and beach culture, which marries health and fitness with fashion. Health and fitness magazines abound. As one surgeon said, "A gym culture demands a tight belly, tight arse—maybe labia don't fit into that," given that labia are not naturally taut. Regarding beach culture, one surgeon who operates on the Gold Coast in Queensland explained:

> There are a lot of things that are different on the Gold Coast. I think because it is a coastal community, people are very body conscious because it is a beach culture. It is the kind of environment that lends itself to, um, wearing as little as possible. Almost all the young girls comment on their look in a bikini. I mean, you just go down to the beach; the girls are wearing bikinis that do not actually camouflage anything that is underneath, so if they have large labia minora they're going to find that it's obvious, you know. I wouldn't be surprised if, per capita, for labiaplasties, we do more here.

All the women and doctors I interviewed came from coastal towns and cities; this is where most Australians live, ensuring that a beach culture and beach fashions are central to summer life. In promoting the fashions of a gym and beach culture, women's magazines construct female genitalia as potentially problematic. At the same time, women are exposed to information in the media that supposedly provides a solution to their problems. Something can be done to assuage their insecurities. The media has the dual role of generating concerns—presenting a look against which to be judged, a stimulus for worries—and providing information about a solution, the surgical "fix."

A study carried out in the Netherlands regarding female attitudes toward labia minora appearance and reduction found that almost all participants (the majority were students) were aware of labiaplasty and that 78 percent had heard about labia reduction surgery through the media. According to the study, "Information may be provided in such a way as to suggest that the 'problem' of unattractive genitalia can be 'solved' by surgery. Some women may tend to feel that they are somehow to blame for having this 'problem' that needs a surgical solution. Moreover, the fact that aesthetic genital surgery has been actively promoted in the media by some medical professionals, along with patient testimonials of positive experiences, has possibly encouraged women to feel that not undergoing labial reduction is a missed 'opportunity'" (Koning et al. 2009, 70).

Certainly, genitalia are construed as problematic in much of the media, and women are influenced by the text and images that appear there, sometimes in subtle, unacknowledged ways and sometimes more overtly. One labiaplasty recipient first became aware of vulval aesthetics from the Australian version of the television program *Big Brother*.

> Ann: I remember there was a thing on the television—do you remember the *Big Brother* show? I think there was one girl in the second one; it was in the news that she said to somebody else in the house, "Do you have an innie or an outie?" Yeah, and I suppose—[*pauses*]
> Lindy: I always thought that was for belly buttons.
> Ann: Yes! Yes! It really hit home to me then. I thought, "I really have an outie, I suppose," you know, [to] a couple of closer friends, well, I said, "Does yours stick out?" And they said, "No, not at all." And I thought, "Well, mine do," and I am always finding myself pushing it all back in to make it look pretty.

On Mamamia, a popular women's website in Australia, articles regularly appear about female genitalia, pubic grooming, and genital cosmetic surgery. A post in 2013, "So I Have an Outie Vagina and I'm Meant to Feel Bad About It?" penned by Rosie Waterland, a writer and public commentator, describes her encounter with a slightly inebriated friend at a party who revealed she had an "outie" and was saving up for a labiaplasty.

> She was actually on the verge of tears as she told me about the day in her late teens she overheard a boy she had slept with refer to her vagina as "weird." Since then, she has obsessively looked at before and after pictures of vaginas. . . . She knew right down to the last detail, how she wanted to improve her lady parts. . . . The labiaplasty was going to transform her "outie" into an "innie." Or basically, a very neat single slit between her legs, not dissimilar to what I assume Barbie has under those plastic knickers. . . . "Innies" are in, "outies" are out. (Waterland 2013)

The purpose of Waterland's article, which reflects the ethos of the website, is to persuade women not to be ashamed of their genitalia, yet the author says that realizing that an "outie" is considered unattractive sent her into a panic about her own genital morphology. "How bizarre, that something I had never known I was supposed to worry about, had now, in less than a week, begun to morph into one of my major insecurities" (Waterland 2013). The fact that discussions of "innies" and "outies" are appearing in the media reflects, but also perpetuates, public concern about vulval aesthetics, ensuring that the possibility of surgery hovers in the background. As *Cosmopolitan* magazine nonchalantly and briefly explains in an article about female genitalia, "The outer labia surround your inside parts: the inner labia, clitoris and vagina. Some 'outies' are self-conscious and suffer chafing. Surgery can be an option" (*Cosmopolitan* 2012b, 83). Although women who resist surgery may be admired, there are others, like Ann, who undergo surgery to alleviate the anxiety affirmed in the media.

Women's magazines are a significant and pervasive source of cultural ideals about appearance, and appearance is frequently construed as a medical problem. This has certainly worked to the advantage of the cosmetic surgery industry. Articles about female genital cosmetic surgery published in magazines often have eye-catching titles, such as "Rough Sex Led to My Labiaplasty," "New Sex Surgeries," "Secret Women's Business," and "The Surgery That Saved My Sex Life." In 2006, *Cosmopolitan's* UK and US editions published sealed sections on designer vaginas. These articles describe the experiences of women who have had surgery, which is usually portrayed as a positive choice. For instance, in an article in *Marie Claire* titled "The Surgery That Saved My Sex Life," a woman explains:

> Then, one day in early 2005, I was sitting in a dentist's surgery waiting for a check-up when I came across a magazine article about labiaplasty, a surgery that reshapes the vagina. In it, a woman recounted how she'd had her labia reduced and how the operation had changed her life and given her the confidence she craved in the bedroom. It was the first time I became aware that I could do something about it, and I decided then and there that one day I would have the operation. . . . I started to seriously research a labia reduction on the internet. . . . From then on, I knew there was no turning back. . . . I was relieved to be starting a new chapter of my life. (*Marie Claire* 2009)

Reflecting prevalent sexual stereotypes, the woman describes in clichéd terms her newfound confidence in the bedroom after having surgery: "With my new, tidy vulva, I felt so much more confident. . . . I felt free, especially now that I was liberated from the self-critical, internal dialogue I had always run through my head during sex. Suddenly empowered, I felt more womanly than ever" (*Marie Claire* 2009).

This woman's surgeon has a link to the article on his website. In 2010, he told me it was not a "good" article and that he had had no editorial control over it. He said he complained to the magazine and asked them to change the article because it did not represent his patients accurately. Although the article describes the woman as suffering extreme pain—"my vagina was burning hot and excruciatingly painful"—and focuses on sexual satisfaction as an ideal, the surgeon claimed these concerns are not routine. However, *Marie Claire* published the article regardless; its sensationalism no doubt made good reading. I was curious to know why the article, which was written in 2009, was still on his website in 2010.

> Lindy: Do you think female genital cosmetic surgery gets negative press?
> Dr. Oliver: Um, I think it does. Look, journalists will do whatever it takes to get a story. The article in *Marie Claire* wasn't done particularly well in that they had ten patients to choose from to interview, and they chose the patient who sensationalized it. The woman had been told by her partner that she had big tissue down there. She is one of very few women who have said that. Also, she found it extremely painful afterwards and the majority of women say it is not painful. Actually, that article would put people off. A lot of people have actually said, "I read that article and I am not sure that I want to have it done now." I actually wrote to *Marie Claire* and said, "Please could you write . . ."
> Lindy: Mmm . . . Is it still up on your website?
> Dr. Oliver: I think so. I do, but it is so old I am not sure it would carry any weight.

The article remained on his website in 2017. Perhaps, for some women, enduring the pain this woman describes is worth it for the confidence and enhanced femininity she professes to experience. Media stories of the experiences of women who have undergone genital cosmetic surgery provide a subtle form of advertising for surgeons.

Ideals are portrayed in the media not merely through images of ideal bodies and information on how to achieve them but also through advertising. We live in what Susan Bordo (2003, xvi) refers to as "the empire of images," in which the media dictates aesthetic ideals. As Jean Kilbourne (2010) suggests, advertising images are processed subliminally, and "they tell us who we are and who we should be." Although women may not acknowledge the power that images exert over them (Bordo 2003), these images enter their subconscious and dictate what ideal beauty looks like. Advertisements for cosmetic surgery are common on the internet. All the surgeons I interviewed in Australia had websites, and many were represented in feature articles and advertorials in newspapers and magazines and on television. Although the Medical Board of Australia has recently adopted detailed advertising guidelines, the rules for advertising vary from state to state. Although inducements such as discounts (often time limited) and free initial consultations for cosmetic procedures are discouraged, gifts and discounts are not prohibited providing terms and conditions are disclosed (Australian Health Ministers' Advisory Council 2011).

There is a more circumspect approach to female genital cosmetic surgery in some sections of the media today, with an increasing number of journalists drawing attention to the lack of scientific studies underpinning the safety of these procedures, the long-term satisfaction levels, the marketing techniques employed, and the lucrative rewards these procedures bring to surgeons. In an episode of the television program *Opening Shot* (2013) titled "The Vagina Diaries," which aired on Australia's ABC 2, the reporter Nat Harris interviewed a number of doctors, patients, sex industry professionals, and men about labiaplasty and vulval aesthetics. Although the program highlighted some of the risks of labiaplasty and the reasons women choose surgery (to increase confidence), it also drew attention to the procedure. Given that the surgeon who was filmed performing surgery on screen posted a link to the program on his website, I assume he feels it will bring patients to his door. Cautionary commentary has to contend with "rational" medical opinion and other compelling visual cues that appear in the media. Discussing female genital cosmetic surgery, even in an informed and critical manner, helps to normalize it, and therefore, any publicity may be good publicity for the practice.

The Medical Profession

The media is increasingly important to the medical profession, and it is where women learn of medical services. By suggesting that female genital cosmetic surgery results in aesthetic improvement—often aided by before and after photographs on surgeons' websites—the medical profession is complicit in generating genital ideals and perpetuating genital anxieties. Medicalization confers an aura of authenticity onto genital cosmetic surgery because of its basis in (supposedly rational) biomedicine. Medical authority and expertise are represented as if they exist outside culture rather than being firmly embedded within it. What constitutes health, particularly in the image-saturated culture of the West, has been broadened to include beauty and sexual satisfaction. This trend generates new opportunities for intervention while constricting the range of acceptable difference for women. Regarding genital appearance, one of the surgeons I interviewed said, "I think people were probably concerned before about it, but they didn't have the avenue to do anything about it. Now, because of the availability of plastic surgery, I think this has become more prominent and people are seeing much more media. Um, they think, oh well, something can be done about it so why should I have to put up with it? The same as you having a big nose or big ears—people are upset about it."

In a media-driven makeover culture that offers ordinary women biomagical solutions, the underlying shame some women feel about their genital appearance can be assuaged. Doctors recognize that their patients are worried about the appearance of their genitalia; however, they typically blame the media for the production of these ideals. Genital cosmetic surgery just happens to be available and what they provide. Although many of the surgeons I interviewed agreed that cultural forces were important factors driving women's choices about their bodies, they did not see medical science as complicit in generating ideals. A concern for genital aesthetics is presented as inevitable given the current cultural climate of depilation and pornography. As one doctor reflected, "Aesthetic and functional labiaplasty is becoming increasingly common as women become more conscious of the appearance of their genitalia and the surgical options available to them. The proliferation of Brazilian waxing and permanent hair reduction treatments—as well as increased exposure to photos and videos online and in magazines of nude models—has made the 'average' woman much more concerned about the attractiveness of her genitals."

It did not seem to worry the surgeons I interviewed that the media generates impossible ideals because images have been digitally altered or, in the case of pornography, bodies may have been surgically transformed. For them, the ideal has been created, women have been persuaded, and they, as surgeons, are merely the executors of their patients' desires. Changing normal bodies to approximate an ideal is the very nature of cosmetic surgery.

Despite rising concerns in sections of the medical profession and among women's health organizations about the prevalence of female genital cosmetic surgery, it is increasingly visible and available. Labiaplasty is one of the least expensive cosmetic surgical procedures on offer, although prices vary considerably. Many surgeons' websites have links to institutions offering financing. If women believe that genital perfection is available, it becomes a possibility, if not an imperative. In a society that has historically represented female genitalia negatively, that is saturated with media images of an ideal body (and increasingly, genitalia), and that has the medical expertise and authority to transform bodies to suit the ideal, it is more difficult for women who can afford it or women who suffer low self-esteem to resist the enduring "quick fix" on offer. This pattern of exploiting feelings of deficiency or anxiety in order to sell medical products and services follows a well-blazed trail adopted by the pharmaceutical industry, where medications such as Viagra® (sildenafil) and more recently Addyi® (flibanserin), which purport to treat male and female sexual "dysfunction," respectively, have found their way onto the market. Pharmaceutical companies no longer only sell drugs; they also promote "conditions" to the level of disease for which they then market treatments.

Similarly, surgeons' websites acknowledge women's concerns about their genitalia, and in so doing, authenticate them: "Physicians have neglected aesthetic surgery of the female external genitalia. However, awareness of female genital aesthetics has increased owing to increased media attention, both from magazines and video. Women may feel self-conscious about the appearance of their labia. The aging female may dislike the descent of her pubic hair and labia. A large pubic fat deposit may be unsightly" (Alter 2008).

Surgeons' websites, such as that of Beverly Hills surgeon Dr. Gary Alter, suggest that surgeons are sympathetic to women's presumably justified concerns. Terms such as *descent* and *unsightly*, expressions echoed by the surgeons I interviewed, strengthen negative impressions of female genitalia. The word *descent* not only evokes masculine sexuality (e.g., the descent of the testicles) but also suggests aging—the sagging of breasts, buttocks, and stomachs, which are all targets of cosmetic surgery. By validating women's concerns about their genital appearance, surgeons reproduce and legitimize women's genital anxieties. The language used to describe procedures, such as *vaginal rejuvenation, designer vagina*, and *female genital enhancement*, suggests an implicit set of desirable or aesthetic standards for female genitalia to which women should aspire—and that female genitalia are inadequate in their natural state. When asked in a live interview what, in his eyes, a perfect vagina looks like, Dr. David Matlock (referenced in chap. 4) replied with certainty, "I know it when I see it" (Good Medicine 2003).[4] Clearly, surgeons are complicit in defining aesthetically pleasing genitalia and creating the ideal—this cannot be solely attributed to the media or pornography. Most of the women I interviewed garnered information about genital cosmetic surgery by visiting doctors' websites, and these sites helped them develop their sense of vulval aesthetics.

One study of the content and clinical implications of doctors' online advertisements for female genital cosmetic surgery concluded, in an open letter published in the *British Medical Journal* in 2012, that "FGCS [female genital cosmetic surgery] procedures were presented on all the provider websites as an effective treatment for genital appearance concerns. . . . There was scant reference to appearance diversity. Only minimal scientific information on outcomes or risks could be identified. There was no mention of potential alternative ways for managing appearance concerns or body dissatisfaction" (Liao, Taghinejadi, and Creighton 2012, 1).

Similarly, in Australia, the medical profession is implicated in the rise of female genital cosmetic surgery as a practice, and surgeons' websites can be profoundly influential in persuading women to undergo surgery. As Braun (2009b, 136) states, "Surgeon website discourse, then, contributes to the ongoing construction of experiential as well as material bodies, to the production of desires, and practices around these desires"—that is, to the choice of surgery itself. Surgeons' websites not only advertise products that they want women to purchase but they also "educate" women about what is normal and desirable (Braun 2009b). Choosing a surgeon is an important part of the process for many women. As one nineteen-year-old labiaplasty informant commented, "Finding the right surgeon can take months of researching. I think I spent about sixty hours on the computer . . . I typed each doctor's name into Google and looked at their website (some don't have one, so I didn't bother much with them as I think the more professional they are, they will have a website)."

A British study by Lih-Mei Liao, Neda Taghinejadi, and Sarah Creighton (2012) found that the websites of surgeons offering female genital cosmetic surgery emphasized both the aesthetic and functional benefits of surgery, mirroring the content on surgical websites in Australia. Surgery was recommended to make labia "sleeker" and "more appealing," although some of the websites also noted that vulval appearance varies widely (Liao, Taghinejadi, and Creighton 2012, 3). Bringing women's attention to vulval diversity, however, does not appear to deter them from choosing surgery. Most women are already aware of the wide range of normal, but mentioning vulval diversity on their websites ensures that surgeons cannot be accused of being dishonest with patients. Rather, by informing women about variation but still offering surgery, surgeons confirm that cosmetic surgery is not about normality. "I change normal all the time," said Dr. Lim, a plastic surgeon based on the Gold Coast in Queensland.

Images on surgeons' websites advertising female genital cosmetic surgery tend to depict demure females from the waist down, their hands (or some other item) placed over their vulvas, or women in snugly fitting white shorts or underwear, implying a perfect, flat V. Some websites have reassuring photographs of the surgeon, or images of a couple, suggesting that surgery can improve intimate relationships. The text on Australian surgeons' websites is also revealing.

Labiaplasty can provide some excellent health benefits in terms of your
physical health and self-worth as well as your emotional well-being. . . .
The decision should be yours and yours only; however, having made the right
decision for you, you will be on the path to joining the hundreds of people
who undergo labiaplasty every year who are delighted with the results.
(Cosmos Clinic 2013)

Are you embarrassed by excess skin in your feminine area? Labiaplasty can
help you. . . . What's more, elongated labia may sometimes also inhibit the
sexual experience, making it more difficult for women to achieve orgasm.
With a labiaplasty, women may experience increased sexual pleasure, as well
as an end to the discomfort of tight clothes. (Nguyen 2013)

It is indicative of a shift from the vulva being a part of women's "natural" body
where modification was not mandated, to being a part almost inherently
inadequate without at least some minor modificatory (e.g. depilatory)
practice. Female genital cosmetic surgery is part of this shift in status [of the
vulva]. (Aesthetica 2012)

Surgeons' websites suggest that genital cosmetic surgery has "excellent
health benefits" and that, although choosing surgery should be the woman's
decision alone, if women proceed with surgery, they will be pleased with the
results, since female genitalia are "inherently inadequate" without at least some
"minor" intervention, such as hair removal. On these websites, altering normal
genitalia is normalized and surgery promoted as beneficial to well-being.

While the allure of increased sexual pleasure may provide an added incen-
tive for intervention, most of the women I spoke with did not suggest this
was their reason for choosing surgery. One woman who underwent clitoral
dehooding reported increased sexual satisfaction after surgery, but most just
felt less self-conscious about their genital appearance. Unhappiness with appearance is a cultural, not a medical, condition. An online poll conducted after
the Channel 4 documentary *The Perfect Vagina* (2008) aired in the United
Kingdom revealed that 48 percent of 14,642 voters said they would consider
labiaplasty, although it may be that women more interested in genital cosmetic
surgery watched the program and participated in the poll. Another UK study
of 135 women found that only 50 percent felt that their genitalia were of normal
appearance, and almost a third believed that "their labia were too large at least
sometimes" (Bramwell and Morland 2009, 22), which is an interesting remark
given that labia do not change in size (in the short term) when not aroused.
Perhaps this remark exemplifies the deeply personal and subjective nature of
body-image issues.

One plastic surgeon, Dr. Romeo, told me that female genital cosmetic surgery "is a field that people get into when they're scratching their heads for
work . . . so, you find that when a market is saturated, you get that kind of funky
behavior going on where doctors may be looking for a little niche that hasn't
been explored yet." This surgeon said that most of his patients were not referred
by their general practitioner and that they did not claim the cost of the procedure on Medicare:[5] "In fact, it's kind of like an underground thing. It's almost
like the drug deal of the cosmetic surgery world; you know what I mean? These
girls come in, they want to pay cash, and sometimes they don't even want to
see me." In his practice, the first appointment is usually with his practice nurse,
who examines the patient and explains the procedure. There appears to be a
disjunction between the information provided on surgeons' websites and their
own beliefs. For instance, Dr. Romeo's website emphasizes that protruding
labia minora can impinge on a woman's self-confidence and personal relationships as well as cause physical discomfort when wearing certain clothes or when
exercising and that surgery can prevent the labia from chafing. In our interview,
however, he said, "Occasionally I see someone who has got extraordinarily
long labia and I think that there is no question that it would be uncomfortable.
But most of the time I think it is bullshit! Most of the time I think it is just an
excuse; they come in and make it sound like a reconstructive problem when it's
a visual thing." On their websites, surgeons include functional, as well as
aesthetic, problems as reasons for surgery because they want to appear sympathetic to women's concerns while simultaneously offering a (surgical) solution.

Some surgeons in Australia promote their practices at annual Sexpo exhibitions held in the main cities. Breast and buttock augmentation and female
genital cosmetic surgery, the latter often advertised as a "designer vagina,"
predominate at such events, with photographs of the various body parts labeled
with phrases such as "enhance your pleasure" (for genital cosmetic surgery),
"enhance your assets," and "tighten your tush." I visited Sexpo on several occasions and was surprised at the ordinariness of the exhibition. The space was
populated by mothers and daughters, groups of youngish women, couples of
all ages, many people with disabilities (mostly male) and their caretakers, and
same-sex couples. There was no feeling of perversity—it was just like any trade
fair, full of a diversity of people inspecting items, looking, and listening—a
commercial celebration of sex. According to the Sexpo website, "The aim of
the exhibition is to provide a fun, vibrant atmosphere for like-minded people
to enjoy and find information on *all things adult. Sexpo* is not just about *sex*;
it is about sexuality and adult lifestyles. At *Sexpo* you will find hundreds of
exhibitors, and there is something for everyone" (Sexpo 2013). The "something

for everyone" described here includes information on female genital cosmetic surgery, along with myriad technologies for pubic hair removal.

One surgeon I spoke with had canvassed both men and women at one such exhibition for their opinions regarding genital aesthetics. According to him, having been shown a variety of photographs of vulvas, (lay) men and women favored surgically altered or naturally occurring neat and tidy genitalia. He suggested that this preference was proof that this vulval ideal is somehow both innate and natural, and therefore desirable. When I asked cosmetic surgeons whether alternatives to surgery were ever suggested, they replied that the only alternative was not to have surgery. This attitude fails to acknowledge the possibility that women could be educated about the wide range of normal and told that pubic hair removal may exacerbate discomfort and make the vulval cleft appear more pronounced.

—⁂—

The women and surgeons who participated in my research appear to have thoroughly internalized the clean-slit ideal, indicating the pervasiveness of the cultural milieu in which this preference has emerged. The existence of a genital ideal is taken for granted, as is the notion of an ideal face or perfect body. A narrowly defined ideal is identified as "natural," making the raw (presurgical) body appear deformed (Adams 1997). Protruding labia are thus perceived as ugly. Cosmetic surgery has become normalized as a solution to bodily anxieties, and the vulval ideal is defended as a functional, comfort-inducing, and feminizing benefit for women. The current era, which Bordo (2003, xvi) refers to as the "empire of images," is also the empire of information, consumerism, and medicalization. Some media sensationalize female genital cosmetic surgery to sell copy, and surgeons use the media to disseminate information and promote their businesses. The media, therefore, both shapes ideals and makes certain bodily choices more accessible. Some women choose to pursue the clean-slit ideal through surgery simply because it is available.

To infer that pornography and pubic grooming are the sole drivers of female genital cosmetic surgery is simplistic and convenient. While these are undoubtedly contributing factors, the burgeoning media landscape—particularly the internet—and the medical profession's use of digital media to promote surgery also contribute to the increase in interest in these procedures. The introduction of Brazilian waxing to New York by the J Sisters in 1994 (J Sisters 2012) and its popularization through the television program *Sex and the City* (1998–2004) coincided with the rise of the internet as a public medium that has facilitated the increasing reach and commercial interests of biomedicine, thus creating a rhizomal effect whereby many factors and discourses have coalesced to make the clean-slit ideal desirable (Deleuze and Guattari 1987). The clean-slit ideal exists whether or not women choose to consume pornography or have a Brazilian wax. The visual erasure of female sexual characteristics has been eroticized, making the look desirable while diminishing the true markers of female sexuality.

Tradition and ceremony as transmitters of culture and purveyors of ideals have been replaced by the more insidious mass media, which communicates to women what is desirable, appropriate, and ideal. In this environment, new rituals focusing on health and beauty have emerged. However, the media cannot be divorced from culture, because they inform each other. The two exist in a symbiotic relationship. Although it may be convenient to point to pornography and depilation as the main reasons for the clean slit surfacing as the genital ideal for women, they are merely components of a broader cultural web that informs contemporary embodied desire for women. Culture itself is transmitted through the media, and with the rise of social media, culture has become more pervasive and less unidirectional, thereby disguising its omnipresence: "In the post-modern world, culture is produced, transmitted, recepted and re-signified through mass communication and within mass communication. No social sub-system can function outside the mediation provided by mass communication. But this is not only a simple channel through which cultural symbols circulate, it is the very system that produces culture; media are substituting traditional forms through which culture is generated and, through their ubiquity and power, they take over the culture's functions from the pre-modern societies" (Coman 2013). Rather than the media producing culture, the two are interdependent. The media gives expression to culture at the same time as it informs it. There can be no understanding of female genital cosmetic surgery without considering the profound role of the media in society today. Culture is, after all, a semiotic process.

History, art, and language have also contributed to the construction of female genitalia as problematic. Second-wave feminism sought to dislodge many women's feelings of shame about their genitalia, thereby empowering them. Although women can now speak more freely about their genitalia and their sex lives, they do so in a media-driven milieu. In this media landscape (which includes soft-core pornography and consumer medicine), the naked female form and its desexualized genitalia are widely trafficked, ensuring the creation and eroticization of a certain ideal. The historical antipathy between feminism and pornography has largely disappeared. As a culturally informed aesthetic ideal, the clean slit combines appearance with hygiene and notions of appropriate femininity. This ideal is an extension of the smooth, hairless ideal that abounds in the visual media. It is also about ease; women want to look good and partake in normal activities without discomfort. Perhaps not surprisingly in our highly medicalized and commercialized world, biomedicine—the biomagical—is able to help women achieve the ideal and assuage their genital anxiety (for a price). Although female genital cosmetic surgery is taken up by only a small number of women contemporarily, many women now remove their pubic hair to achieve a smooth, clean appearance.

Bodily ideals are always evolving, but for now the clean slit is the dominant ideal for female genitalia. Most genitalia in the media are minimalist because this look is what society deems attractive and appropriate. Perhaps, therefore, it is inevitable that women will aspire to a neat, tidy, hairless aesthetic. Just as the Barbie doll is bereft of genitalia presumably to render her nonconfrontational for children (an adult decision), the full range of genital aesthetics for women is considered too real and too scary (and too desirable) for public viewing. In the mainstream media, the erotic is applied to every sign of femininity except its primary essence—the genitalia. The contemporary vulval ideal also enables women to escape the pathological or grotesque, which has historically been projected onto the "other," thus rendering Western women less abject. Social control is nowhere more profoundly worked than through sexuality, and the clean-slit ideal represents a minimization of marginal zones, one that reinforces acceptable modes of femininity. It is an ideal about youth, smoothness, neatness, and safe, anodyne sexuality—perhaps sexuality with less lust and passion but a (visual) sexual ideal that has been adopted by many women themselves.

NOTES

1. See Barnes and Lumsden (2010); Blank (2011); Dodson (1996); Karras (2003); McCartney (2014); Robertson (2011); and Werner (2013), who have all published or exhibited works affirming vulval diversity.

2. "Fanny" is a colloquial Australian term for female genitalia.

3. In Australia, some publications are classified as unrestricted. These publications may contain content that is not recommended for children under fifteen and are labeled accordingly. Restricted publications are for adults only and cannot be sold to minors. They contain content that may offend some sections of the adult community, for example, nudity or explicit sexual content (Australian Government, Department of Communications and the Arts 2015).

4. On October 14, 2003, MSN closed all Australian chat rooms (known as NineMSN), including Good Medicine.

5. Medicare is the Australian federal health care system providing primary health care to all Australian citizens and permanent residents.

TWO

—⚏—

NORMATIVITY AND THE
CONTRADICTORY NATURE OF NORMAL

IN HIS RICHLY ILLUSTRATED TOME the *Atlas of Human Sex Anatomy*, first published in 1949, the obstetrician-gynecologist Robert Latou Dickinson attempted to depict the average shape and measurements of the vulva as a "basic form to which the others can conveniently be referred without any claim that it constitutes the *normal* anatomy of the parts" (Dickinson 1949, 42). Figure 2.1 depicts protrusion of the labia minora through the labia majora: "Thickened, elongated, curled on themselves, thrown into tiny, close-set, irregular folds, as in a cockscomb, the lesser labia protrude, in all positions, through the larger labia. The pigment deposit varies with the general type of coloring. One labium is sometimes greater than its fellow. Sebaceous follicles are often conspicuous as whitish spots. The prepuce commonly, and the fourchette occasionally, participate in the corrugation and duskiness, or one of these alone may be affected. At times a wrinkled band runs off to the labia majus" (Dickinson 1949, 53).

While Dickinson used the term *hypertrophy* to describe larger labia minora, he did not classify them as abnormal, although the medical definition of *hypertrophy* is "abnormal enlargement of a body part or organ" (Princeton University 2013a). Dickinson found that more than one-third of women "showed two or more of the various vulvar hypertrophies," which he both illustrated and described in detail (Dickinson 1949, 55). In 2013, more than sixty years later, Vincenzo Puppo (2013) concurs: "There is great variation in the size and morphology of the labia minora. They may be almost unrecognizable or may protrude from the labia majora ('hypertrophic' labia minora should not be considered a malformation). In addition, they can be asymmetrical or doubled on one or both sides" (Puppo 2013, 140).

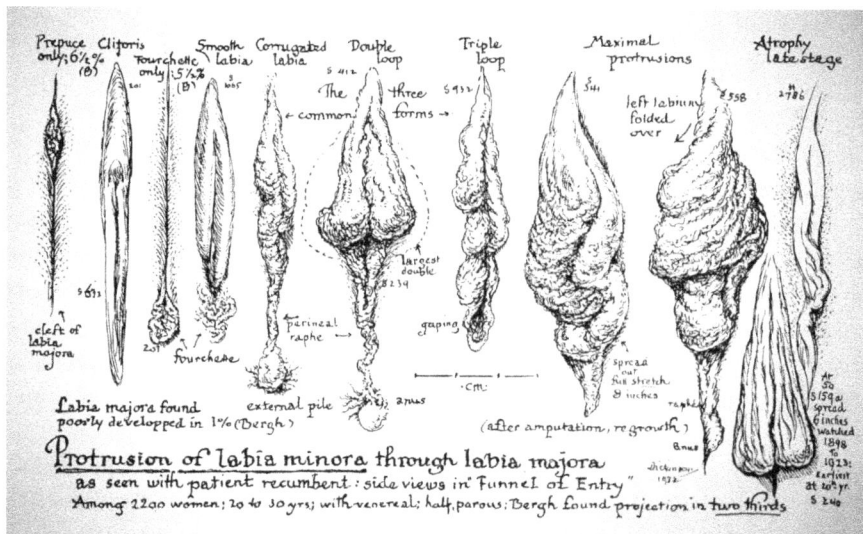

Figure 2.1. Protrusion of Labia Minora through Labia Majora. *Atlas of Human Sex Anatomy*, Krieger Publishing Company, Dickinson 1949, figure 80. Reproduced with permission from Krieger Publishing Company.

Despite this affirmation of diversity, a vulval ideal has emerged today that does not include the "irregular folds" or "cockscomb" aesthetic described in Dickinson's early writings. Instead, a language of normality and abnormality permeates contemporary discourse around labial dimensions. Such discourse implies that, although variation is to be expected, a limited amount of variation is considered acceptable, and once this (indeterminate) limit is reached, labial size becomes a treatable pathology (Malone 2013). This chapter is based on the narratives of three women who felt that their labia minora were not normal before surgery because they protruded past their labia majora or were asymmetrical. A fear of not being normal emerges as a common trope when discussing female genital cosmetic surgery. Women want to be what they consider normal, despite the reassurance from both Dickinson and Puppo that hypertrophy is not abnormal. However, employing the medical term *hypertrophy* signals that protruding labia are undesirable.

Although some women *do* aim for vulval perfection, most of the women I interviewed chose to have surgery in order to feel less self-conscious. Some women have other body-image issues, while others do not. The women I spoke with described how they wanted to fit into society and be like (imagined) others—normal, but not necessarily perfect. However, as the women's stories in this chapter reveal, what is considered normal also approximates the ideal (clean slit), resulting in most postoperative vulvas being close to "perfection." The women who have surgery to become normal may have different motivations from those of perfectionists (see chap. 3), but the results are similar and, as Jane's story (recounted later in this chapter) demonstrates, there may be slight disappointment if the finished look is less than perfect. The desire to be normal is therefore defined by cultural expectations rather than by natural physical attributes, and this affects the decisions women make about their genitalia. Women not only want to look what they consider to be normal, but they also expect to be able to wear current fashions, participate in popular exercise regimens, undergo beauty routines, and engage in sexual activity without constraint or embarrassment.

The media and medical science shape what constitutes normal genitalia. As ideals become normalized, they influence women's perceptions of genital normality. What is anatomically natural and a part of standard human physical variation is often perceived or represented as abnormal or, at the least, mediocre and undesirable, and is therefore increasingly altered for the "better." In an era of constant innovation, the body has become a commodity, and a normal or "average" body is often no longer sufficient for happiness. Bodies are upgradable. As Emily Martin succinctly puts it, "We are not seeing the end of the body, but rather the end of one kind of body and the beginning of another kind of body" (Martin 1992, 121)—a body much more likely to be touched by the biomagical.

IN SEARCH OF NORMALITY

The women whose stories follow chose to undergo labiaplasty because they felt that their genitalia were abnormal, and this affected their confidence and well-being. Tara and Nell are young women but older women, such as Jane, also can be subject to genital anxiety and concerns about normality. While Tara and Nell were beginning their sexual lives, Jane was reentering the sexual market, thus making surgery a rite of passage into a more confident sexual life for all three women.

Tara: Crying in the Bathroom

Tara, a bright and bubbly student, was twenty-two years old when I met her, and she had recently undergone labiaplasty. She had decided to have surgery to "correct" her protruding (not asymmetrical) labia while she was still "single and young." Tara denied being a perfectionist and said she was not obsessed with her appearance. In fact, she stressed that she was the opposite: relaxed about her looks. However, she said she had recently been watching her diet (despite her small build) and endeavoring to improve her fitness. She said she goes to the gym, does not dye her hair, and likes to get a fake tan from time to time. Before her labiaplasty, Tara had used depilatory cream to remove her pubic hair because she was too embarrassed to go to a beautician, but since her surgery, she had been regularly attending a waxing salon. Tara said she comes from a middle-class background and is the youngest of three girls. At the time of the interview, Tara was living at home. She denied that her notion of an ideal or normal vulva (and the two are conflated) had been influenced by images found in the media or pornography—she said she preferred to watch homemade pornography, which tends to depict genital diversity—rather, her ideal arose after comparing her genitalia with those of family and friends. This is Tara's story:

> First of all, I'll give you a little background. I noticed that when I went through puberty, at about thirteen, my labia grew heaps and started to poke out. My mum saw this when I was in the shower one time, and she had a look and seemed concerned about it, um, and then she asked if I wanted to go to the doctor about it, and I said, "Yeah, sure, I will go." I was terrified. Mum just booked it, and we went to this doctor, a GP, who my mum already knew.[1] My sister came too. I was really nervous about showing a doctor my private parts. It wasn't exactly fun. She just had a quick look at it and said it was perfectly normal, labia develop during puberty, and that some labia are just bigger than others, the same way that people's noses, eyes, and ears are different sizes. It wasn't something to worry about.
>
> However, I was super self-conscious about it, even before my mum took me to the doctor. I didn't like it, but I did manage to have sex with a few guys. If you want to keep your kid a virgin for a long time, get them to be self-conscious about the most intimate part of their body. I only had sex with boys for the first time when I was drunk for years because I needed the alcohol to work up the courage to let them see me naked. It sounds terrible saying that, even as a fit and healthy young girl, I didn't feel comfortable being naked in front of anyone. I never heard anything bad from any of these guys. In fact, the one boyfriend I talked to about it said it was no big deal and I shouldn't even be thinking about surgery.
>
> Fast-forward a few years. Now I am twenty-two, and I'm at a party and one of my friends tries to come into the toilet while I'm peeing. This may sound weird, but me and my friends often pee together, saves time, you can chat while you're on the toilet, it's never been a big issue, and none of my friends really watch you while you're actually on the toilet, they're just in the same room.

Well, I must have been in a weird mood (and drunk) because I freaked out about her coming in and said I didn't want her watching me pee. She said something along the lines of, "Well, we're all the same so I don't get what the big deal is all of a sudden," and it spiraled from there. So, it ended up being my friend and my sister (who came to see what was taking so long) listening to me drunkenly cry about my large "flaps." Now my sister knew this was an issue 'cos she'd been to the doctors with me all those years ago, and I'd asked her about it since then, but we hadn't really talked about it in detail.

My poor friend was taken aback because she had no idea what I looked like down there (although she did ask if she could look while we were in the bathroom and I said no) and had no idea this could be an issue for someone, but both my sister and my friend dealt with it really well and told me that if it's upsetting me this much then I should do something about it.

Crying in the bathroom about it at a party was actually the best thing I've ever done. Now I had two people who were asking me what I was doing about it. I finally got up the courage and, after some Googling, rang a cosmetic surgeon, and had a consult with him.

Tara's sense of shame affected her ability to have sex with new partners—she could not do so unless she was inebriated. The fact that her friend said, "We are all the same" glossed over the possibility of genital diversity. Tara did not feel she was the same as her sisters and mother. Tara's concerns about the normality of her labia were reinforced by her mother, who took her to see a general practitioner, where Tara (and presumably her mother) was reassured that her genital appearance was normal. However, as Tara matured, she was still unhappy with her labial appearance. It was an issue for her, and confiding in her friend and sister was an impetus for biomedical intervention, not social acceptance. Under the imperative of working on the self (a recurrent theme that emerged in the research; refer to chap. 3), Tara was determined to take (biomedical) action in an effort to feel normal.

Tara chose her surgeon based on his website, which she described as "nicely set out and informative," but she said that even if there had been only one surgeon available, she would have gone ahead with surgery. The doctor asked her whether she wanted the labia minora flush with the labia majora.

Tara: He asked me if I wanted it all gone or a bit still showing and I just said, "Yep, whichever." I know there is no normal.
Lindy: So, do you think you left the decision up to him a bit then?
Tara: No, I knew what I wanted. I just wanted it all gone.

As Tara relates it, it appears she was rather disempowered and indecisive in her interactions with her doctor. She wanted the aesthetic that is portrayed as normal in the media, one where the labia are "all gone," but she did not articulate this clearly to her surgeon. However, she did achieve the desired result. At the end of the consultation, the surgeon asked Tara whether she wanted to go away and think about it for a while or whether she was sure she wanted to go ahead with surgery. "I almost told him that I would not be here, having cried in the bathroom, if I was not sure about the surgery, but instead I just said yes, and he took a quick peek down my pants so we were all on the same page about what he would be dealing with."

Tara said most of her consultation was a verbal exchange, with her surgeon imparting information and outlining the risks of surgery. The physical examination was a brief affair at the conclusion of the consultation. Whether or not Tara's labia were in fact abnormal was irrelevant to this conversation because her quest was not for normality, although initially it was framed in such language. What Tara was seeking was the clean-slit ideal. Women use the language of normality when expressing their anxieties about vulval appearance, but their surgeons are not concerned with normal because they are being asked to produce the ideal. Tara's surgeon did explain that there was a possibility of irreparable nerve damage that could lead to painful sex in the future, but this did not deter her. With the decision to have surgery finalized, Tara now had to tell her parents.

> I printed off information from my doctor's website about the procedure and went to the lounge room, where my parents were watching TV. I had already told my sister to be around, so I had support.
>
> So, I walked in and I wasn't really sure what to expect. My mum is really against plastic surgery, mainly because it's a lot of money to spend on something when there are starving children in the world (her words), so I was a bit nervous about telling them but had sorted out in my head that I was not asking their permission, I was simply letting them know out of courtesy that I was having surgery.
>
> So, I walked in and turned down the TV—bam—had their attention, and then I announced with a nervous giggle that in two weeks, "I'm having surgery."
>
> Mum asks, "On what?" and for some reason I wasn't really prepared for this, so I answered, "My lady bits," with a giggle.
>
> Dad gets up and leaves.
>
> I show Mum the printout I had and she says, "I'm not surprised— remember when I took you to the doctor about it? I think it's good you're doing something about it."
>
> So, that was easy, plus my parents loved the fact that I told them what was going on. They hate lying and people avoiding the truth, so they were happy.

So, it was quick and painless telling my parents. I left Mum with the printout and retreated to my room, and just before I went to bed Mum knocked on the door. She asked about prices, and I said that I'd already paid the surgical fees, and she said that she and Dad had some money set aside for me and my sisters and that they'd give me the money for the operation from that, so I wouldn't have to pay for any of it, which was really nice.

She also said that Dad got up and left because he figured it would be easier for me if he wasn't there and figured Mum would tell him what was going on anyway. That was fine. My Dad's not much of a talker; he's more of a listener, silent observer.

Tara received family support for her decision to have labiaplasty; even though her mother was generally disapproving of cosmetic surgery, she was pleased Tara had decided to have surgery. Despite her father being "not much of a talker," he did confide in Tara that he had read a book about women being teased if their labia protruded, so he was sympathetic to Tara's concerns. With the sanction of her parents, Tara went ahead with surgery, and she is happy with the results.

The day before surgery, Tara went in for her second consultation with the surgeon to ensure she was still determined to go ahead with the procedure. The doctor said she looked relaxed, unlike some of his patients, who require seda- tives the night before surgery to settle their nerves. Tara said, "It might sound silly, but I wasn't nervous at all; I was really excited. It had got to the point where I was so happy I was finally doing something about it that I couldn't wait to have the surgery and get it dealt with so I wouldn't be crying in any more bathrooms, or being really nervous when hooking up with a new guy, or not being able to get a spray tan or wax because I was too embarrassed."

Tara had made her decision before she booked the first appointment with her surgeon. Because of her internet research, she felt she already knew ev- erything there was to know about labiaplasty and vulvas. She was aware of genital diversity and that most people might not think her genital morphology was unattractive or abnormal, but for her, it was embarrassing and shameful and precluded her from participating in certain activities. "I had surgery to make my labia look better, so they were nothing special. Having unique eyes or a unique smile is good. Having a unique vagina, unique labia, is not," she said. This comment highlights the tension that exists between fitting in—or "passing," in Sander Gilman's (1999) terms—and standing out. With labia, it appears that fitting in demands the ideal rather than uniqueness or normality. In response to whether viewing a wide range of normal genitalia would have influenced her decision to have surgery, Tara replied:

I don't think that seeing the wide range of normal would have helped at all, because I knew that other people looked the same as I did but that didn't make me like it any more. I could have gone through life, I would have been okay, but I just did this because I wanted to be a bit happier about it. It's not as though if I didn't have this done I wouldn't be able to find a husband or boyfriend or anything—it only would have impacted me. And I assume that, for whomever I am intimate with, it would not be one of their biggest concerns either, because guys probably don't care. That's why I realized I was doing it for myself. I did it for me because I didn't feel comfortable with it, not because someone else didn't.

Tara was grateful for the biomagical "quick fix" that labiaplasty provided—the one cosmetic procedure that she desired. As she explained, "Now I have had the operation, I don't really have anything else to do. It is very different to putting moisturizer on your face. It seems quite drastic, but now I can understand why people take drastic measures. It all happened in a short time frame; one month, and everything was back to normal."

Many women view cosmetic surgery as a quick and permanent fix, and this is the impression given by before and after photographs on surgeons' websites (see chap. 3). Not only was "everything back to normal" in the sense that Tara had no pain or concern about her genitalia at the time we spoke but she had also achieved what she perceived as aesthetic normality. Vulval aesthetics are important to certain women and their feelings of self-worth, normality, and inclusivity.

> Lindy: Your vulva is a very intimate thing. Why was getting this surgery so
>   important for you?
> Tara: Yeah, it is quite strange, um. The number of people who are going to see
>   that area is not very many.
> Lindy: Maybe they are important people?
> Tara: [laughs softly] It just comes back to doing it for yourself. Even if no
>   one were ever going to see me naked again, I would still want to get this
>   surgery done. Logically, I knew it wasn't a big deal, that everyone is
>   different and things and all that, but it was still affecting me.
> Lindy: Mmm.
> Tara: I think when it got to the point that I wouldn't have a spray tan or bikini
>   wax by anyone, I think when it gets to the point that it starts impacting
>   you . . . So, I just kind of thought if it was impacting me in so many areas
>   of my life, then I should do something about it. I've always been quite
>   fit and healthy, and I guess, like, I am sporty but not obsessed. My
>   labia never interfered with my wearing swimsuits and things. I never
>   considered that.

Tara was happy to admit that her concerns were about aesthetic normality and that shame, not discomfort, drove her to surgery and precluded her from feeling comfortable naked. Her story demonstrates the power of the invisible, intimate vulva—there is a fascination with what we cannot see, and this creates desire. Women rationalize that they are making decisions independently by invoking the invisible intimate. They are "doing it for themselves." This is obvious to them, because they are prepared to alter a part of their bodies rarely seen by others, thereby confirming their agency without acknowledging that their ideas of normality and aesthetics are formed subliminally through immersion in a certain cultural milieu. Labiaplasty makes them feel normal and happy, even if most people are unaware of the aesthetics of what Natalie Angier (1999) calls their "intimate geography."

Nell: The Labia I Saw Were More Normal Than Mine

Nell was an eighteen-year-old student when we spoke, and her experience echoed Tara's in many ways except that she blamed her vulval abnormality or asymmetry on what were most likely labial adhesions, a condition where the labia minora stick together as an infant. Nell could not name her condition except to say that she had had skin covering her vagina that had required medical treatment. Labial adhesions are quite common, affecting almost 2 percent of girls aged three months to six years, with a peak incidence of 3.3 percent between the ages of thirteen months and twenty-three months (Neill and Lewis 2009). The condition is thought to be caused by irritation to the delicate membranes of the external genitalia. In most cases, labial adhesions resolve without the need for medical treatment. As she matured, Nell became concerned about her labial asymmetry and sought advice and, eventually, surgery.

> The reason I had surgery was due to the fact that I had an extra-large right labia; the left was normal. This really affected my confidence, especially when it came to wearing bathers at the beach,[2] getting changed in front of other girls, and intimacy, and because it was always in the back of my mind, I was self-conscious even *talking* to guys! I had not been sexually active, because I felt abnormal. It was uncomfortable doing some sorts of exercise, like horse riding and cycling. Also, urinating was messy, and it was difficult inserting tampons.
>
> I guess I was always aware of my labia, but I really started to notice one wasn't normal going through puberty, learning about genitals and stuff in sex education and human biology at school. I knew my labia weren't quite right. It was really easy to tell.

But it didn't really affect me until I was about fifteen, when I told my mum. We went along to the GP, who referred me to a gynecologist, who said she wasn't the one to speak to about it, and she referred me to a plastic surgeon. Only being fifteen, I was quite afraid of the idea it was plastic/cosmetic surgery, so I just left it. But over the years, I grew more self-conscious of it, so when I turned eighteen, I started researching into it again, looking up side effects, other people's experiences, methods, and what a pretty, normal labia looks like. I know there is no normal, but the labia I saw were more normal than mine were.

I'm a very sporty, outdoor person. I play hockey and netball. I love to go to gym class and for runs outside. In summer I almost live at the beach too, but before I had surgery, I was always a little self-conscious of wearing plain-colored bathing suits that showed curves, especially sunbaking because I felt like I was exposed! I don't think I have ever had a negative comment from anybody directly, but then again I kind of avoided intimacy and dressing in front of people. I never compared myself to any other person, although I did show my mum and she said it was a bit abnormal but that is about it!

When I went to my GP first, when I was fifteen, she inspected me and said my labia were quite asymmetrical and bigger than normal, but she also assured me that everyone has different sizes and shapes, et cetera, and that there are no perfect labia. My surgeon also explained that all labia are unique; no two people have the same. He also mentioned that a couple of years ago the rule was that they could only operate on labia larger than 4 centimeters, which my right side was. The reason my right labia was over 4 centimeters and my left side was quite normal is because when I was a baby, I had a flap of skin covering my vagina. With therapy, it eventually split but obviously not evenly—one side was larger than normal. Since the surgery, there is not such a big difference between right and left, and they tuck into the larger lips and don't show little bumps through my bathers.

Nell felt that her genitalia were abnormal prior to surgery and stressed that she did not want to be perfect—she just wanted to look normal. I explained that some women *did* aim for perfection, the ideal clean slit. Nell replied:

Well, my labia were so disproportional, over 4 centimeters on the right and maybe only 1 or 2 centimeters on the left side. It was actually quite ugly and embarrassing. It is quite hard to explain but, say, if I had been born with 2 centimeters on the right and 3 centimeters on the left, for example, I would be okay with that. But, obviously, because I was getting correction surgery, I wanted a good job done, so, more even and close to perfect, since I was paying thousands of dollars for it! But I was going to be happy with anything more even and smaller, even if they didn't quite match up. Although I am

only eighteen and people may say that I am still immature and stuff, I knew
I didn't want this to hold me back in life or for me to miss opportunities
anymore because of it.

Nell's concerns were both functional and aesthetic, and they highlight that
normality is culturally, not biologically, determined. Like many of the women
whose stories inform this book, Nell thought her labia were precluding her
from certain activities. She believed that her labia were abnormal because they
were asymmetrical, which she had not seen depicted in educational reference
material. Helena Howarth, Volker Sommer, and Fiona Jordan (2010) studied
available visual depictions of female genitalia and discovered that they varied
depending on the source, with the widest variety found in feminist literature
and the highest conformity found in pornographic material. Anatomy textbooks depict the components of female genitalia in smaller proportions overall.
As their study explained, "Medical illustrations are constrained by their educational function of detailing the anatomy of the vulva: the labia minora must
protrude from the labia majora in order to be labeled, but not so much that they
obscure other features" (Howarth, Sommer, and Jordan 2010, 77). Nell sought
information on what "pretty, normal labia" look like, demonstrating that norms
and ideals are conflated. Both her mother and general practitioner concurred
that her labial proportions were not normal.

Although a cosmetic surgeon performed her procedure, Nell felt that her
problem was medical, despite having little knowledge of her childhood morphology. Medicine often works to justify social decisions. I have been unable
to find any reference suggesting that labial adhesions result in labial abnormality or asymmetry, but asymmetry is a common phenomenon (Neill and
Lewis 2009), something that doctors frequently consider pathological. Nell
wanted "a good job done . . . close to perfect," despite her general practitioner
assuring her that "there are no perfect labia." After all, as Nell rationalized,
she was paying for the surgery and could therefore fast-track from "abnormal"
to ideal.

In many respects, the two narratives discussed to this point are remark-
ably similar. Both these young women described the genital anxiety they experienced prior to having labiaplasty, and in both cases, their mothers were
involved in their perceptions of how a normal vulva should look. Despite
being aware that the size, shape, and color of labia vary enormously, Tara and
Nell used vocabularies of normality and aesthetics to explain why they were
unhappy with their own vulvas. The language of normality is also the language
of biomedicine. To be normal is the ideal state.

Daughters, Mothers, and Normality

As described in the narratives above, mothers are often concerned about their daughters' vulvas and whether they are normal because mothers care about their daughters' well-being. The age at which cosmetic surgery can be performed is a sensitive topic, and I describe a particular encounter with a cosmetic surgeon here.

I arrived early for many of my meetings with surgeons, and given the nature of the medical encounter, I often had to wait for a considerable time before the doctor was free to see me—appointments can easily run overtime, and sometimes emergencies arise. Dr. Silver's surgery occupies a pretty weatherboard house near the bottom of a hollow in a residential area. The rooms are light, airy, and far less clinical than many of the other surgeries I have visited. I have noticed, over my years of visiting doctors' offices, that female surgeons tend to have more comfortable, less modern, or less opulent spaces than those of their male counterparts. They emanate a slightly different atmosphere. On this occasion, the staff members were chatty and relaxed. As I sat waiting, activities continued around me. The telephone rang. Someone was calling from out of town inquiring about labiaplasty. The receptionist explained that she could arrange a Skype appointment with Dr. Silver and that the prospective patient would have to send some photographs (of her vulva): "Dr. Silver does lots of them, honestly. She just does so many of them," the receptionist said reassuringly. "Obviously, being a woman, she knows the female form." I found this comment interesting. One of the concerns about the rise of female genital cosmetic surgery is that many women are ignorant of the diversity of female genitalia; therefore, being a woman does not necessarily connote expertise in genital aesthetics (if such a notion were to exist). It would be just as plausible to claim that gynecologists, men, and women who have sex with women are the arbiters of vulval normality.

Finally, Dr. Silver emerged, wearing a bright floral sleeveless dress and strappy sandals. With her blond hair perfectly bobbed, she looked just like the photographs posted on her website, a fact I found quite unusual. Throughout my fieldwork, I was struck by how different surgeons look in the flesh (usually older) than they do on their websites. Whether this is due to their busy schedules or is a strategic practice remains a mystery. Dr. Silver was bright and breezy, and I immediately liked her. She apologized for running late, and we went into the kitchen area at the back of the clinic, which made our conversation feel less formal and somehow more "girly" than the usual office interview across a solid desk. A tall stainless-steel table in the middle of the room was covered in a jumble of used women's clothing and underwear. Dr. Silver explained that the all-female staff brought their old clothes in from time to time to swap items. There was a definite air of female inclusiveness here. Laughing, she picked up a black bra from the pile and asked me if I needed one. It was an overly supportive push-up style, and I politely declined. We stood around the table chatting over a cup of tea. It was lunchtime.

After a lengthy discussion on training and other issues, I raised the subject of patient age. Surgeons often seem wary when it comes to discussions about the age of their patients. Queensland, where Dr. Silver's practice is located, is the only state in Australia where the legal age for cosmetic surgery is eighteen years. If doctors are found to be operating on patients younger than this, they may be jailed for two years. In other Australian states, guidelines require minors considering surgery to have a three-month cooling-off period before another consultation, and a referral to a health professional for assessment is recommended. In reality, the lines are more blurred, particularly if surgeons note "pathology" such as hypertrophy or asymmetry. Dr. Silver asked me to leave some of her statements off the record, and then she continued.

> Lindy: What is the minimum age at which you operate?
> Dr. Silver: The minimum age is eighteen.
> Lindy: Is that the legal age?
> Dr. Silver: No. You can have an abortion at sixteen without your parents' permission. Essentially, in the state of Queensland, there is legislation preventing anyone from performing cosmetic surgery on anyone under the age of eighteen. Is labiaplasty cosmetic surgery? In some cases no, it is not. In some cases, it is gynecological.
> Lindy: Because there is so much tissue?
> Dr. Silver: Um, if someone presents . . . I think my cutoff is something like 8 centimeters. If you are sixteen, and you have labia minora that are 7 or 8 centimeters, each one, in width, I will photograph that and will operate on you. I hate the idea of young girls being sexually active at sixteen, but it is something that happens regularly. I think more than anything . . . I have never operated on anyone under the age of eighteen, but I would consider someone at sixteen if they presented with their mother and if they got a tick in every single box. I would never do any cosmetic surgery on anyone under the age of eighteen, because it's against the law, for starters. There is legislation protecting patients. I think a reconstructive labiaplasty on a sixteen-year-old girl who has gross hypertrophy of the labia minora is not cosmetic surgery. I think it's a reconstructive gynecological procedure.

Lindy: That they could get done by a gynecologist?

Dr. Silver: Absolutely. The youngest girl I have operated on, who was eighteen, would not get undressed in the gym in front of all her girlfriends, would not have a shower at the pool or put on her togs,[3] or when they all went camping she would go and get dressed somewhere else. She was totally inhibited and completely insecure and it affected every aspect of her life— with her girlfriends, whenever they had sleepovers at each other's houses, you know—everything. The rest of them would all be running around naked like they do—not her. Every element of her life . . . She just was permanently self-conscious. She wouldn't wear bikinis. All sorts of things.

This conversation highlights how a language of normality and pathology can be manipulated so that surgery is constructed as a valid medical intervention even for young women. The hypothetical case of a sixteen-year-old described by Dr. Silver affirms that sometimes labial reduction may be a reconstructive or gynecological procedure; certainly, labia as long as 7 to 8 centimeters fall outside the normal or average range as described in the (limited) literature (Lloyd et al. 2005). However, my conversation with Dr. Silver also illuminates the ambiguities inherent in categories of the normal and the pathological and issues of who decides these arbitrary values when there is a dearth of scientific data determining statistical norms. The subject of age is also addressed on some surgeons' websites.

Question: Is it better to have labiaplasty done at an early age if there is a need, or is it better to wait until one gets older?

Answer: In almost every case, it's better to have labiaplasty done when it's needed. If large labia bother you either physically, or emotionally—then it simply doesn't make any sense to live with these physical or emotional pains. Only five years ago, few patients knew of labiaplasty surgery to correct problematic areas. Today, with a heightened awareness of the problem by both young girls and parents, many are now turning to the surgical methods available to correct these problems. The reasons are that young women today are more physically active and armed with the knowledge that there is a simple, one-hour surgery to correct the problem—thus many women are moving forward with labiaplasty while still young. As far as any medical reason for delaying a labiaplasty, there simply isn't one. Whether or not a young woman decides to have the minimal procedure performed, or not, is up to how she feels about herself. In those cases, women and young girls who have an actual physical problem with their labia—such as large, or asymmetric labia—having labiaplasty performed early can result in an anatomical correction that results in greater patient self-esteem as they mature. (Esteem Cosmetic Studio 2013)

Here, metaphors of need and action—"turning to," "moving forward with labiaplasty," resulting in "anatomical correction"—combine with a trivialization of the risks of surgery, which is described as a "simple" or "minimal" procedure. There "simply isn't" a reason for delaying labiaplasty. At the same time, the expression "armed with" references the common medical metaphor of the human will at war with the transgressive body. These metaphors firmly position young women "as fighting the good fight by siding with civilization against the wrongs of the natural and therefore imperfect body" (Moran and Lee 2013, 382). Such language underpins the rhetoric of choice that surgeons manipulate in such a way that the choice to have labiaplasty appears reasonable and empowering, made independently of culture and coercion, as though language such as "problematic," "large," and "asymmetrical" were neutral terms.

Apart from its illegality (if the procedure is done for cosmetic reasons), Esteem Cosmetic Studio's claim that no medical reason exists to not operate on adolescents is contested by many gynecologists, who argue that the labia can develop unevenly throughout puberty, making surgery before puberty is complete inadvisable. As one gynecologist explained to me:

> The thing is, particularly with adolescents there is often uneven growth, so one side grows first; then the other side grows. There was a case presented in New Zealand where someone had a grossly abnormal labium on one side and they got rid of it, and then she came back and the other side had grown and they got rid of that! But, in fact, probably if they had left it . . . Sometimes it grows so quickly, and then often one area grows first and then the rest of the vulva grows over afterwards, so, you, when you're in early adolescence, it might be more prominent, but then at eighteen or twenty you grow into it. A little more estrogen, and then they [the labia majora] become fuller and it's less obvious. So, to jump in too early is really a concern because that whole area is very, er, it is rapidly changing and very stimulated by the hormonal environment, which is completely skyrocketing in adolescence.

Obviously, there are medical contraindications for performing surgery on adolescent girls, but more troubling is the fact that many adolescents are extremely self-conscious about their vulvas, and their mothers sympathize. One gynecologist commented, "An image is being set that something is wrong with them, when it's highly likely that they're completely normal."

As occurred with both Tara and Nell, mothers of adolescent girls are sometimes responsible for them presenting to general practitioners and gynecologists with concerns about vulval normality. Dr. Sonia Grover, a gynecologist who specializes in adolescents, said, "These requests come from a lack of understanding of what is considered normal and this is found across all age groups of both men and women" (quoted in Jemison 2012). The following year, speaking on Australian radio, Dr. Grover said that a quarter of the patients who present to her clinic anxious about the normality of their labia come with their mothers, who say things such as "She'll never be able to have sex when she looks like that" and "She'll never get a boyfriend" despite the daughters' genitalia looking perfectly normal (*Radiotherapy* 2013). Dr. Grover argues that it is often not the daughters approaching their mothers asking whether they are normal, but the mothers seeing their daughters and becoming concerned because they themselves are unaware of the wide range of normal vulval morphology.

Neither Nell nor Tara had surgery until they were eighteen and twenty-two, respectively. One plastic surgeon I interviewed willingly discussed performing a labiaplasty on a twelve-year-old girl, and several others said they routinely operate on sixteen-year-olds who present with their mothers. In a study by Naomi Crouch et al. (2011), the youngest female presenting for labiaplasty was eleven years old, and children as young as nine are now requesting labiaplasty in the United Kingdom (Mackenzie 2017). In a Greek study of sixteen girls between ten and seventeen years old presenting to an adolescent gynecology clinic, four had obtained information on genital normality from their mothers, and in four cases, the girl's labia had been described as hypertrophied by specialist doctors (Michala, Koliantzaki, and Antsaklis 2011). Under such circumstances, it is understandable that young women may begin to think their genitalia are not normal. However, girls do not always confide in their mothers. One gynecologist, when describing teenagers who present about vulval normality to an adolescent gynecology service in New South Wales, Australia, offered an explanation.

> Elise: I mainly see young women because that's what I do. Girls come in through the clinic as teenagers, and over two and a half years we had probably twelve or fifteen come through with their mothers—sometimes not telling their mothers the reason for the referral. And then, of course, we had our clinic in this area where pregnant women came, antenatal sort of stuff. Their mothers were completely panicked thinking, "Oh my God! My daughter's pregnant, that's why we're here! Tell me what's going on!" And then you have to tell them what it's all about.
> Lindy: Do their mothers always come with them?
> Elise: Well, if they're, if they're younger than thirteen, the mother should be there. If they're over fourteen—fourteen to sixteen—you make an assessment as to the maturity of the patient and you, er, um, it's a bit of

a gray area. As a doctor, you can decide whether you would treat or, um, require consent from a guardian or parent to treat someone. But, and it would depend upon what you're doing, so, something like this surgery [labiaplasty] would normally require consent from the guardian. And then, over sixteen, they're entitled to come by themselves.

It is evident that young women are becoming concerned about the normality of their vulvas at increasingly younger ages and turning to the internet and the medical profession for assurance and help. At times, this leads to the decision to have surgery. Both Tara and Nell are examples. Their mothers supported them. Although their vulval appearance may not have been statistically average, it was probably normal given the wide range of genital morphology. However, they were unhappy with the aesthetic appearance of their vulvas and experienced physical or psychological discomfort.

Jane: Norms Persist

The interconnectedness of functional and aesthetic motivations for surgery is also borne out in the following narrative of an older woman who felt that her vulva was abnormal before surgery. Jane, a fifty-nine-year-old woman, was happy to share her experience of labiaplasty with me; in fact, she was extremely animated and frank. At the time, Jane had three jobs (one in administration) and a boyfriend. She rarely had sexual intercourse with her boyfriend but they "hung around together." Jane, a keen cyclist, had had several cosmetic procedures in the past, including a breast reduction, liposuction, and laser skin resurfacing. Jane said she believes that more women should be made aware of the availability of solutions to their genital "abnormalities." She had been due to have a thyroidectomy and decided to have a labiaplasty at the same time to avoid requesting additional time off work for the second procedure and being interrogated about her decision to have genital cosmetic surgery. Jane had had her only child, a son, at the "tender" age of sixteen and was wondering whether having a child so young had caused her "problem." The surgeons I interviewed were divided on whether childbirth alters labial morphology in the absence of overt tearing or trauma. Certainly, surgeons' websites regularly give age and childbirth as causes of protruding labia.

Jane realized at about age eighteen that her labia minora protruded outside her labia majora.

When I stood there [my protruding labia made it look like] I had my tongue sticking out of me, which I didn't like the look of very much. I realized I was exposed, but not from looking at other girls. I didn't know if that was normal.

It didn't worry me. I would jump up [on the couch] for any doctor. It didn't worry me what I looked like. I just didn't think all that flesh was normal, but it wasn't until fifteen years ago when I started doing different sports and different things that I became concerned. I don't think anything changed down there, but my tolerance to being uncomfortable changed.

Jane described her suffering in terms of discomfort and embarrassment. As she grew older, the latter prevented her from going to a male doctor for her Pap smears or having a Brazilian wax. She said, "It really stops your life. You just can't do what you want to do. You've got to be selective. I had some spray tanning done, and when I leaned over I thought, 'Gosh, she will see everything sticking out.' She probably wouldn't care, but it is me, yeah, I did it for me, so now I can wear my uniform pants and they look wonderful, no bulges, and I can sit down and stand up, down, up, down, up, down. I have a very mobile job." Like Tara, Jane was convinced that she had labiaplasty solely to please herself, so that her vulval look would be more in keeping with the norm and she would feel comfortable in her daily activities. I was curious about her increasing intolerance of her vulval appearance as she aged and that this had coincided with her discovery that something could be done about it.

Jane: When you are younger, it is not an old part of your body, but when you get older, you have an old-looking part of your body, and you think, "Oh, hang on." If I had known that this operation was possible twenty or thirty years ago, I would have done it sooner, no two ways about it. I just thought I had to put up with it.

Lindy: If the doctor had said you were normal and showed you lots of pictures of a wide range of vulvas, would that have made any difference?

Jane: I tell you what would have made a difference. A lady doctor I used to go to for my smears; I asked her if it was normal and she said, "Oh, yes, that is perfectly normal. Don't worry about it." But if she had said it was normal but I could have an operation [to change it], I would have known earlier, and I would have jumped at it. I just didn't like it. It was like I had a great big earlobe jutting down, so I think GPs, I think it would be good if they said there is . . . But you've got to be careful, you know. "You've got exposed labia here; do they worry you?" And, if they do, that's fine. "Here is what is available." If you gave women that option, it would be nice. Anything that is protruding when you are standing normally, well, yes, I think that is certainly qualified for removal.

What Jane describes is an ideal aesthetic rather than normal variation, further confirming that the ideal and the norm have drawn closer together despite surgeons and women acknowledging a wider less-ideal range of normal. The idea that GPs should be critiquing women's genitalia and discussing labiaplasty is disturbing; however, with a reliance on the internet and social media for information about vulval aesthetics and labiaplasty, surgical solutions are only a click away for many women. Of course, aging is normal, but its effects are often considered unacceptable. Body parts droop and become less aesthetically pleasing. As Dr. Silver stated, "Age is bad for everything—it really is. The labia minora tend to become more friable, the tissue becomes more friable with the lack of estrogen, and the mucosal cells tend to become a little bit longer and droopier, and they have less integrity in terms of their normal sort of architecture and function, um, so I don't think any of the changes are good, you know." Dr. Silver mixed medical jargon with lay terms in a persuasive fashion, making aging appear an abnormal rather than natural process: older women's labia have "less integrity" and the changes are not "good."

Viewing the wide range of vulval diversity is not an attractive proposition for some women who have chosen labiaplasty. One woman commented that if she were encouraged to view vulval variety in the form of artwork, coffee-table books, or websites, it would wear her down. She explained, "I don't want to be persuaded not to have surgery. It would be annoying if I were persuaded to conform. I don't care what other women look like." Jane expanded on this theme:

> It would be great if on morning TV shows they could have a doctor explain about labiaplasty. I think that would be great. You don't have to have anybody there, not a patient, but they have doctors come and do little talks about things, and I am quite sure some of these women presenters should put it out there. "Some women have this condition; it is quite normal, but guess what girls, if you don't like it, you can get rid of it." Then they can do their own research. And at least if you plant the seed . . . I would love to be a spokesperson for it, but I couldn't do it with my face. I couldn't do it. It just wouldn't work with the sort of work that I am doing. I am in a high-profile thing; it just wouldn't work. My son would not want me to be famous for that. It would reflect on him.

Jane was adamant that labiaplasty is a legitimate, empowering procedure that women should be made aware of even though she acknowledged that protruding labia are normal. For Jane and many other women seeking genital cosmetic surgery, to be normal is not sufficient criteria for self-esteem and happiness, as she explained when describing some of the functional difficulties her longer labia posed:

Jane: The other thing too, I can tell you, was a big problem for a while there. When you are single and you have a new man, it is very hard for them to find their way down there if they are using their fingers or anything. You just—they could never find their way. I would say, "Excuse me, I just have to rearrange things here." Like that is just hideous! It is so wrong. It only happened twice though. Being in a permanent relationship, it is not a problem, you are with the same guy. And my second husband thought it was great. He said, "All the more to wrap around me."

Lindy: Yes, a lot of men don't really seem to care, but you are vulnerable with a new partner.

Jane: Yes, well, that is where I am now. I do and I don't have a partner, but potentially I could end up with others, and at my age I wouldn't want to feel like an old girl down there, so now at least I feel a bit more—not so much younger—but yes, maybe normal. I look better, and the whole process of having sexual relationships should be a bit smoother. I feel more confident.

Lindy: Mmm. Are you back on the sexual market, would you say?

Jane: Yeah, yes. There is still life in the old girl yet. It is not as though I am a young girl going out looking for different partners. I did it more for just how I look, I guess, and how I feel more than to enhance my sexual satisfaction. You don't want a couple of tongues sticking out all the time. It was dark, it didn't look very pretty, yeah, nothing very pretty at all down there, but now I am a lot prettier looking.

We both laughed. People were filtering back into Jane's workplace, so the conversation was curtailed. Jane had escaped having "ugly" (normal) labia, and with surgery had been able to attain a "pretty" vulva. However, she was not a hundred percent content with the results: "The end result, to look at, is good, but one side is different to the other, but everyone says that is how you look anyway, it's normal, and I don't regret doing it because now I can . . . I haven't been on a pushbike yet, but even wearing my uniform is more comfortable." Although Jane was happy with her decision to undergo labiaplasty and she acknowledged that labial asymmetry is common, she had expected a slightly more perfect, symmetrical result.

Despite her advocacy and enthusiasm for labiaplasty, Jane had suffered considerable pain and had felt rather disempowered throughout the process of her transformation.

It took two full months for me to be able to be comfortable and to realize that this pain will go away. It was quite a drastic procedure. I envisaged that it would only be about a week of discomfort and then I would be right, but this was *two full months* of, not pain, but I kept going "OUCH," and I had to be careful how I sat.

I was aware that quite a bit had gone on down there . . . and I think she [the doctor] should have explained it better. I have not actually spoken to her in person [since the surgery]. I have been back, but you only get to see the nurse, not the doctor. The nurse is very nice. I have no complaints, but for the first few weeks I felt so mutilated and mortified that I was thinking, "Oh God, what has gone on with you, woman?" I thought that I won't be able to have sex anymore, and I felt all different and that I would be too small and that I've got funny bits here and there, but I am okay now.

When I asked the nurse to explain what they had actually done, it still seems, for some reason, to be difficult for them to explain. I think they cut bits off and wrap it around or something, but the result is good to look at. I got a shock when I looked in the mirror the next day. I had stitches on the outside of my labia area and up around the clitoral area and down on the side, and then later I realized they were actually going inside as well, and I am thinking, "My God! What has happened? I hope she was not experimenting on me" [*laughs a little nervously*].

I really don't know what she [the doctor] has done—that's sort of a bit of a mystery.

I mentioned to Jane that sometimes surgeons do take skin off the clitoral hood and that doctors are constantly tweaking their techniques to get what they consider a better result. I was astounded at Jane's faith in her doctor, her amazing trust in medical "science," and her lack of knowledge of the details of the procedure itself. Although Jane yielded to the magic of biomedicine, her recovery involved considerable discomfort. However, her choice to have labiaplasty was a "now or never" decision. She said, "For once in my life I just wanted to do something for me, by me, and not have to explain anything to anyone."

Both Jane and Tara expressed a certain lack of agency in their quest for vulval normality. They appear to have largely surrendered to the authority of biomedicine when choosing surgery. Along with being potentially painful, surgery can usurp women's agency and place them in a vulnerable position vis-à-vis their surgeons, thus taking some of the magic out of the biomagical. Both Tara and Jane referred to labiaplasty as a "drastic" action, and Jane in particular felt "mutilated and mortified" and was concerned that she may have lost normal sexual function, thereby confirming the "drastic" nature of surgery. The sacrifices paid for normality (vulval minimalism) are, therefore, not trivial.

THE MEDIA'S DEFINITION OF NORMAL

The media wields enormous influence in the construction of ideals and perceptions of what is normal. What is deemed appropriate femininity and desirable physical appearance is generated and disseminated in the media, and the range of acceptable physical difference is often narrowed in this environment. Women's genitalia and sexual needs have historically been constructed as an area of concern, a trend that continues unabated and more publicly today (Wilding 2001). In the problem pages of women's magazines and on the internet, women seek to confirm that their genitalia are normal. For example, in a special edition of Australian *Cleo* dedicated to sexual matters, "Cleo Clinic" provides information on normal genital size, shape, smell, color, and discharge.

> Question: "Is it normal to have one vaginal lip smaller than the other?"
> Answer: "Yes, it is quite normal to have one labia that is a different size from
>   the other."
> [And with regard to color]: "It's an individual thing, but any of the warmer
>   shades such as pink, red, or even purple, are totally normal."
> [And smell]: "A normal vagina smells a bit like vinegar but can change
>   depending on your diet and hormones" (*Cleo* 2008, 105).

Although it is reassuring that a wide range of normal is acknowledged (for white women), the media is also instrumental in producing conformity.

In the same edition of *Cleo*, an article, "The Vagina Files," includes photographs of eight naked women. The photography spread is titled "What Other Women's Bodies Look Like: If Hollywood Has Got You Feeling Slightly Paranoid, It's Time to Take a Good Hard Look in a Real Woman Mirror." The women range in age from twenty-five to thirty-two years. All have altered pubic hair, and three have genital piercings. The article does not discuss cosmetic surgery, nor does it acknowledge that these images may have been digitally altered to remove genital "detail" as required by the Australian censorship classification system (discussed in more detail in chap. 1). All eight women have uniform clean slits with no dangling labia visible, which appears to conflict with the typical range of labial size described in the medical literature and reiterated in the health pages of glossy magazines. These images would scarcely be reassuring for women whose labia minora protrude beyond the labia majora. All the women in this particular article have altered genitalia, but they are presented as completely normal women. To have altered or groomed genitalia is thus portrayed as not only acceptable and common for this age group in Australian society but also, by association, desirable. All the women are white, presumably reflecting the magazine's target audience, and this, too, is portrayed as normal. Although women are told that variation in genital proportions is to be expected and a body positive image is invoked, the genitalia shown differ only marginally. Claiming there is a wide range of normal and then presenting a narrow, altered sample as the example of that range may fuel body-image issues. It appears that the days of (Western) women paying little or no attention to the grooming (and perhaps shape) of their genitalia is over.

Jean Baudrillard (1994), in *Simulacra and Simulation*, describes postmodernity as a realm of hyperreality, in which representations of reality in the media and in public spaces, such as Disneyland and shopping malls, appear more real than reality itself, thereby fooling the viewer and ensuring that the models and images seen there come to control thought and behavior, how we believe life to be. Virginia Blum (2003, 56) also suggests that the visual media has contributed significantly to what we have become: "Visual media seems to stand for something fraudulent, a lure away from what really counts in life, or in print culture, or in the good old body prior to its reinvention through camera angles, airbrushing, and surgery." We infer value from the two-dimensional images in the visual media and act accordingly. "Much of our information, especially our entertainment, is now conveyed through glossy, high-quality pictures. We tend to forget that this was not always the case; globalisation and digitalisation have infinitely sped up the production and dissemination of images in the past two decades" (Jones 2012, 199).

The proliferation of "glossy, high-quality pictures" influences our notions of what we consider normal and desirable in ways that often go unacknowledged. As an examination of notions of normality (real as opposed to ideal bodies) demonstrates, we may have lost a sense of the original, of our authenticity. What we consider real has already been transformed, making cosmetically altered bodies simulations in themselves (Baudrillard 1994). Individuals in a postmodern world are strongly influenced by the media, technology, and the hyperreal. When notions of normality are gained primarily from hyperreal images, the real body and real female genitalia drift further apart: "It is the generation by models of a real without origin or reality: a hyperreal" (Baudrillard 1994, 1). Blum (2003, 259) concludes, "The plastic surgery of the multitudes could be read not only as the culmination of the incursions of star culture but also its ultimate undoing. . . . Just as the television watches *us*, perhaps we are now the models—or rather, models of models, whose thoroughly internalized two-dimensionality functions as the ever-receding basis for 'human' performances." Hyperreal images of vulvas involve the erasure of body parts, skin folds, and protrusions, and this visible lack is evident in the images in the

Cleo article, an article that could be expected to espouse a sex-positive and women-centered perspective on vulvas. Instead, such images present a visible bias, further influencing women's feelings about their vulval aesthetics and reinforcing genital anxiety.

Young women in particular are concerned with issues of normality, but they are not alone. Older women (such as Jane) have similar worries. The internet provides an easily accessible, discreet source of information about genital norms. The example that follows is from Somazone, an Australian website published by the Australian Drug Foundation, which claims that "Somazone aims to empower young people to address their physical, emotional and social health needs in a way that is relevant and non-judgemental, by providing free and anonymous access to reliable health information" (Somazone 2012). On the site, stories and experiences are shared and advice offered. In these ways, Somazone provides "confidential advice and information for young people about drugs, sex, mental health, body image and relationships" (Somazone 2012). One example regarding vulval morphology reads:

> I'm a 16-year-old girl and I don't mean to sound conceited but I know I am quite sexually attractive. I've got an hourglass figure, long legs, large breasts and a pretty face. I have a boyfriend, and other admirers. But I have a secret that no-one knows about, not even my boyfriend. I have the world's absolute ugliest vagina. I am not even kidding, it is hideous. Both my labia minora are larger than the labia majora, but the one on the left-hand side dangles down about three centimeters. It's brown and wrinkled on the end and can smell really bad.
>
> The funny thing is, until recently I didn't even know that it was ugly. I guess I thought I was normal, or maybe I just didn't ever look. I'd even experimented sexually with a guy and he hadn't said a thing. But then I was here on Somazone and read a story from a girl with the labia issue. I started wondering if I had it too, so I got a mirror and had a look.
>
> Now I am in a very difficult place. I'm a flirt, I'm a tease, I pride myself on being attractive. And yet, in the most important place, I'm as unattractive as can be. I'm terrified about my boyfriend ever seeing or touching it, so essentially even though I am a quite sexual person, I have to shut myself down and act frigid. I know that plenty of women have labia minora that stick out and that it's perfectly normal. However, I am really insecure about my vagina.
>
> To begin with I am sure that mine is even longer than most long labia. Furthermore, there is certainly a very negative perception of this issue in pop culture. Just like I don't want to have cellulite or a saggy stomach (even though those things are perfectly normal and blah, blah, blah), I really don't

want to have an ugly vagina. I am aware that there is a procedure called labiaplasty you can have to correct this issue.

So, my questions are: how can I get my parents to take me to a gynecologist? Is labiaplasty usually pricey, and is it covered by any health funds i.e. Medicare?[4] Is this procedure generally regarded as safe? And finally, can teenagers have this procedure?

Oh also, I suppose I had better ask: in real life (yes it would help if you were a man answering this, or a gay woman) how much does vagina attractiveness really matter? Is it about on a par with "size" for guys (i.e. the accepted truth is that "size doesn't count" but there are some people who believe it does)? (Somazone 2012)

The author of this extract is clearly anxious about her genital appearance and the implications this holds for her sexuality. She acknowledges that normal variation exists but believes that protruding labia are not ideal, and she is "sure" that hers are "even longer than most long labia." The intimate and invisible nature of genitalia (what I refer to as the "invisible intimate") does not protect them from scrutiny, because they are "in the most important place" as identifiers of sexuality, hence the concerns about labial morphology—the "labia issue." Rather than alleviating genital anxiety, discussions in the media about normality can create new concerns, despite sites such as Somazone providing an anonymous medium for young women to discuss intimate issues. Anxiety is particularly likely to occur around puberty, when the genitalia are changing and new bodily norms emerge. Values and notions of beauty or ugliness are attributed to certain morphology. The clean slit, the look most commonly seen in the media, is considered desirable and assumed to be the norm. Beauty is then aligned with normality, and ugliness with pathology—the grotesque.

The final comment in the Somazone query ("How much does vulval attractiveness matter?") demonstrates the affiliation between ideals and notions of normality. This inquirer's original concerns about normality are revealed as concerns about aesthetics and desirability and about fears of discovery, exposure, and revulsion in others. There is a slippage between norms and ideals—normal as both desirable and beautiful (ideal) and normal as not good enough. Although the reply to this query suggests the girl see a counselor to help her with her body-image issues, it continues as follows:

If you want a medical opinion, you could first go to your GP and ask them to take a look at your vagina to see what they think. (You can ask to see a female GP if you like.) If they see anything to worry about, they can refer you to a specialist (most likely a gynecologist and/or a plastic surgeon) who knows about labiaplasty (plastic surgery to alter the appearance of the inner lips of the vagina). Your GP can also help you involve your parents in the process.

For some women, labiaplasty is a valid surgical option that allows them to improve their body confidence, and also reduces the discomfort that may come from having these sensitive body parts irritated by tight clothing, etc. To answer your questions about this procedure, it's best that you talk with someone who knows a lot about this and has done many of these procedures before. (Somazone 2012)

Although the teenage inquirer does not mention discomfort as a concern—her anxiety is about aesthetics only—the response cites discomfort as a justification for labiaplasty. In addition, by suggesting that surgical intervention is a valid way to improve self-esteem, the response promotes a narrow definition of normal as acceptable, indicating that the "labia issue" is less about vulval normality than vulval aesthetics.

On Scarleteen, an American website developed expressly to provide sexuality education for teenagers and young men and women, a questioner asks for advice.

I've read a lot of your articles on labia but I still can't seem to get the thought of my own out of my head. Mine are big and noticeable which I know are normal but [they] still bother me. I think it looks gross in certain underwear and I am very insecure about it. At times I even try to tuck them in so you can't see them. I am 16 and started noticing this about a year or so ago. I am not sure if I was always like this or not. I've been with this guy for about 8 months and he's been down there with his hands and what not but I am a virgin and I was very skeptical about even letting him perform oral sex on me because of the reaction that he might have [been] thinking it's disgusting. About a week ago at his house things started to get serious but [I] kept my hands covering my vagina because I was nervous. He was confused at why I would do that and told me he really wants to give me oral sex and I really wanted to. I eventually let him and he did not say one thing about my larger labia. I was very surprised and pleased but couldn't shake the idea of what he really thought. I [will] still consider surgery when I turn 18 for myself. I just cannot get the thought that I look gross out of my mind. I really need help on what I should do. (Corrina 2008)

Again, ideas of ugliness, grossness, and disgust are evoked and linked to certain normal morphology. Both of these requests for advice demonstrate the persistence of genital anxiety among young women despite their awareness that protruding labia minora are normal. For them, vulval aesthetics remain important, even when their labia do not draw negative attention from sexual partners.

The actual incidence of labial protrusion is contested and remains undefined. One cosmetic surgeon I interviewed insisted that 15 percent of women have this morphology. However, Dickinson (1949) suggests that 33 percent of women have labial protrusion, and in some accounts, the suggested rate is closer to 50 percent (Corinna 2008; Moen et al. 2006). Despite the many websites dedicated to educating women on the wide range of normality, some women and girls continue to consider their vulvas ugly or abnormal because they differ from the images they see in the popular media. Normalizing is not only about providing a norm; it is also about erasing, occluding, and "disappearing" an element of what is within the normal range of genital morphology. A girl or woman who finds her genital appearance unsatisfactory may feel uncanny, inauthentic, or unfeminine, given that body image is defined by what is *not* represented as much as what *is* represented: "The cultural obsession with improving or 'normalizing' the female body does not stop at the visible/public body. The notion of a perfect vagina, and its corollary, an imperfect but perfectible vagina, is evidence that such norms extend to the private/hidden domain as well" (Braun and Kitzinger 2001a, 263). Some young women embarking on their sexual lives are concerned about their vulvas. This concern is heightened because of the intimate nature of genitalia. Simply because the vulva is not on public display does not mean it escapes normalizing forces, particularly given the hyperbolic visual milieu in which desirable femininity is defined.

Women are more susceptible than men to oppressive norms regarding body image and have historically been more vulnerable to extremes of body manipulation (Bordo 2003). They are more easily persuaded by the images and discourses supporting the "mythical norm" that underpins the beauty industry in Western society. Audre Lorde (1990, 282) describes this norm as "white, thin, male, young, heterosexual, Christian, and financially secure" and therefore unattainable for most. However, this norm serves to define a cultural body-image ideal that is taken as a point of reference. Heterosexual women want to be desirable to men without necessarily listening to what men consider attractive. Although men (or women who have sex with women) may not be demanding featureless genital uniformity, some women have adopted this aesthetic as the norm.

I was unable to ascertain whether women who have sex with women may have different perspectives on what constitutes a normal vulva, as I spoke with very few of them. Those I did speak with, however, were concerned about their own vulvas. I asked all the doctors I interviewed if same-sex-attracted women sought labiaplasty, and responses varied from "I don't ask about their sexuality" to "Yes, they often come with their partners." Lesbian women speak about vulval normality on message boards and in magazines where it seems that aesthetics are not a major issue, and it appears that these women are aware that morphology varies. Although heterosexual women may not frequently see the vulvas of other women in the flesh, there are increasingly more websites and other resources (artworks, books, photographs) that women can access if they are concerned about vulval normality. The Labia Library (2017), created by Women's Health Victoria, with images by Katie Huisman from *I'll Show You Mine* (Robertson 2011), is an example.

DEFINING NORMAL IN MEDICINE

Annemarie Mol (1998) highlights how norms and ideals in medicine are conflated. Normalization as a process, she explains, ensures that medicine is disciplinary in nature and therefore entwined with political, economic, and technological imperatives, not merely the parameters of scientific normality. "A society *with* a medicine striving after the normality of its people differs from one *without* such a medical effort—which is what Michel Foucault has shown us in so many ways. And thus it is *his* work that turned the term *normalization* into a word for the way in which modern medicine helps to govern the society of which it forms a crucial part: by ordering; by holding up *normality* as a norm, a standard, an ideal for each and everybody (every *body*) to attain" (Mol 1998, 280, italics in original).

The comments of the doctors I interviewed reveal the contradictory nature of the category *normal*. "Normal—where do they [the patients] get the idea from? There is no such thing as normal," said one. Surgeons acknowledge that there is a wide variation in genital size and shape but stress that this variation is not acceptable to their labiaplasty patients. Social ideals regarding desirable genitalia appear to conflict with the norms acknowledged in medical discourse. What is considered normal is not what is physically manifest but what a particular society dictates, and these culturally produced norms are constantly changing. As one plastic surgeon ruminated:

> How do we get to the idea of normal? I had one patient, a thirty-eight-year-old that I operated on—not shaved, and her labia were hanging down. She was a totally normal female. Surgeons shouldn't operate on something that is normal. That is almost contradictory to the Hippocratic Oath, for me to be doing surgery on someone who is normal. I think they have convinced themselves by looking at women in magazines—pornographic magazines

have these images on every page—that they are abnormal. They are looking at women who have either been airbrushed or somehow modified to look like this.

This surgeon's statement highlights the tension between aesthetic norms generated by the media and the attempt by medical science to define the normal (as opposed to the pathological). Although this surgeon made it clear that enlarged labia are not inherently abnormal, the premise of cosmetic surgery is to alter the healthy body for aesthetic purposes in an endeavor to improve self-esteem and facilitate social inclusion. Medical surveillance therefore extends beyond the pathological to the social being, and cosmetic surgery defies destiny by physically rectifying a psychic, and therefore cultural, problem (Edmonds 2009): "Implicit in a woman's desire to alter her genital appearance may be that her genitals are not normal, that there is such a thing as normal female genital appearance, that the operating surgeon will know what that is, that he or she will be able to achieve this for the patient and that this would somehow improve the patient's wellbeing or relationships with others" (Lloyd et al. 2005, 643).

Normality and the patient's happiness are contingent on a complex succession of events. First, the category *abnormal* needs to be created because the body that has arisen without intervention is deemed unsatisfactory. Second, the patient must become convinced that she falls into the category of abnormal and that the surgeon has the expertise to make her normal and the foresight to see that such an intervention will make her happy. It is thus implied that happiness is wedded to being normal, even as the category remains elusive and undefined. Furthermore, the possibility of fast-tracking from abnormal to ideal is increasingly likely with surgery.

Hypertrophy

To legitimize surgical intervention, in some medical literature, women's labia have been classified according to size, with larger labia being labeled *hypertrophic*, a term suggesting abnormality. No agreed-on definition exists for hypertrophy of the labia minora. The condition is variously classified as anything greater than 5 centimeters (Mass and Hage 2000) or 4 centimeters (Rouzier et al. 2000), or divided into Types I to IV, with Type I less than 2 centimeters and Type IV greater than 6 centimeters (Franco and Franco 1993), or only nonexistent if the labia minora "are concealed within or extend to the free edge of the labia majora" (Chang et al. 2013; Davison and de la Torre 2011). While the frequently used descriptor *labial protrusion* "invokes abnormality, the label or diagnosis of 'hypertrophy' locates certain genital appearance *firmly* within the realm of the medical and the pathological" (Braun and Tiefer 2010, 3). Naming the condition *hypertrophy* medicalizes it and makes it a disorder in need of attention rather than a normal variant.

A study conducted by Jillian Lloyd et al. (2005, 645) challenged the idea of hypertrophy, arguing that "previous work has defined the labia minora as hypertrophic and thus deserving of corrective surgery if the maximum distance from the base to the edge is greater than 4 cm." Their research demonstrated that labia are more diverse in size and shape than previously documented, and none of the women in their study had expressed concern about their genital appearance or sought genital cosmetic surgery. The width of the women's labia minora ranged from 7 to 50 millimeters, with a mean width of 21.8 millimeters. Based on this group of fifty premenopausal women, the researchers concluded that hypertrophy of the labia minora is merely an anatomical, and quite common, variant of female genitalia. They found no statistically significant association between genital dimensions and "age, parity, ethnicity, hormonal use or history of sexual activity" (Lloyd et al. 2005, 643). Despite such findings, the doctors I interviewed were sympathetic to their patients' aesthetic ideals and bodily anxieties. When asked whether such a condition as labial hypertrophy exists, one surgeon replied:

> I would label it *hypertrophy* if there is a clear indication in the history that there has been a change or growth rather than, you know, a variation of normal. If somebody comes in with enlarged labia with no clear history of an episode that caused the enlargement, then that's a variant of normal, but should you operate on that? Well, I often do, you know, and again, it always comes down to . . . what I then fall back down on is, can I make the labia smaller, can I do it safely, and do I think the patient has a reasonable expectation . . . It's a subjective call, you know, there is no measurement for that.

Another said, "Yes, I have seen it. I would agree with you that there is no standard for measuring the labia from where to where and what have you. I would agree with that, but when you have seen hypertrophic labia, you know it. You don't really expect the labia minora to protrude to the level of the majora. You don't really expect it to do that. It should be about that [not protruding]. If it is getting any longer than that, then you know you are dealing with hypertrophy, and these are the people you operate on."

Interestingly, the second surgeon was adamant that he only operates on women with functional problems and turns away those whose vulvas are normal. Yet his criteria for judging normal vulval morphology is extremely narrow.

These two definitions of hypertrophy, "change or growth" on the one hand (reflecting the more accurate medical definition) and protrusion beyond "the level of the majora" on the other, are examples of the way the term *hypertrophy* is used without specificity.

What people refer to as *labial hypertrophy* is treated not because it is physically abnormal but because it is aesthetically displeasing and affects patients' psychological well-being. Similarly, the gynecologists I interviewed considered labial asymmetry a pathological condition. It is not clear why asymmetry is considered pathological, although, of course, symmetry has long been associated with aesthetics. *Hypertrophy* and *asymmetry* are descriptive terms that, when used in medicine, imply abnormality and can be used strategically to validate medical intervention. If normality were accepted to mean having healthy and functional genitalia, a broad range of labial dimensions would be considered normal (Malone 2013). This, however, is not the case.

REASONS FOR LABIAPLASTY: BECOMING NORMAL

Surgeons give two main reasons for performing labiaplasty: functional (discomfort) and aesthetic. Whether performed for functional or aesthetic reasons, labiaplasty is purported to have positive psychological effects. No doctors mentioned that they had operated for medical (or clinical) reasons to repair obstetric trauma, even though some had allowed their patients to claim a rebate for the operation from Medicare, Australia's federal health care payment system. Most women had aesthetic concerns, and even when discomfort was given as a reason for surgery, women were happy with their new vulval aesthetic postsurgery. As with aesthetic preferences, functional concerns are informed by societal norms. Although both functional and aesthetic motives for seeking genital cosmetic surgery are normalizing, they carry a different valence. If surgery is performed for functional reasons and not merely for vanity, it is perceived as a more legitimate and rational choice. In one study of 163 patients who underwent labiaplasty for supposed hypertrophy, 87 percent of cases were motivated by aesthetic concerns, 64 percent by discomfort in clothing, 26 percent by discomfort while exercising, and 43 percent by entry dyspareunia—that is, the labia being caught during penile penetration, causing pain (Rouzier et al. 2000). Although most women told me they wanted surgery for purely aesthetic reasons, they often raised functional issues as well, making it impossible to sustain a clear separation of these two motivations for surgery.

The surgeons I interviewed believed surgery was mostly an aesthetic choice. One suggested that as many as 90 percent of requests were for aesthetic reasons, saying, "Certainly, sex and the genital area, this is quite a private thing. People get embarrassed quite quickly, especially on seeing someone for the first time. If it's not quite normal, a lot of people think, so they are hidden, their genitals, they can hide it but, you know, with your clothes off, they may get embarrassed. And, um, and I think people are more concerned about their own, their own, what I am trying to say is, it's more in someone's head. It's people's self-image that they think there is something wrong, and so they want to change it."

Here, the male surgeon uses the term *normal*, implying that some women's genitalia are abnormal, while suggesting that surgery is performed to improve the patient's self-esteem rather than to correct a physical defect. However, what some women are searching for is not normality but invisibility. One surgeon explained that women "don't like seeing the lips of the vagina hanging down—they can see something hanging below the pubic hair." Another said that women say things such as "I hate the way my vagina looks. I hate it, it sticks out and I get very self-conscious." These statements describe women who are seeking medical intervention not for their labia to become normal but to more closely approximate the clean-slit ideal.

A study by David Veale et al. (2014) found that approximately a third of women seeking labiaplasty recalled being subjected to negative comments about their labia (mostly from ex-boyfriends). The study found no correlation between childhood sexual abuse and women seeking labiaplasty. However, the authors did point out that "body shame, from abusive experiences, is often associated with vulnerability to body image problems" (Veale et al. 2014, 58). Mandy, whose story opens this book, described a "bad experience with a boy" when she was eighteen as the root of her genital anxiety and other body issues. After the incident, which she did not elucidate, she thought she was "wrong," "ugly," and "abnormal," and the experience had a substantial impact on her confidence. Her husband also commented once on her protruding labia minora, and it was these incidents that led her to consider labiaplasty. Mandy's experience is echoed in other women's stories, demonstrating that it is very difficult for women to forget past negative comments made by sexual partners.

One woman said she had suffered sexual abuse and had chosen labiaplasty to erase her memory of that experience. Another had a partner she described as narcissistic and very controlling. Four surgeons told me they thought women who requested labiaplasty may have had a traumatic or violent sexual experience in the past, such as child abuse or rape. One (female) surgeon said she encouraged women to talk about their past before undergoing surgery and explain why altering their genitalia may provide a break with past trauma.

When I asked one plastic surgeon about the likelihood of past sexual abuse, he replied:

> Yes, I have had somebody who was abused as a teenager. She had the surgery in her twenties; I think just to try and change things somehow and get on with life. But that is only a small ... I have only had one of those who said anything. But then again, a lot of people who have been abused never say anything to someone who they meet for the first time, like me; that would be very unusual. You know, most people wouldn't even discuss it with their GP, who they have known for twenty years, let alone someone they have just met!

Another said:

> I have had quite a number of girls who have been in abusive relationships, and part of their healing process is to come and have some genital enhancement [he prefers this term], not just for the new partner but psychologically. They want to surgically excise the area—they have to do something so they can move on. And I had one woman who scrimped and saved for ten years or even longer so that she could leave her abusive husband, who kept pulling on her labia and nipples, and finally she left him. The first thing she did was come to see me to have the nipples reduced and the labia tightened. It was part of the healing process after an abusive partner.

For such women, there is a significant psychological component to surgery. They may perceive the excision of parts of the genitalia associated with past abuse as a new beginning. Having female genital cosmetic surgery in an attempt to erase histories of abuse therefore renders more complex the aesthetic–functional divide as the reason for choosing surgery. As Virginia Braun (2010, 1399) notes, cosmetic surgery is often justified on moral grounds, because it allows recipients to "move beyond bodily distress," giving surgery a (psychologically) functional role.

The functional reasons given for labiaplasty are primarily directed at relieving discomfort experienced when wearing certain fashions or when engaging in sports and other physical activities, such as sexual intercourse. Women who have labiaplasty for functional reasons want to participate in the everyday activities that society offers. Particular fashions are routinely worn for certain activities, such as in the gymnasium and for swimming and cycling, and women seem loath to forgo these tight garments for something looser and more comfortable. The desire to be normal in a fashion sense means the body must conform to the demands of contemporary styles. It is the body, rather than the clothes, that must change, reflecting a long history of female bodies being forced to conform to fashion.

Poor genital self-image can contribute to painful sex, providing further justification for labiaplasty. Although long labia can interfere with sexual intercourse, one surgeon explained that, in his experience, this was more likely to be a psychological issue—with anxiety causing dryness—rather than any physical impediment. According to Els Pazmany et al. (2013, 1006), "Women with dyspareunia [painful sexual intercourse] have less positive feelings and beliefs about their own genitals compared to women without dyspareunia." Given that sex is both a central aspect of sexuality and a private matter (what actually happens in the bedroom is not usually open to medical scrutiny), mentioning problems with sex is a powerful motivator for intervention. One woman confided that when she was seeking labiaplasty, "I just said they were uncomfortable and causing me sexual issues to make sure he agreed to operate." Before surgery, Tara, Nell, and Jane all had issues with sex because of self-consciousness or physical difficulties.

Patients often feel they have to convince surgeons that their problem is serious enough to warrant surgical attention, and to facilitate this, they stress functional concerns. Some men have queried the necessity of undergoing labiaplasty for functional reasons, pointing out, quite rightly, that having protuberant genitalia is not physically restrictive. In fact, for most men, protuberant genitalia are desirable. In response to a woman complaining on the internet about her long labia, one man responded, "As a man my genitals sometimes get rubbed when walking, but I'm not cutting them off. There has to be a better way for you to deal with your labia" (Joe 2013).

However, this practical, pertinent advice fails to recognize that women participate in daily bodily activities guided by strict codes of femininity that few women choose to ignore. Norms are social as well as physical. As Thomas Laqueur (1990) has shown, bodies and body parts are social entities that receive their meaning not from their inherent physicality but from the set of discourses through which they are understood. The language of science has determined our understanding of sexuality and what is considered normal. Changing individual bodies in an endeavor to be normal is easier than changing the social attitudes and discourses that make healthy individuals psychologically distressed and thus unable to engage in normal activities. Desirable genitalia are therefore a social construct, and the two reasons given by women for opting for surgery—functional and aesthetic—collapse into each other as women attempt to attain a normal genital appearance, one that allows them to engage fully in society—both functionally and aesthetically.

NORMS, IDEALS, AND THE POWER OF LANGUAGE

Language is an important indicator of how lay and medical people approach
and rationalize notions of normality. All three women whose narratives are
presented in this chapter tend to use the pronoun *it* when referring to their
medical experience and use the noun *problem* rather than being specific or
descriptive: Jane: "*It* took two full months . . . *It* was quite a drastic procedure.
I envisaged that *it* . . ."; Tara: "I knew that other people looked the same as I did,
but that didn't make me like *it* any more . . ."; Nell: "*It* didn't really affect me
until I was about fifteen." In all these instances, the "problem," the presumed
abnormality, and the solution are referred to only obliquely. This language contrasts with that of surgeons, who use terms such as *hypertrophy* and *asymmetry*
in the medical literature. However, on many of the surgeons' websites, which
are designed for women, surgeons eschew medical terms and instead use terms
such as *excess, elongation, large, protruding*, and *irregular* to describe undesirable
labia. Either way, such terms conjure up notions of abnormality.

In some areas of medicine, "Health professionals are becoming increasingly
attentive to language and culture in an attempt to understand and provide
better health care to patients" (Wynn, Foster, and Trussell 2010, 12). However,
many plastic and cosmetic surgeons use particular language (on their websites)
to persuade women that they are abnormal and that medical intervention is
justified. Health professionals and lay people use different language when discussing sexuality and aesthetics (Wynn, Foster, and Trussell 2010). The women
I observed used the evasive *it* along with words such as *pretty* and *ugly* when
discussing surgery and their vulvas, whereas surgeons choose terms that more
clearly imply abnormality. Their language stresses pathology over aesthetics
and abnormality over ideals. The language used by the medical profession is
in no way value-free, and it feeds into women's concerns about normality and
abnormality. However, "Health and disease know no sharp boundary. They
could only do so if it were possible for biology to adopt the dictionary definition
of normality. But variability, both in time and in the species, is one of the most
distinctive and necessary attributes of life, which thus admits no constant and
no norm" (Ryle 1947, 5).

There is no single, static norm. Normality is a multiple concept. Norms
"coexist in tension" (Mol 1998, 283). There is a (largely undetermined) scientific average size for labia minora; there is the ideal portrayed in the media as
normal; and, more importantly, there is the norm that any individual woman
feels is acceptable to her personally—that is, her experience of normal. The
language of health and, by association, normality is political because it "frames

issues and problems," ensuring they are understood in specific ways that then shape possibilities for intervention (Wynn, Foster, and Trussell 2010, 2). Both the language of medicine and the language of aesthetics draw on notions of the normal and the ideal state, but the manner in which they do so differs. In medical terms, one should be normal (that is, healthy), whereas in aesthetic terms, one should be better than normal. Both states are ideal. In the realm of health, these two languages (of medicine and of beauty) coalesce in a "medical border zone" (Edmonds 2013a, 234) where the link between the two is redolent with ambiguity. People are persuaded to be both normal and ideal, and negotiating these two imperatives is not simple: "The body, in short, has become a 'project,' one which is reflexively open to control amid a puzzling diversity of imperatives, choices and options. This, in turn, sets up something of a paradox, namely: the more control we have over our bodies, the less certain they become" (Williams 1997, 1041), and the more we try to be normal, the less normal (more ideal) we actually are. "The price of normalcy and the cost of avoiding what is not normal are high, especially when surgical procedures, often repeated, are intrusive, painful, time-consuming, emotionally wrenching, minimally helpful in improving the body's functionality (and sometimes, as in the case of genital surgery, impede function), and expensive. Against all these material and emotional costs are placed the advantages of normalcy, or at least the appearance of normalcy" (Kittay 2006, 90). Eva Kittay is referring here to surgery to "correct" ambiguous genitalia (rather than female genital cosmetic surgery) and other physical abnormalities— the art of using surgery as a normalizing tool. Normalcy is highly valued, and many sacrifices are made to obtain a semblance of normality.

Cosmetic surgery, the biomagical, introduces the "charm" of surgery to attain "normalcy" in much the same way that Sjaak van der Geest and Susan Whyte (1989) speak of the "charm of medicines." In both instances, doctors manipulate language through metaphor, thereby making it purposeful. Both *normal* and *ideal* are metaconcepts—they have no meaning in themselves. They only have meaning when used in conjunction with a noun: the normal vulva, the ideal vulva (Hacking 1996). "The point is that nothing is normal, full stop" (Hacking 1996, 61) or, conversely, everything is normal. Anomalies, however, are weighted; some are admired and others abjected. As George Lakoff and Mark Johnson (1980) reveal in their seminal work *Metaphors We Live By*, metaphors are used subconsciously to mediate an understanding of the world, to help make sense of experience, not merely to describe it. "Our conceptual system thus plays a central role in defining everyday realities. If we are right in suggesting that our conceptual system is largely metaphorical, then the way we think, what we experience, what we do every day is very much a matter of metaphor. . . . *The essence of a metaphor is understanding and experiencing one kind of thing in terms of another*" (Lakoff and Johnson 1980, 3, 5).

Women understand what is not ideal in terms of what is not normal, and this persuades them to act. The average or typical state is not always ideal. Medicine conflates health with normality, although it is also normal—but less ideal—to be unhealthy. In Australia, for example, it is statistically normal to be obese (Australian Bureau of Statistics 2012), but this is not a healthy condition. The normal and the ideal are thus fraught with ambiguity. However, in the same way that the "metaphoric objectifying of illness fulfills the expectations of medicines" (Geest and Whyte 1989, 356) by making illness a concrete entity that can be acted on, defining some labia minora as abnormal makes treatment both possible and desirable. The ideal then becomes the norm, the expectation. "A common assumption would be that some concept of the norm must have always existed. After all, people seem to have an inherent desire to compare themselves to others. But the idea of a norm is less a condition of human nature than it is a feature of a certain kind of society" (Davis 1995, 24).

We live in this "certain kind of society" today. In *Enforcing Normalcy: Disability, Deafness, and the Body*, Lennard J. Davis (1995) contrasts the norm-based society of modernity with the ideal-based society of antiquity, in which the ideal (beautiful) body belonged to the gods and mythology. This ideal was beyond the reach or expectation of mortals. The relationship between the ideal and the norm has become more complex in today's environment, in which cosmetic surgery is normalized and the biomagical embodies the desire to make the ideal (which is everywhere visible) attainable. A desire for normality and a desire for the ideal are therefore not mutually exclusive (McMahen 2012).

In *On the Normal and the Pathological*, Georges Canguilhem (1978) presents the classical history of normality, describing how the idea of norms emerged in the nineteenth century in medicine as part of the binary normal–pathological, with the normal being that which is usual, typical, and healthy, and the abnormal being that which is considered pathological. In medicine, the normal physiological state is both the habitual state of organs and their ideal state, thus leading to a conflation of these two terms. However, in the social world, ideals and norms are actively set and given value. Within this paradigm, normativity implies adaptability and action, rather than stasis and averages. Norms are amenable to change, resulting in medicine not merely returning the body to a habitual state, as was the original aim of therapeutics (Canguilhem 1978), but frequently creating an ideal, more perfect state. In nineteenth-century medicine, "the difference between normal and pathological was taken to be quantitative"—that is, measurable and acultural (Mol 2002, 121). However, as Canguilhem (1978) argues, difference or anomaly is not necessarily patho- logical; rather, some anomalies have a positive resonance (perfect beauty or athletic aptitude, for instance). Therefore, "the difference between normal and pathological is of a *qualitative* kind" (Mol 2002, 122). Norms are socially de- termined rather than statistically manifest. Referring to physiological norms, Canguilhem (1978) argues that the clinic, not the laboratory, should determine what is normal and what is pathological, thus highlighting a more subjective form of normality that involves how individuals *feel*, one that has important implications for aesthetics.

Normality as a concept is both contradictory and ambiguous: contradictory because it is accepted that there is a wide range of normal (vulval morphology, for instance) but only the ideal is shown in the media; ambiguous because nor- mality is at once desirable but also increasingly regarded as mediocre or average (as opposed to exceptional and coveted). To be merely normal is insufficient given that value is attributed to body parts; everything is normal, but a particu- lar aesthetic is desirable. This is one fundamental explanation for the popularity of female genital cosmetic surgery: women are not content with being told that their presurgical vulvas are normal. As Kittay (2006) explains, normal is both descriptive, in that it describes what is most commonly manifest, and prescrip- tive, in that it dictates how we ought to be: "Much of the ambiguity surrounding the term *normal* derives from the fact that the descriptive and objective senses of the term are in fact infused with prescriptive and subjective elements—that the notion of the normal is, in short, value-laden through and through" (Kittay 2006, 93–94). Because of this prescriptive force, ideals move from the unattain- able to the attainable, particularly because the biomagical makes the ideal a possibility. Vulval variation is the norm. However, the further labia vary from the ideal (as opposed to average), the less desirable they become.

Although the term *normal* appears to be an objective assessment of what is found in reality, it is in fact subjective because it is a value judgment. "If we ask about the *desire* for normalcy when we understand normal as a judgment of value (of what is desirable), not of reality, the statement that we desire normal- ity becomes a near tautology—for to be normal is to be something desirable" (Kittay 2006, 96). Conversely, to be abnormal is to be undesirable, not valued, resulting in shame and anxiety, as borne out in women's narratives. What is valued aesthetically is what is desirable, thus making assumed norms coercive: "If every woman portrayed in magazine after magazine, image after image, embodies the ideal, then it appears to be the way a woman—any woman— ought to look. To the extent that a woman falls short, she experiences herself as failing to be what she should be—failing to be the woman that other women in fact are and what a woman must be if she is to be the object of desire. Failing to have a normal-looking nose, for instance, then appears to jeopardize even the prospect of being desirable at all" (Kittay 2006, 107). This is also the case with the failure to have a normal-looking—that is, ideal—vulva. Before surgery, Tara, Nell, and Jane were all concerned about not appearing desirable.

Surgeons adopt and invoke the language of pathology and abnormality when referring to labial morphology to justify intervention. Women who find their vulvas aesthetically displeasing wonder whether they are normal. As surgeons are quick to point out, when it comes to physical attributes, medical normality is not always adequate for happiness. Some women are not bothered by large labia, whereas others are very self-conscious despite their labia protruding only minimally. With the increased acceptance of cosmetic surgery, normal variations of the body become undesirable. As Kathryn Morgan (1991, 41) states, "The naturally 'given,' so to speak, will increasingly come to be seen as technologically 'primitive'; the 'ordinary' will come to be perceived and evaluated as the 'ugly.' . . . the technological beauty imperative and the pathological inversion of the normal are coercing more and more women to 'choose' cosmetic surgery." In this paradigm, the normal, or average, is considered not merely ugly but also pathological and therefore no longer normal.

Disciplinary power, as defined by Foucault (1977), works in subtle and dynamic ways, resulting in "self-surveillance and self-correction to norms" (Bordo 2003, 27). As Foucault reveals, normalization both constrains and enables because it requires members of society to conform to certain acceptable states, both physical and psychological, while allowing some room for individuality. "The judges of normality are present everywhere. We are in the society of the teacher–judge, the doctor–judge, the educator–judge, the 'social worker'–judge; it is on them that the universal reign of the normative is based; and each individual, wherever he may find himself, subjects to it his body, his gestures, his behaviour, his aptitudes, his achievements" (Foucault 1977, 304).

Many of these normalizing forces are subsumed and naturalized in everyday experience. They act in subtle ways that persuade us to conform. Therefore, pressures to fit the norm also come from within: "In general, individuals are complicit in the process of their self-formation and they learn to normalize themselves. Indeed, normalization does not suppress individualization, but produces it" (Hoy 1999, 9). Although female submission to normalizing trends can be both physically and emotionally degrading, women are directly implicated in the proliferation of these discourses, because feelings of power and pleasure can be experienced through control of one's destiny (Bordo 2003). Agency is always filtered through normalization, and every society produces aesthetic ideals that place normalizing demands on bodies (Heyes 2007c). These imperatives must be continuously considered and negotiated. Women who alter their genitalia see these alterations as worthwhile because sexuality is pivotal in determining identity, and compliance to gender norms informs the decisions women make about genital modifications. However, cosmetic surgery also feeds into "a cycle of suffering and desire that normalization is capable of endlessly perpetuating" (Heyes 2007c, 60). In this sense, cultural (not anatomical) norms influence the individual choices women make about their bodies.

Paradoxically, although individualism is valorized, individuals all desire the same thing. Notions of normality and individualism have arisen together. The twin desires of individuality and normality, although contradictory, produce a powerful impetus for cosmetic surgery, and they drive the discourse harnessed by surgeons and the media to persuade women to comply with current bodily ideals. Although parents state that they love their children for their individuality, they also want them to be the same as other children, to be normal (Kittay, 2006). Mothers of young women seeking labiaplasty, as described in this chapter, are concerned that their daughters are not normal, and they turn to the medical profession for help. Such individual problems or concerns, however, have their origins in wider social phenomena, as the rise of female genital cosmetic surgery demonstrates. Supposed aesthetic bodily defects are not merely personal problems; they reflect a society's values, connecting the physical body to the social body (Edmonds 2007). Alexander Edmonds (2007, 376) suggests that cosmetic surgery works "on the borders of proper medicine, it not only medicalizes the body but also in a sense 'de-medicalizes' itself." Medicine has a new social purpose in this paradigm.

A second paradox is that, although Canguilhem (and a phenomenological approach to medical anthropology) argues that it is important that patient experience of illness be considered when determining normality and disease (i.e., normality cannot be reduced to mere biological statistics), when women's experience is foregrounded, surgical intervention becomes more likely. Canguilhem "defines health as the ability to adapt to challenges posed by the environment, to create new norms for new settings (Horton 1995, 317)." Taking into account the experience of women rather than being bound by measurements works in favor of cosmetic surgery because it is driven by social, as opposed to medical, norms. Abnormality is not simply an excess or a deficit of a particular variable. Women are creating "new norms for new settings" in an environment where the settings are imposed by ideals found in the media and where attaining the new norm involves surgery. Aesthetic normality is experiential—that is, how women feel about their genitalia—ensuring that statistical normality is no longer desirable, because the intervention of medicine in nonpathological conditions has become normalized. The biomagical nature of cosmetic surgery renders medicine less objective, exactly what Canguilhem called for. Medicine no longer merely addresses scientific normality. However, it *does* invoke the pathological in order to validate surgical intervention, perhaps because there is unease in acknowledging the full cultural embeddedness of medicine. Science is not meant to be subjective: "Canguilhem's appeal to doctors to exercise their subjective judgement when evaluating disease might sound like nebulous anti-science to some readers" (Horton 1995, 319). As such, what *does* define (dis)ease when health, beauty, and medicine coalesce? How paradoxical that Canguilhem's more holistic and affective form of medicine has, with cosmetic surgery (in which the lines between aesthetics and reconstruction or disease are blurred), become a kind of antiscience that subjects women to unnecessary pain and risks in the name of conformity.

Recent discussions in the academic literature have revolved around the role of biomedicine in influencing subjectivity and altering normality as well as the way in which capitalism and medicine have become intertwined in advanced liberal democracies. Advanced capitalism requires continual expansion and the creation of new needs and desires, medical as well as material (Sontag 1978). Consequently, disease categories and those who suffer them materialize together (Petryna and Kleinman 2006). This is not to say that individual suffering is trivial or not authentic, but as Arthur Frank (2002) suggests, the broader social causes of suffering and anxiety are frequently left unexamined. Consumerism and the increasing medicalization of the body create new individual needs but fail to acknowledge that all needs are socially mediated (Frank 2002). In this milieu, biomedicine has expanded from the treatment of abnormalities to the alteration of normality itself (Rose 2007). Medicine (surgical and pharmaceutical) has the ability to create new norms, a type of medico-normality that becomes routinized, and what was considered natural is no longer necessarily normal (Rose 2007). Instead, "the cultural 'ideal' becomes the cultural norm and the request for intervention becomes the request to be normal" (Tiefer 2008, 471).

—∞—

The relationship between norms and ideals is both contradictory and ambiguous: contradictory because while the wide range of normal is acknowledged, only the ideal image is shown, and ambiguous because although to be normal is desirable, it is increasingly considered suboptimal, particularly when normative judgments are applied to the body, fitness, and aesthetics. Language and metaphor twist these notions into a tautology that is both political and coercive. Language is manipulated in order to authenticate intervention; it is therefore political. Language is also employed to undermine the confidence of women, rendering it coercive. The term *normal* is polyvalent: nothing is normal, or everything is normal; normal is desirable but not good enough; normal is how we hope we are or what we aspire to. We want to be individual, authentically ourselves, but at the same time we want to be normal, like everybody else. Furthermore, medicine struggles between being driven by an adherence to verifiable norms and reflexivity; doctors are urged to view their patients holistically and to take account of their experiences and how they personally perceive their bodily concerns (as opposed to being slaves to statistical norms), but with cosmetic surgery, such a stance makes intervention more likely. If women *experience* themselves as abnormal, it becomes more legitimate for them to undergo surgery. Since Dickinson intricately described human genital anatomy in 1949, there has been little medical interest in the normal range of female vulval morphology. However, as Canguilhem (1978) argues, normality is not created by science alone. Rather, it is created by society, and today we live in a society where images of the (often medically enhanced) ideal proliferate.

Being complicit in correcting to norms, be they behavioral or physical, serves to reinforce them. As more women choose to have genital cosmetic surgery, the acceptable range of normal will continue to narrow. This could lead to an increased demand for surgical intervention. Hairless genitalia are already the norm for many women. The desire to achieve a clean slit could lead to female genitalia becoming eerily similar. Normalization can invade new spaces and become hegemonic, thereby disallowing other ways of being and constricting the possibilities for anything but minor difference. For example, in a makeover culture where it is normal to alter the body for aesthetic purposes, to resist this trend could be perceived as laziness (as it is with the fitness industry), something that is increasingly stigmatized. Although pubic grooming comes under this rubric, currently, only a small (albeit increasing) number of women undergo genital cosmetic surgery. Symbolically, however, the activities of this small number of women represent the tip of a broader cultural trend toward biomagical transformation, beautification, and bodywork.

Kathy Davis (1991) argues that women subject themselves to cosmetic surgery not for reasons of aesthetics or for the pursuit of beauty but in the hope of becoming normal. However, if women perceive the ideal to be the norm, they are achieving a close-to-perfect aesthetic, not normality (the topic of chap. 3).

The beauty industry and the medical industry work both independently and together to define acceptable norms. Each of these industries actively sustains its own commercial interests, which are fueled by the images and ideals that the other generates, without (necessarily) perceiving how they are increasingly working in concert to discipline women's bodies. This tendency is heightened when new technologies bring medical possibilities into the lives of a greater number of people. Discourse, not science, decides what is normal and acceptable in society, and powerful institutions, such as the media and medical science, are extremely influential in producing normalizing cultural forces that women (and men) must negotiate daily. What is normal embodiment is always changing. It is important, however, that "normalization does not assert norms as necessary, natural or universal" (Hoy 1999, 9). If men and women become accustomed to seeing the clean slit as normal, it may become more difficult for women to resist the desire for a more thoroughly (and culturally produced) medically enhanced body. With the normalization of cosmetic surgery, it is perhaps inevitable that the ideal becomes the norm, rather than the norm remaining the ideal.

NOTES

1. *GP* is a general practitioner, a community-based doctor.
2. *Bathers* is a term used for a swimsuit, swimming costume, or bathing suit.
3. *Togs* is a colloquial term for a swimsuit, swimming costume, or bathing suit.
4. Medicare is the Australian federal health-care system providing primary health care to all Australian citizens and permanent residents.

THREE

―ᴍᴍ―

SEEKING VULVAL PERFECTION

CERTAIN VOICES IN THE MAINSTREAM and social media promulgate a notion of vulval beauty that is difficult for some women to resist. The following
quotation from an online forum demonstrates this.

> Question: Is there a beautiful vulva and an ugly vulva? What does a perfect
> vulva look like?
> Answer: Perfect cleft, nothing hanging or sticking out, or even showing
> between. Straight line, with curved perimeter. The perfect vulva does
> exist, but it is not common. From what I've seen on TV, a surgeon is
> certainly capable of producing a perfect one from an imperfect one.
> (Dissident X 2010, gender unknown)

Such statements are prescriptive and are reinforced by practicing physicians'
notions of vulval beauty (see chap. 4) and images of female genitalia found in
the media.

Mia and Kylie, whose narratives inform this chapter, have chosen to alter
their vulvas not in a quest to become normal but in search of vulval perfection.
Drawing on a satirical work of fiction that portrays female genital cosmetic
surgery as ridiculous—*excess*, in Michael Taussig's (2012) terms—I theorize
that the pursuit of perfection is a moral project of "care of the self" in a culture that values self-transformation (Foucault 1988). Self-enhancement can be
viewed as a form of optimization, which now extends to the invisible, intimate
vulva, and with this, medical technologies have become technologies of life
(Rose 2007).

Within this paradigm, cosmetic surgery is offered as a biomagical solution to perceived shortcomings of the flesh. However, as Salvador Dali

famously said, "Have no fear of perfection—you will never reach it." Despite this sentiment, women are increasingly choosing cosmetic surgery in their search for vulval perfection. Striving for vulval beauty is not merely about conforming to the wide range of normality. For many women today, particularly younger women, normality is deemed unattractive and "just not good enough." "I had a labiaplasty in order for my genitals to be aesthetically pleasing rather than normal," said one woman I interviewed, and another said, "I had surgery to make my genitals look attractive, not just normal. There is obviously a greater emphasis these days on how all parts of your body look. Health is important and a primary concern, but attractiveness is also very important." There is an increasing desire for genital "perfection" made possible through consumerism and medical technology and fueled by the neoliberal imperative of self-enhancement or transformation. Although not all women choosing genital cosmetic surgery are in pursuit of perfection, even those who seek normality are, in reality, striving for an ideal form. Perfection per se is, of course, not commensurate with consumption, because an endpoint negates the desire for further improvement. Once perfection is reached, consumption should theoretically stop. Fortunately, for projects of corporeal self-improvement, bodies are living flesh—always aging, forever changing—making them an ideal site for intervention and ensuring that the promise of enduring perfection remains elusive. In *Unbearable Weight*, Susan Bordo asks, "When did 'perfection' become applicable to the human body? The word suggests a Platonic form of timeless beauty—appropriate for marble, perhaps, but not for living flesh. We change, we age, we die. Learning to deal with this is part of the existential challenge—and richness—of mortal life" (Bordo 2003, xvii).

Bordo questions whether cosmetic surgery is hubris. Certainly, for detractors of cosmetic surgery, there is always the specter of too much surgery resulting in a wholly unnatural look. Such vanity is ridiculed, as are botched operations that leave patients dissatisfied. The media runs these stories as a warning to those considered excessively vain or arrogant—the hubris of cosmetic surgery. In the many internet communities dedicated to so-called labiaplasty nightmares, women recount their sad tales of disfigurement, and internet photography galleries show surgically damaged vulvas. In the United States, surgical revision of unsatisfactory procedures has become the specialty of some surgeons. Despite these disturbing signs, the quest for bodily enhancement remains contagious and ripe with promise as women imagine gaining a more perfect, biomagical vulva through cosmetic surgery.

STORIES, BOTH IMAGINARY AND REAL

Mia and Kylie were in their early thirties when I met them. Both had had a breast augmentation as well as genital cosmetic surgery. Mia was in search of a quick and permanent fix for her aesthetic concerns; however, Kylie had embarked on a focused self-enhancement project using cosmetic surgery to define both her identity and physical appearance. For these two women, regimens of beauty and health were central to their presentation of self.

In the fictional narrative *White Girl Problems* (discussed later in this chapter), seeking perfection, particularly of the vulva, is portrayed as obsessive and ridiculous, the ultimate form of vanity and excess. Given that a woman's genitalia, unlike her breasts, are not on public display unless she is wearing particularly tight or skimpy fashions, to be overly concerned about their appearance is presented as unnecessary. Genitalia are, however, prime indicators of femininity, and an outright dismissal of the legitimacy of female genital cosmetic surgery (and pubic grooming) as worthwhile body projects fails to consider the experiences of women who choose to undergo these procedures. In this chapter, I focus on that experience and show how women make sense of their encounters with cosmetic surgery through their narratives. I draw on women's stories to demonstrate that cosmetic surgery is "both an occasion for autobiographical accounting and is itself a particular kind of account of the self" (Gimlin 2000, 80). Because the body is a primary symbol of identity, women reveal aspects of themselves through their use of cosmetic surgery; at the same time, cosmetic surgery constitutes personhood and enables women to express themselves in this era of self-enhancement. Kylie and Mia are adamant that they are "doing it for themselves" and that because they already maintain a fit and healthy body, they are deserving. Their new bodies, their new vulvas, reflect their willingness to work at being feminine and presentable. Both Kylie and Mia want to be a particular kind of woman: the type of woman who, through her bodywork, commands the respect and acceptance of others. For them, the employment of cosmetic surgery shapes their identities as better people.

Cosmetic surgery recipients use narratives to find meaning in their experiences and to tell a story about what type of women they are. Their narratives also serve to justify their decision to have surgery, because cosmetic surgery, as a practice, remains socially problematic despite its increased prevalence. This is particularly true for genital cosmetic surgery. After all, what sort of woman would choose to alter a part of her body, one central to pleasure, when it is not on public display? The cosmetic surgery experience lends itself to storytelling: it comprises a beginning (the desire for surgery), the procedure itself, and a transformation—it has a narrative quality. Narratives assist women in "making biographical sense of the transformation of the body and self through cosmetic surgery" (Davis 1995, 98). Things are different in the end for Kylie and Mia; their vulvas are perfect. Rebecca Huss-Ashmore (2000) argues that women's accounts of cosmetic surgery *constitute* their experiences, rather than merely reflect them. Women rationalize their choice to have surgery by narrating their stories: "The cosmetic surgery process is like other ritual events, from religious observances to the Fourth of July: we have a special story about who we are (Americans, the Children of God, etc.) and we act it out on these occasions to experience it as true" (Huss-Ashmore 2000, 32). The therapeutic narrative in cosmetic surgery tells a story about identity, not necessarily an authentic self, but a created self, and this becomes apparent through recounting in words the emotional experience of surgery.

Kylie: Determined to Be Perfect

Kylie was a recently single thirty-one-year-old when I met her. She described herself as a perfectionist in all areas of her life. She said that she watched her diet and exercised assiduously. Kylie had had a breast augmentation and three operations on her vulva over a twelve-month period. She was an especially willing participant in my research. Like many of the women I interviewed who had undergone surgery, Kylie appeared self-confident, bright, happy, and ambitious, but also reflective. She was petite, with self-described "big boobs," and her hair, replete with caramel-blond highlights, fell midway down her back. Although she said she loved fashion, Kylie indicated that she dressed a little conservatively at times as she did not want "to offend other women by flaunting my boobs." Kylie had experienced other women feeling threatened by and being extremely critical of women who have undergone cosmetic surgery, even though they are, according to Kylie, "gorgeous-looking girls themselves." Thus, Kylie intimated that there is a price to pay for having an assumably perfect feminine physique.

Cosmetic surgery can be divisive: its benefits are considered by some as "inauthentic and, therefore, undeserved" (Gimlin 2000, 81). Critics of cosmetic surgery describe its users as vain, shallow, and beholden to consumerism. They argue that beauty should be a gift, not something manufactured (Sandel 2004). Kylie felt that some women are jealous of her, but among her friends who have also had surgery, there was mutual understanding and solidarity. She said, "We always talk, we always chat, touch, talk about it. I think it is just people who don't believe [in] or don't approve of cosmetic surgery. I don't want to upset other people. I don't want them to feel uncomfortable. I want them to like me for who I am, not what I look like."

For a woman who had invested so much time and effort into producing the perfect feminine body, Kylie's desire to not be judged on her appearance seemed paradoxical, yet she rationalized this by insisting that her self-en-hancement strategies were purely for her own enjoyment. Women employ their narratives to account for their actions. Kylie's story of cosmetic surgery is a narrative about her search for perfection, but it is also a narrative about countering charges of inauthenticity and emphasizing that her use of cosmetic surgery was deserved and part of a much more extensive project of working on the self, "good vanity," and "socially responsible self-care"—attributes that are valued in the makeover culture of the early twenty-first century (Tanner, Maher, and Fraser 2013, 179).

When we met, Kylie was working in the then-booming Australian min-ing industry, which meant she had money to spend on cosmetic surgery and other self-improvement practices. She was planning to spend a few more years "setting herself up" so that she would always be able to take care of herself and further her career and self-development. She said she had been on a "steep learning curve" over the previous few years (since breaking up with her long-term partner). Her experience of labiaplasty was an integral part of that journey.

> At first, I didn't know how to function. I did everything for him; I didn't care about my career when I was with him. I was so fixated on him and making him happy that I lost myself, and I lost my happiness. I knew halfway through the relationship that it wasn't working, and I wanted my independence, so I started to pull my finger out and do things with drive and determination, as I had seen other women left without a career, with kids, etc. I said to myself, "I am going to achieve so much more than you ever thought I could." I haven't stopped; like, I am nearly at the peak, I am sure, but I have another two or three years in me yet, and then I think I will be at a more content place.

Kylie's focus on self-improvement involved more than her body. It extended to her state of mind, her career, and her social life. She wanted to be in control of her life and was ambitious about her career as well as her appearance. She said she aimed to earn "great money" and to enjoy the freedom that it can offer—the freedom to travel but also the freedom to spend on bodywork. Kylie noted that, perhaps subliminally, the emotional pain she had experienced be-cause of her breakup had driven her to alter her body through cosmetic surgery, saying, "It was more about 'It is time to make me happy,' and I was trying to search for what made me happy, and I said to my mum, 'I know that getting a boob job is not going to make me happy.' Like, I have to be happy within myself, but I just feel like I want it because I can, because I have the money, because I want perfection, and why can't I?"

Kylie's self-transformation was to a state of independence as well as perfection, a quest for self-love, strength, and individuality as a guard against future emotional vulnerability. Kylie believed that to avoid being in a compromising position in the future, she needed to take control of many aspects of her life. As a woman, she saw the perfect feminine body as a tool in this endeavor. Her narrative focused on "loving herself," thereby placing responsibility for her future happiness on herself as an individual, a central trope of late modernity. Whereas women in the past were expected to be beautiful but not independent or career-oriented, Kylie aspired to be all these things, and happy. The paradox here is that Kylie's way of expressing her independence after the end of her long-term relationship was to use her wages to buy into the feminine ideal of big breasts and a neat vulva.

Kylie said that no one had ever commented on her vulval appearance. She had never suffered from genital anxiety, nor had she felt acutely embarrassed about her vulva. Despite this, images in pornographic material triggered her desire to alter her genitalia. She explained:

> Women want to be perfect, and if we see trim and tidy vaginas in pornographic material, magazines, movies, and adult videos, we start comparing our own, and [if] it doesn't look as good as theirs, then of course we're going to want to change ourselves. Initially, when I read about genital surgery in magazines, I dismissed it as I wasn't overly concerned, but as the past couple of years went by I noticed my labia were changing from what they used to look like. I then started to become more of a perfectionist in all aspects of life and myself. It wasn't until I got a fantastic job this year with great money and a separation from my partner that I actually made the decision to go ahead with it. I like the look of neat, tidy, and trimmed vaginas; they are just perfect in my eyes.

Kylie assumed that all women seek perfection. From her perspective, it is a natural feminine attribute. Although acknowledging that she desired the genital look most frequently displayed in the media, Kylie's emphasis on autonomy ("It is definitely just fully my thoughts and my decision") implies that her individual choices were made outside culture rather than in the image-saturated milieu from which she garnered her idea of what constitutes a perfect vulva.

Kylie decided to have a labiaplasty procedure because she was not a hundred percent happy with how her labia looked: "I'm a perfectionist and wanted it to look perfect, and in turn that would give me more self-esteem, make me feel confident with a future partner. I wanted to be happy with every part of my body." On reflection, and having considered the matter further, Kylie realized that her presurgical vulva fell well within the normal range. To explain her decision to have surgery, she emphasized her perfectionist nature. Although Kylie was concerned with only minor imperfections—her labia protruded only a "teeny, tiny bit"—the first surgeon she consulted was happy to operate without any psychological counseling. Kylie proceeded with surgery with this surgeon, primarily because the nurse who ran the clinic helped her feel confident about her decision. She was not unduly concerned about the risks of surgery or with the details of the procedure. Kylie's initial written response describing her experience with surgery was poignant, and I include it here.

> I couldn't be happier with my result now. I was devastated beyond belief after my first two operations. My previous doctor didn't care. With my first op, the sutures fell out, and my labia didn't heal on both sides. The second op, they cut out too much skin on one side, and I was honestly preparing myself to never be intimate with a guy ever again. I've purposely pushed guys away, as I didn't want anyone to be near me. My mum has helped me through this the entire way, and it was a hard thing to even tell her in the beginning. I never actually uttered the words *labiaplasty* to her until after the first op failed. She eventually cottoned on to what op I was doing as she's a nurse, but she knew how private I am, and it was such a personal thing to go through. One doctor even told me to use Restylane injectables on one side of my labia to puff it out and try to mask where too much skin was cut out.[1] I knew I didn't want a temporary measure for this. So, I tried another male doctor, and he took twenty seconds and said, "No, I cannot do anything for you whatsoever; you'll never fix it." At this point, I was preparing myself for injectables. Then I researched more and more. I was even prepared to go to Melbourne, Sydney, or anywhere to fix what went wrong. And then I came across a female doctor who continually reassured me and said she believed she could make quite an improvement in what my vagina looked like. There was no guarantee it would ever look perfect in my eyes, but she thought she could improve on what the previous doctor did. We spoke a lot over the phone and through Skype, and I told her what every other male doctor said. It wasn't until I got to the city a day before my operation that she sat me down and said she'd do a whole vagina [vulval] reconstruction, and if I wanted a clitoral dehooding, she would go ahead with that also. The end result is a billion times better than I ever could have expected. Honestly, you have no idea how happy and in

love with life and my vagina I am now. Since May, I've constantly been sick and cried myself to sleep, taken time off work, honestly fearing I was going to be (in my eyes) "deformed." And now, I am so utterly grateful for what my last doctor has done for me. She has given me so much more confidence than I ever could have imagined. I feel truly blessed.

Kylie's story is one of loss and disfigurement, a struggle to find help, and then restoration at the hands of biomedicine; it is a narrative of work, sacrifice, and perseverance, fear of lost sexuality, and then a magical transformation to perfection. Because of the intimate nature of the procedure, Kylie felt somewhat ashamed of her decision to have surgery initially, hence her reluctance to discuss it with her mother. However, her perseverance was finally justified, and she was grateful to the very system—biomedicine—that had caused her disappointment in the first place. At last, the magic of cosmetic surgery to produce happiness had prevailed. Kylie's narrative is also one of finding gendered sympathy from a female surgeon after her unsatisfactory experience with several male surgeons. She was not only grateful to biomedicine but also to a specific, understanding, and capable surgeon. However, Kylie did not reflect on the fact that biomedical intervention had caused her suffering in the first place.

Sander Gilman (1999) contends that happiness is a result of "passing," which cosmetic surgery enables. He describes passing as crossing the boundary from one group of people to another and uses race as an example. Similarly, Eugenia Kaw (1993, 74) describes how Asian-American women choose cosmetic surgery to disguise their natural facial features that are associated, in the West, "with dullness, passivity, and lack of emotion." Passing is "rooted in the necessary creation of arbitrary demarcations between the perceived reality of the self and the ideal category into which one desires to move," and happiness is contingent on attaining the ideal (Gilman 1999, 21–22). Partakers of cosmetic surgery cross the boundary into a desired group. Although Gilman says that passing allows a subject to become invisible within the desired group, he stresses that that group is socially constructed, not natural. In Kylie's case, she has moved into an enhanced, hyperfeminine group, one with perfect vulvas and breasts. Consequently, Kylie wrote that she is now "happy and in love with life and my vagina." As Gilman explains, aesthetic surgery is associated with the erotic; it is employed to enhance femininity, and this is particularly true for breast and genital surgery. "The wish to be erotic is the desire to 'pass,' not to 'pass' as unnoticed, but to 'pass' as desired, to 'pass' into the group that silently acknowledges itself as erotic. It is to identify so intensely with the idealized image of that group that you will yourself to become one of them. Indeed, 'passing' is never vanishing, but rather merging with a very visible group. The boundaries between the beautiful and the ugly, between the happy and the unhappy, are also those between the erotic and the unerotic" (Gilman 1999, 206). Kylie's aim was to pass as desirable through her display of (erotic) femininity, and her happiness was the consequence of having found a female surgeon willing to rectify earlier unsatisfactory surgery as well as the better than expected result. The group that Kylie now belongs to is not only the height of femininity but also the group of people who take care of themselves, who are always striving to be better.

Kylie explained that her female physician did not discuss clitoral dehooding over the telephone. She raised this possibility when Kylie presented in her office immediately prior to surgery. The doctor suggested removing skin around the clitoral folds because it had become more prominent with the reduction of Kylie's labia. Kylie said, "Once my second op was completed, my clitoris stood out in a way I had never seen before, and I was going like, 'Why didn't I see this before?' So, my third op was a dehooding and to fix up what went wrong with the first op. It looks better than I had ever thought I could have expected. My last doctor was fabulous. I have a whole new vagina. No extra skin hanging down, and with the dehooding of my clitoris it looks trim, taut, perfect."

As far as influencing patients' aesthetic choices was concerned, the surgeons I interviewed were divided. Some were adamant that they only alter the labia and will not encroach on the clitoris, whereas others, including Kylie's surgeon, view the entire genital region as a piece of architecture, an aesthetic whole to be artfully fashioned. Kylie reported increased sexual satisfaction since her clitoral dehooding: "It comes easier to me; it is more exposed and it is just [speaks slowly] ten times better." In her narrative, Kylie emphasized her delight and her indebtedness to biomedicine rather than the fact that her first operation had resulted in severe pain because the wound hadn't healed properly and that the initial revision had been unsatisfactory, leaving her feeling "deformed," constantly sick, and crying herself to sleep. This is the magic of biomedicine as perceived by women who choose cosmetic surgery. Through narrative, cosmetic surgery is constructed as transformative, and this transformation is more than corporeal; women express their identities through their bodies. Altering the body is about more than its appearance. It is also about how the body is experienced, and narration is the vehicle through which cosmetic surgery is inevitably understood. "Changing one's body allows the self to enter into situations with an increased sense of efficacy" (Budgeon 2003, 46); therefore, as well as being a superficial change, cosmetic surgery also has symbolic meaning, and this is particularly true for genital surgery because the actual physical change goes largely undetected due to the invisible, intimate nature of genitalia.

Despite her satisfaction, reflecting on her experience, Kylie stated:

> I would like to also add, I wish sometimes women (myself included) didn't feel the need to always make ourselves perfect, but this world just seems to concentrate more and more on our looks. A character trait of mine is trying to achieve perfection, and I have to admit I believe I will always try to improve myself in any way that I can. Some days I wish I wasn't like that as I don't want people to think I'm so vain, but I also don't really care what other people think of me. I guess even though I'm told I am pretty, I still suffer self-esteem issues, and really I am only trying to make myself feel happy. But I have also learnt that fixing minor imperfections isn't always going to make me happy. I have to be happy and in love with myself as a whole, and that is something else I'm trying to work on.

Kylie's narrative is conflicting. She recognized her desire for perfection but did not want to appear vain, which is difficult when we live in a world where we are judged on our appearance and where "our exterior is a medium of expression, the outward representation of the inner self" (Holliday and Sanchez Taylor 2006, 186). Therefore, as Carl Elliott (2003) suggests, we have become more narcissistic, but less out of personal vanity than out of anxiety about the opinions of others regarding our appearance; Kylie said she had "self-esteem issues." The choice to undergo cosmetic surgery is about social relations, not only appearance and individual ambition. Kylie acknowledged the enormous pressure to conform to exacting health and beauty standards contemporarily and that some people may have considered her vain because she was focusing so resolutely on taking care of herself. Control is important to perfectionists like Kylie, and as Linda Hogle suggests, "The phenomena of enhancement technologies may not be so much a pursuit of perfection or immortality as much as a way of controlling, designing, and planning the body as an integrated unit of biology and technology. . . . Enhancements are upgrades. Upgrades support scientific research agenda and the ongoing production of goods and services that suit the needs of global exchanges. At the same time, the ability to engineer bodily functions gives currency to the illusion of controlling predictability in an unpredictable world" (Hogle 2005, 703–4). Of course, the world has always been unpredictable, but over time, the tools at hand to counter that unpredictability have become less spiritual and more medical. The salvational quality of biomedicine

(Good 1994) affords it almost magical powers. Kylie was working on all aspects of her life, gaining biomagical control, to best prepare herself for an unpredictable future.

After three operations on her vulva, Kylie believed her pursuit of perfection had paid off: "I swear to God, now it is the best vagina I think I have ever seen. And I am probably biased because it is mine. My last doctor took me further than I ever thought I could go." On describing her involvement with genital cosmetic surgery, Kylie noted in an incredulous tone that the past year had certainly been an experience, largely undertaken because her job in the mines meant she could afford surgery. The pursuit of perfection, for Kylie, was also a pursuit of personal happiness. She was adamant that she could not rely on anybody but herself to make her happy, and she equated happiness with being a better person: "How I look is not about other people and what they think; it's about how I feel about myself and all I care about. So, if I am happy with my-self, then I can make everyone else around me happy too." Like many who seek perfection, Kylie said she could always improve and that perhaps her journey with cosmetic surgery was not yet complete: "Yeah, I could always improve [*laughs briefly*]. I am definitely, like, a thousand times happier now. I cannot rave enough, like, I am truly grateful, I am, but, um, I am a perfectionist as well, so I would never say I could never improve, but, granted, I swear I am so, so grateful. I am so happy." Kylie's pursuit of perfection (and happiness) was constant, even as she realized the elusive nature of both. Although she tried to be self-accepting and achieve a balance in all areas of her life, her desire for perfection simmered beneath the surface. Kylie was content with the decisions she had made. She did not begrudge the money she had spent on cosmetic sur-gery; it had given her a nascent self-confidence expressed through her newfound independence.

Mia: Cosmetic Surgery Is Not Abuse but Care; It Is Not Mutilation

Although her circumstances were different from Kylie's, Mia also admitted to being a perfectionist. For her, bodily appearance was a potent indicator of a desire to "bring happiness to other people." When we met, Mia was thirty-four years old, married, and the mother of two children aged fifteen and twelve. She was a petite woman with a broad Australian accent and a generous, down-to-earth nature. She worked full time. Mia had filled out my online survey, and despite working long hours, she was happy to meet with me one evening. While we were speaking, her husband and son arrived home, and she asked them to leave us alone, requesting that her son close the door behind him. Mia seemed to relish the opportunity to chat about her private decision to undergo labiaplasty and her satisfaction with the procedure. She described how she had used the internet to research labiaplasty extensively and had telephoned several surgeons' offices for information before deciding to proceed with surgery: "Yes, so then I thought I better get real."[2]

Mia had previously had a breast augmentation because her breasts had shrunk after breastfeeding her two children for four or five years, and she had been unhappy with their appearance. Mia's decision to have labiaplasty was rather puzzling given that she had not historically been concerned about her labia.

> Mia: I just sort of . . . Everything was fine, perfect, nothing from the sexual point of view. Like, I only did it for myself, obviously.
> Lindy: What I am trying to work out is why did you suddenly decide to have this surgery?
> Mia: [laughs softly, then more raucously, and I join in] I think it is the internet. Like, if you can improve something—I must say, it seems so wacky! Like, it is just the internet; if you can improve something, why not do it? [laughs] So that's it!
> Lindy: What was wrong?
> Mia: Just a little inner bit sticking out, just a little bit more on one side. Yeah, I thought, if you can trim it all, trim it, well, it is all nice and neat for life. One little thing, and it is fixed. It is all good for life now—it is all perfect.

Mia had been seduced by the perception of cosmetic surgery as a permanent quick fix for bodily "defects," particularly quick when compared with the ongoing nature of other beauty regimens, such as dieting, exercise, and the application of cosmetics. However, the permanency of cosmetic surgery is not guaranteed, because genitalia change with age and with fluctuating hormone levels. Mia attributed her choice to undergo labiaplasty to the power of the internet and of the media more generally. The capacity of these mediums to influence individual choice is reflected in statements from other female informants: "To be honest, I never thought that I needed it. But I read about the procedure in a magazine," said one woman. Another commented, "I knew I wasn't born this way. I accidentally discovered the procedure on the internet when I was searching for eyelid reduction. I noticed the before and after photos, and that helped me decide to have the operation." These decisions to have surgery seem almost whimsical—the result of stumbling across the possibility for "improvement" during media and internet browsing—and yet they are predicated on the underlying premise of a deficient or flawed female body in need of improvement and on the possibility of perfecting the flawed body through biomedical means, a form of biomagical perfection.

The internet has become a primary source of information particularly for younger women researching labiaplasty. The information found there is extremely diverse, reflecting both popular and medical opinion. This is highlighted in the (hyperbolic) quotation that opens this chapter, "The perfect vulva does exist, but it is not common." Given that speaking about genitalia, particularly female genitalia, is still taboo in many contexts, the anonymity of the internet is appealing; women can carry out research in the privacy of their own homes. All my informants used the internet, not only for accessing surgeons' websites but also for joining message boards and weblogs to seek information and share their experiences. There is no scarcity of opinion in this virtual space, but as Nell (the eighteen-year-old woman we met in chap. 2) said when I asked her why she had posted on MakeMeHeal, a plastic surgery message board, "MakeMeHeal helped me in my decision to have surgery. You can ask questions there and get more information than from the doctor, and there is no reason for people on those message boards to lie. They are not going to get anything out of it. The doctor can tell you whatever, but to actually hear someone's firsthand experience is really helpful." In a world of social media and reality television, it has become normal for these mediums to influence the decision-making process.

Paradoxically, Mia was adamant that she had had labiaplasty for her own satisfaction while admitting that her decision was sparked by information she accessed on the internet. Reflecting on her decision to have surgery, Mia explained, "I had surgery to please me alone, not my partner, as he didn't want me to do it. But it was my money, my idea and wants, so my choice. And my right for myself. I had surgery to enhance the look of my genitals mostly for my own satisfaction, of course. I did it for myself only. If a person wants to do it for the fun of it, which affects the rest of their life, only beneficially, and it is done for them only, very important, well then that is good."

After surgery, Mia received a positive response from her partner, who commented that her vulva was "nice and smooth," which made me wonder what he had actually thought of it before surgery. Perhaps he was merely being supportive of her decision. None of the women I spoke with had been encouraged to have surgery by long-term partners; obviously, to do so could jeopardize the relationship. However, this does not mean that their partners are not happy with the results of surgery.

Mia did not feel that the effects of childbirth had influenced her decision to have labiaplasty. She had had one natural delivery and one cesarean section, and she said, "I have never noticed a difference in look at any time in all my life."

She also stated that the reason for her cesarean had not been to avoid damage to her vagina and vulva: "I have never been embarrassed at any time about the appearance of my genitals. I have always been happy; I only wanted to improve my genitals, if possible, for myself. I like to improve. It is fun." Unlike for many women who explained their decision to have surgery in terms of their embarrassment about their vulvas before surgery, Mia's decision to have labiaplasty must be understood as part of her project of self-improvement, from which she gained pleasure. Mia denied she had surgery to make her genitalia more normal. Instead, she said, "I had surgery on my genitals to make them awesome and to give myself a new thrill, for the rest of my life. Mine have always been normal. I think everyone's are normal, or most of the population's." The pursuit of perfection is about enhancement, not normality; however, it is not the permanent solution to bodily imperfections that Mia suggested. Mia obviously gained pleasure from "improving" her body. By using terms such as *fun*, *awesome*, and *thrill*, she downplayed the risks and pain of surgery. These terms fit with her narrative of a quick fix and the permanency of her operation. Unlike breast implants, which women realize may need replacing in the future, women assume that labiaplasty is a permanent solution to their aesthetic concerns. This belief persists despite there being no long-term follow-up (to date) of female patients who have had genital cosmetic surgery and the likelihood that genital morphology, whether surgically altered or otherwise, will change with age.

When I asked Mia in what way she looks different in her genital area, she responded that there were no inner pieces of labia minora protruding and that it was neat and trim and felt cleaner. "It is lovely and neat, but it is also, you know, when you touch yourself, you go for a wee, and you dab it there, it is all really neat now. It is clean [*giggles*]. It is the smallest change, it is the smallest little thing, not a massive thing." Here Mia conflated two aspects of the clean slit. Her altered vulva not only conformed to the desired visual aesthetic but was also cleaner in a sanitary sense. Despite extolling the virtues of labiaplasty for reasons of cleanliness, Mia denied having any issues with hygiene before her operation.

> No, nothing. It wasn't anything from childbirth or anything from comments from another person; it wasn't anything from uncomfortable, nothing. I just did it to trim it and make it neat and [all] that. I did it for myself! My husband was fully against it and he was a bit angry at first; he didn't want me to do it. And then I just thought, well, I want to have it done. Well, he really loved all the little bits, to be disgusting about it. It was definitely not to do with any commentary from another person. I am happy with it now; it is so neat. The scar is just a lovely little plain invisible line, like—amazing [*laughs*].

Mia denied that exposure to pornography, or to the media more generally, had influenced her desire to have surgery. She said that she does not believe that the media necessarily influences individuals, because people can choose the visual material with which they engage. However, she did use the internet and visual representations she discovered there, in the form of before and after photographs, to inform her decision-making process. Although asserting her agency and independence, Mia decided to conform to the ideal: "I am pretty grateful, basically. People—as your questions indicate—have surgery for different reasons other than for themselves, but I am just in a different category." Women who choose to undergo cosmetic procedures "engage in distancing or boundary-work that delimits their involvement in a practice that remains socially problematic even as its prevalence increases, and referencing the imagined other in cosmetic surgery is an important means of doing so" (Gimlin 2010, 74). In her narrative, Mia referred to imagined others who possess less agency, her purpose being to distinguish herself from women who perhaps, in her eyes, are more persuaded by outside influences.

Mia told me she was not planning to have further surgery. When I pressed her to explain her motivations for labiaplasty and her desire for a quick fix, Mia became slightly defensive.

> It wasn't like that; it wasn't like that for me. Like, it's just like trimming your hair or something—I just did it for myself, but it is permanent, and it is really awesome, and it is all done now, so I am happy. I think it is all set now. I am a bit of a rebel and I just did it for me. It's like getting your hair cut. I am just making this up, but your partner might think your hair is lovely long. "Don't cut it." He might think it is nice, but you want to cut it. You like it short. You are an individual. It's your choice and like, well, this is my life and I want a funky short haircut, and you just do it, you know, despite your partner's disapproval, and that is all I did [cut my labia] and now I am happy!

Mia justified her choice to have labiaplasty by recounting it as a trivial matter, and she downplayed the risks of surgery even though she said the recovery process was "full on." She had been unable to do any activities for the initial couple of months postsurgery, and she had thought it might take a year before her genitalia were completely healed. Mia explained how she had had no functional problems with her labia: "It was just like a little, you know, like something private. I have never been embarrassed about the appearance of my genitals—no way, no, no way!" Mia stressed her agency and individualism despite conforming to an ideal she had gleaned from the internet. She saw herself as a rebel who chose surgery despite her husband's reticence. Although her partner had not influenced her decision to have labiaplasty, she had not been immune to other external pressures. When I asked about her desire for self-improvement, Mia responded, "Well, I have just got to be presentable in general. I don't want to look like a slob or anything." For her, having cosmetic surgery was part of showing respect for her body more generally. She viewed her surgery as an individual choice, and an agentic one at that. She was a woman bent on improving herself.

Mia was critical of people who do not show respect for their bodies, who perhaps consume too much alcohol or have an unhealthy diet, thereby making them "feel terrible and bad." She said, "You know, you have got a life, and you need to be really grateful for who you are and treat your body with respect and then bring happiness to other people with your attitude to life, like, pick them up and make them, you know, proud of who they are, and everyone then feeds off each other. You know, give each other some happiness and zest for life. Cosmetic surgery is not abuse but care; it is not mutilation."

Mia's reference to cosmetic surgery as a tool that can be employed for the social good through the positive effects of bodily care, as opposed to mutilation, reflected her awareness of current debates about the growing popularity of cosmetic surgery as an acceptable instrument for bodily management. Perhaps, also, although she did not mention it directly, her use of the term *mutilation* reflected her awareness of the comparisons made in the popular press (and some medical circles) between female genital cosmetic surgery and female genital cutting (FGC). Mutilation suggests a lack of technology (and agency) and therefore is generally represented as the antithesis of biomedicine and cosmetic surgery. However, one surgeon (and we had not mentioned FGC) said, "We are all social animals. Cosmetic surgery is a mutilation. I do mutilate bodies, for the better, but it is still a mutilation, if you really think about it that way." The actual physicality of cosmetic surgery may be a mutilation because all surgery is mutilating to a degree, but proponents of cosmetic surgery, including Mia, do not see it as mutilation, because it comes under the rubric of biomedicine, which is associated with healing and rational science—mutilation "for the better." Much FGC discourse revolves around the alteration of perfectly healthy genitalia for cultural reasons; Mia claimed that her vulva had not been defective, yet she had chosen to have labiaplasty. Many of the controversies that surround female genital cosmetic surgery are thus underscored by the contradictions inherent in Mia's account.

The notion that a presentable body acts as a social good, that beauty and neatness (extending to the genital region) and a display of pride in one's appearance facilitates social relations, was expressed by both Kylie and Mia. Mia employed cosmetic surgery to ensure she was presentable rather than glamorous, accessible rather than assertive. In doing so, she was reinforcing specific (perhaps outdated) gender stereotypes, even as she defied them by insisting on her right to decide to have surgery despite her husband's discouragement. As with Kylie, Mia saw cosmetic surgery as an extension of caring for the body and as a source of happiness: "Well, it isn't necessary, is it? But if it is safe and it's a quick healing process and it lasts forever and it will make you a little bit happier, well, that's all right [*sighs*]. I had surgery on my genitals to make them look awesome and to give myself a new thrill for the rest of my life." Mia explained that having a breast augmentation and labiaplasty had made her feel more feminine. When I asked her if she would consider more surgery, she replied that she might consider fillers or new technologies as she ages but that she was content for now. She said, "I think the most important thing that I am working on now is my heart. I just want to be a good person and make other people feel happy. That's all I really care about." Both Kylie and Mia used cosmetic surgery as part of a wider self-enhancement project, one harnessed to make themselves, and consequently others, happy. By narrating their experiences of cosmetic surgery in this way, Kylie and Mia were able to justify their choice to undergo surgery and to deflect any criticism regarding (bad) vanity or lack of authenticity.

A Parody: White Girl Problems

The fictional author and heroine of *White Girl Problems*, Babe Walker, describes in her mock autobiography the occasion when she first realized her vagina (vulva, in anatomical terms) was not to her liking, perhaps not normal. *White Girl Problems* is also the name of a Twitter feed, weblog, and Facebook page ostensibly run by Babe, who is a privileged, twenty-something white girl residing in Los Angeles. She is the creation of three authors—two brothers and a female friend. Babe, according to one of her creators, is a self-possessed socialite college graduate who is "an amalgam of everything that is going on right now in pop culture, all the socialites and real housewives and these women that we kind of aspire to, but we also think their lives are ridiculous. She is an accumulation of all of that in one explosive package" (Schoenhals, quoted in Sinha-Roy 2012, 1). As Babe states regarding her vagina:

> This is difficult to admit, because I've always taken pride in my body or
> whatever, but here's the truth: my vagina was forged in the depths of
> Hades and sent to me as a sick joke by Beelzebub himself. It wasn't a fair
> representation of who I was as a person, and I wasn't whole until I had it
> fixed when I was eighteen. The entire experience really grounded me—now

> I totally know what people go through when they feel like they were born with the wrong nose, or born obese, or born with a crippling birth defect. I empathize. I mean, my vagina looked like it had Down syndrome. (Walker 2012, 47)

The book is a lighthearted, amusing parody; however, it trivializes the experiences of ordinary women, such as Kylie and Mia, who understand their search for bodily perfection quite differently. I mention the book here to bring attention to the fact that female genital cosmetic surgery is dismissed by some critics as excess and that this fails to acknowledge the very different meanings that surgery has for perfectionists like Kylie and Mia (and other women who just want to feel normal). A dismissal of genital cosmetic surgery is harder to defend if surgery allows women to engage more fully in social life.

In her "memoir," Babe reveals the daily obstacles she has overcome to achieve physical perfection. She is self-absorbed, extremely vain, concerned about her weight, and fanatical about fashion, and her language is peppered with expletives. Babe is a woman obsessed with bodily control and with her exteriority—the presentation of self for the self and for others. As Babe explains, there are enormous societal pressures to conform to a particular bodily look. In her words, before her labiaplasty, she "was obsessed—consumed by the idea of transforming my wanton vagina into a *perfect* beauty" (Walker 2012, 50; italics my own). Babe says her vulva was not a "fair representation" of who she is as a person; the surface of her body was not aligned with how she felt herself to be on the inside, a condition often offered as a reason for women choosing cosmetic surgery. Babe's obsession with her appearance is portrayed as ridiculous and narcissistic, making it difficult to empathize with her, particularly given that she is a financially privileged woman. The parody is glib and meant for entertainment, but it also depicts Babe (and by extension, other women choosing genital cosmetic surgery) as vapid. However, Babe differs from Kylie and Mia, who were essentially making what they deemed to be good choices as part of their self-improvement projects. Cosmetic surgery renders them "good citizens," happy, independent, and presentable. *White Girl Problems*, the brand, has been criticized for assuming that only white women are sufficiently affluent or of a suitably high social standing to be focused on physical perfection (Brookman 2011). In many Western countries, however, "ordinary" women seek perfection and choose to discipline their bodies in ways not dissimilar to Babe. The cult of the celebrity and the affluent, so prominently displayed in the media, makes some women feel that perfection is within their reach and worth striving for.

Female genital cosmetic surgery has also been sensationalized and parodied on American reality television programs, such as *Plastic Wives*, which looks at the lives of women married to some of Los Angeles's most successful cosmetic surgeons (one is the wife of Dr. David Matlock, referred to in chap. 4). In one episode, a woman produced a clear jar containing morsels of flesh suspended in fluid and presented it to the camera. "This is my labia," she said nonchalantly. "I think she looks better in the jar than hanging down there," pointing to her crotch.

What can a blending of parodic fiction and reality television tell us about female genital cosmetic surgery or about cosmetic surgery and self-enhancement technologies more generally? The lampooning—for entertainment purposes—of women who have genital cosmetic surgery demonstrates that such surgery, as a practice, causes cultural unease. This may be because genitalia are central to sexuality, and their alteration therefore falls into a unique category, or perhaps it is because striving for a perfect body, particularly an invisible, intimate body part, is considered hubris, as Bordo (2003) suggests. The women are depicted as ridiculous and vain, and their experiences are presented as absurd. The parody also implies that there is a gendered, racial element of class privilege that authorizes painful and expensive projects of self-perfection while simultaneously parodying the self-loathing of the privileged. Such a perspective fails to acknowledge that genital anxiety is not confined to those who may be judged as having nothing better to do with their lives. Rather, it is part of a much wider set of societal concerns about the physical body.

NARRATIVE REVELATIONS: STORIES OF VULVAS, STORIES OF WOMEN

Although considered only one interpretation of reality, narratives give meaning to experience. Kylie's and Mia's narratives each tell a story of who they are as individuals as well as a story about cosmetic surgery. Unlike Babe and the women in *Plastic Wives*, who are portrayed as inhabiting a hollow fantasy world lacking in authenticity and emblematic of excess, Kylie's and Mia's narratives reveal a more nuanced form of being and meaning-making. Kylie and Mia are grateful for having had female genital cosmetic surgery. They are somewhat surprised at how perfect the results are and, although they believe they did it for themselves, it is apparent that their decision to have surgery was part of a much wider project of self-transformation. In *White Girl Problems*, labiaplasty is trivialized and portrayed as an absurd choice for a (albeit fictional) narcissistic and privileged woman who has nothing more serious with which to occupy her time than seeking physical perfection. Genital cosmetic surgery is therefore presented as morally reprehensible—a poor choice. Conversely, Kylie and Mia's narratives of self-transformation involve more than aesthetic enhancement. They have embarked on what they believe to be a virtuous project; they are striving to be better people, and they believe that their exteriority—how they look—reflects their personalities. For them, neglecting the body is "laziness, a sign of low-self-esteem and even moral failure" (Hogle 2005, 702). This makes the striving for perfection less ridiculous. Personal happiness with their individual feminized bodies has enabled Kylie and Mia to imagine themselves as more-engaged citizens. Cosmetic surgery works by aligning surfaces (outsides) with emotions (insides) to improve self-esteem or, in Mia's case, for a "new thrill"—the promise of pleasure and happiness. In transforming appearance, cosmetic surgery also transforms identity—how women envision themselves (Davis 2003).

In Kylie's case, the prime catalyst for surgery was money and her newfound single status; she could suddenly afford surgery. For Mia, discovering the possibility of surgery on the internet spurred her to action. One of the major differences between the two women's experiences is a temporal one. The attractiveness of labiaplasty for Mia was its supposed permanent nature and its ability to provide a quick fix to a bodily imperfection, which she said was "one little thing." Kylie's experience of genital cosmetic surgery was much more dramatic because of the unsatisfactory nature of her first two procedures. However, both women emphasized their pleasure with their perfect vulvas and, in doing so, glossed over the risks of surgery and the prolonged recovery phase. They considered any suffering they endured an acceptable component of their self-enhancement experience. Perfection takes work. Kylie appeared more reflective than did Mia, perhaps because of her repeated surgeries, but she had no complaints. Unlike Mia, who appeared to have approached surgery more opportunistically and described having a labiaplasty as "fun" and a "new thrill," Kylie appeared to be the ultimate perfectionist for whom control is paramount. As she said, "God, if I've got a problem, I try and fix it and make myself happy because no one else can do it for me." In both cases, genital cosmetic surgery was an aesthetic choice, and such cosmetic intervention demonstrates how even the invisible, most intimate part of a woman's body has increasingly come under scrutiny—the private has become public. Female genital cosmetic surgery is discussed in surgeons' offices, in the media, in documentaries, on the internet, by regulatory and government bodies, and in fiction. Perhaps, then, it is not surprising that, for perfectionists, vulvas can also tell a public story about what sort of woman one is, even when the genitalia are hidden from the majority of people with whom these women interact. Through their narratives, Kylie and Mia rationalized their choice to have genital cosmetic surgery. They could afford it, and rather than considering themselves narcissistic, they believed in the salvational nature of biomedicine, its magical ability to make people feel better about themselves and hence more fully engaged with society.

PERFECTIONISM, BODY DYSMORPHIC DISORDER, AND THE DOCTOR–PATIENT RELATIONSHIP

While biomedicine is increasingly employed in the pursuit of perfection, it also defines obsessive concern with perfection, or anxiety about particular bodily features, as a medical problem. Good candidates for surgery must be separated from bad (mentally disturbed) candidates. Although I am not suggesting that either Kylie or Mia have body dysmorphic disorder (BDD), I include a discussion of it here because there is an obvious tension between cosmetic surgery as a practice and BDD as a psychological condition, and this tension is often glossed over by cosmetic surgeons. Cosmetic surgery candidates should not only be sufficiently concerned about their appearance to request surgical intervention but also psychologically resilient. As Cressida Heyes (2009) suggests, any attempt to separate a normal concern about appearance from a psychopathological concern is, in part, an effect of disciplinary power: "Although often presented as a way of making cosmetic surgery more ethical and restrained, this epistemic project inadvertently defends cosmetic surgical interests" (Heyes 2009, 73). The paradox implicit here is that cosmetic surgery candidates simultaneously subject themselves to the magic of biomedicine and risk being labeled by the very same institution as mentally unstable. The relationship between cosmetic surgery and BDD, therefore, is not straightforward. "When pathologizing comes too easily, we put the burden of the industry's problems disproportionately on the psyches of individuals. This is not where most of the problems of cosmetic surgery belong. . . . And the solution often focuses on sorting the good from the bad patients, with the former wanting the right surgeries, at the right times, and knowing how to find good surgeons, the latter pushing the envelope of normalcy in various ways" (Pitts-Taylor 2007, 127).

Appraising individuals such as Kylie and Mia as overly fastidious fails to emphasize the cultural pressures that make cosmetic surgery an attractive proposition to them and highlights the moralizing discourse that surrounds cosmetic surgery. Concern with physical appearance "describes a certain norm of femininity" (Heyes 2009, 75); that is, women should, to an acceptable

extent, be interested in and acting on their exteriority but not be obsessive—
something of a balancing act.

The discourse around personal agency and choice for women who undergo
cosmetic procedures has been appropriated by surgeons to validate their decision to perform genital cosmetic surgery. Choice is pivotal to the acceptance of
cosmetic surgery as a legitimate practice, and this is particularly true for emerging procedures such as female genital cosmetic surgery. A closer look at how
choice operates exposes some inconsistencies and challenges within the medical profession, many of which revolve around the doctor–patient relationship.
With cosmetic procedures, individual choice is central to the doctor–patient
relationship, a relationship that is changing as patients become better informed
and more demanding in an increasingly commercialized medical milieu. Doctors fulfill their patients' desires, providing patients' requests are reasonable
(Braun 2009a). Patients need to be "informed, realistic and prepared to have
genital surgery for themselves" (Braun 2009a, 239). Unrealistic expectations
result in unhappy patients; therefore, surgeons use their discretion when deciding whether to operate. Of course, surgeons employ this discretion to their
own advantage. Unhappy patients are bad publicity and may result in decreased
business or litigation. As one surgeon I interviewed said, "How big does a labia
have to be before you can do it? Well, it's up to the person, and if they are—I
suppose—if their expectations are realistic, we can do it for them." Surgeons
who encounter "suitable" patients are able to make women happy without compromising their medical integrity. Surgeons, perhaps understandably from a
medical but not a social point of view, frequently emphasize the ordinariness
of labiaplasty. "Whether it is labiaplasty or rhinoplasty, it is the same deal,"
said one.

Some surgeons describe themselves as responding to women's desire for
surgery almost reluctantly, and they often highlight what they perceive to be
the more assertive attitude of women today, one that puts doctors in new situations where they may feel uncomfortable. That surgery is performed to please
the patient (almost against the surgeon's better judgment) is borne out in the
following description. A patient, whom the surgeon described as "elfin" and
"very beautiful," came to him requesting labiaplasty. He performed the surgery and felt the results were good, but the patient kept returning. She was
fastidious and convinced him to reoperate to improve the symmetry of her
labia. On revisiting the surgery one day, she did not wait for the nurse to be
present (the accepted procedure) before she undressed. This put the surgeon
in a difficult situation. He felt the patient was an exhibitionist and wished he
had not agreed to operate on her. The usual caring, but authoritative, relationship between surgeon and patient had been disturbed, and he contacted his

medical insurance company in case there were any repercussions. This woman was considered too demanding. She behaved in a manner not in keeping with established medical protocol.

More revealingly, perhaps, in stressing the agency and demanding nature of their patients, surgeons are justifying their own actions and distancing themselves from their patients' decisions. Increased access to information about cosmetic surgery has resulted in women presenting to surgeons with their own definite requests; everyone is an expert on cosmetic surgery because of access to reality television programs, the internet, and media articles (Jones 2008). This can bring tension to the doctor–patient relationship. At the same time, doctors frequently project themselves as responding to their patients' desires, and their websites often cloak their consumer-driven agendas in terms of empowerment and choice for women. The discourse of choice therefore deflects any ensuing criticism of cosmetic procedures, unless, of course, patients can be labeled as sufferers of BDD.

Clear links exist between BDD and perfectionism. According to the *Diagnostic and Statistical Manual of Mental Disorders, 5th Edition* (or *DSM-5*), BDD is "associated with high levels of anxiety . . . neuroticism and perfectionism as well as low extroversion and low self-esteem" (American Psychiatric Association 2013, 244). Individuals with BDD are characterized by "perfectionist thinking and maladaptive beliefs about physical attractiveness" (Buhlmann, Etcoff, and Wilhelm 2007, 546). BDD sufferers experience extreme dissatisfaction and preoccupation with the perceived appearance of a particular body part, or parts, and this can result in significant functional impairment and negative emotions. As described on the website Better Health Channel (2012), a popular source of public health information in Australia, "A person with low self-esteem who has impossible standards of perfection judges some part of their body as ugly. Over time, this behavior becomes more and more compulsive. Western society's narrow standards of beauty may trigger BDD in vulnerable people," and even the less vulnerable are profoundly influenced by highly prescriptive beauty ideals.

Although BDD is a distressing disorder that can cause significant impairment rather than what we might popularly term *simple vanity*, many psychological disorders tend to highlight the extreme end of what are often everyday, mundane pathologies. The desire for bodily perfection on which BDD is premised can be persuasive in a culture that expects individuals to look after themselves. Mainstream Western culture is saturated with images of desirable bodies, making it difficult to ascertain at which stage perfectionism becomes maladaptive as opposed to an admirable, or even rational, strategy to promote social inclusion and success. In our discussions, Kylie reluctantly referred to her low self-esteem. As she explained, "I guess even though I am told I am pretty, I still suffer self-esteem issues, and really I am only trying to make myself feel happy." At the same time as BDD has arisen as a medical condition in the West, so too have concerns about physical attractiveness and perfection.

According to Katharine Phillips, a professor of psychiatry and human behavior at Brown University, cosmetic treatment is usually ineffective for BDD and may even worsen BDD symptoms because the preoccupation with appearance may simply relocate to another body area following a cosmetic procedure (Phillips 2012). Alternatively, Merle Spriggs and Lynn Gillam (2016) have argued that labiaplasty may be ethically justified for adolescents with BDD as long as parents and doctors are involved in the decision-making process. Surgery could ensure the well-being of sufferers by averting distress and suicide. Although, according to Canice Crerand, Martin Franklin, and David Sarwer (2006), the prevalence of BDD symptoms in patients seeking cosmetic surgery (estimated to be between 6 percent and 53 percent) is higher than in the general population, the surgeons I spoke with were largely dismissive of the notion that BDD has a role in the desire for female genital surgery. Some proponents of female genital cosmetic surgery have made a concerted effort to prove that undergoing surgery reduces the incidence of body dissatisfaction in BDD patients (Goodman et al. 2016). Of the more than forty doctors I interviewed, only one acknowledged refusing to operate on a woman who presented requesting genital cosmetic surgery. Nevertheless, many stated that patients with BDD more generally are "problem" patients because they are rarely satisfied with their surgical outcomes and are best avoided given that they could bring the surgeon into disrepute.

Surgeons made it clear that they rarely refer their patients for psychological assessment before performing genital cosmetic surgery; instead, they rely on their own judgment in screening patients for BDD. One surgeon, Dr. Marcos, expressed her particular interest in the intersection of psychology and surgery. She believes they are closely affiliated, and she is interested in the context of people's lives and in how people believe surgery will change things for them at the emotional level. She said, "I feel I have an instinct as to how people will cope with surgery and can tell if they have BDD. Surgery is a journey you embark on with the patient, and you both have to be able to see it through to the end even if there are complications and setbacks, [if] things aren't perfect. So, you must have a feeling of how a patient will cope if complications arise, and I stress these things in the consultation."

Here, Dr. Marcos highlighted that cosmetic surgery requires an affective investment from the patient and surgeon in ways that other procedures may not, and her intuition flies in the face of evidence-based medicine. However, while surgeons are wary of women who display perfectionist traits, being a perfectionist does not necessarily lead to disappointment. For instance, Kylie was willing to undergo three surgical procedures, and she was happy, indeed ecstatic, with the final results. Certainly, there are increasing reports of unsatisfactory results with female genital cosmetic surgery, as there are with all cosmetic surgery procedures. However, this could be due to a range of factors, such as more doctors with inadequate surgical training carrying out these procedures, a greater number of surgeries being performed, or the unrealistic expectations of patients.

BIOMAGICAL SCIENCE

Enhancement technologies such as cosmetic surgery alter the body for social reasons. "The work that goes into both identifying and amplifying certain characteristics as being amenable to change and constructing certain traits as desirable does more than essentialize them as preferred human traits. Rather, it forms a circuit of enterprise, biology, medicine, and culture in complex relations to each other. In this sense, the traits being enhanced are not inherently natural but cultural" (Hogle 2005, 702).

A complex set of influences has created the clean slit as the desirable vulva— a thoroughly cultural, aesthetic ideal (see chap. 1). Unlike other procedures and habits such as dieting, going to the gym, having one's hair cut and colored, applying creams to the face and body, and having fillers and botulinum injections to smooth out wrinkles, cosmetic surgery is understood as a quick fix to a particular area of the body—a more permanent transformation. Nothing but surgery will stop the labia minora from protruding past the labia majora. The "magic" of cosmetic surgery as a technology is its portrayal as "production minus the disadvantageous side-effects, such as struggle, effort, etc." (Gell 1988, 9), the everyday drudgery of most beauty practices. While many women with whom I spoke were constantly seeking self-improvement in other areas of their lives (and their bodies)—including through repetitive behavioral and beauty rituals—for them, cosmetic surgery held the promise of a more magical transformation. In this paradigm, the desire for enhancement is, for some, more an imperative than an aberrant disorder despite the fact that the long-term benefits of female genital cosmetic surgery have not yet been scientifically verified. If technology (including cosmetic surgery) makes life more satisfactory, then it is self-evident that people will use technology to enhance lived experience. Many previously described factors coalesce in neoliberal societies, in which the individual is expected to be "hyper-responsible" (Braun 2009a, 236) for her own maintenance. These influences persuade some women that their vulvas may benefit from enhancement.

More than thirty years ago, Alfred Gell drew attention to the symbiosis between the technical and the magical: "And if we no longer recognize magic explicitly, it is because technology and magic, for us, are one and the same" (Gell 1988, 9). Technology, according to Gell, is not just about the tool itself but also the ability to master the use of that tool, or technology, to certain ends. Gell identified three forms of technology: that of production, reproduction, and enchantment. Following Gell, doctors practice the technology of enchantment, one that "human beings employ in order to secure the acquiescence of other people in their intentions or projects" (7). Attracting other people, according to Gell, is the most sophisticated human technology. Physicians do this through the use of advertising and the promotion of female genital cosmetic surgery as a legitimate practice. Gell says that "technical innovations occur, not as the result of attempts to supply wants, but in the course of attempts to realize technical feats heretofore considered 'magical'" (8). As a technology, biomedicine has magical (and enchanting) properties, and developments in technology drive new desires.

In an environment in which enhancement or transformation of the body is valued, the biomagical is increasingly bringing the biomedical and beauty industries closer together through the medium of cosmetic surgery. Although, as Taussig (2012) suggests, cosmetic surgery can be critiqued as excessive consumption, the magic of cosmetic surgery works through both science and consumption, and nothing could be more conspicuous than the body as a vehicle for the biomagical. Alexander Edmonds (2009, 162) finds "the figure of the fetish" useful when attempting to understand how "the magic of the modern can work both in the dream worlds of consumption and medicine," thereby creating desire. The fetish suggests an emotional relationship with medicine that the biomagical articulates. Magic requires faith, hope, and desire—emotions that women invest in their surgeons and new medical technologies. Technology sustains magic—it is imaginatively compelling—and magic inspires novel technological innovations, such as female genital cosmetic surgery. Magic, along with ritual and sacrifice, has not disappeared; rather, it has been redirected to enchanting practices, such as advertising, social media, and intelligent technology. The biomagical (in which the imagination shapes the use of technology) and consumerism blend with "technologies of the self" (Foucault 1988), allowing new, "improved" ways of being. Women undergoing cosmetic surgery look to the magic of biomedicine to cure their perceived imperfections and often stress the permanency of surgery, something that is far from assured. In a world of imagined futures in which more-perfect selves can be envisioned, cosmetic surgery has a major role to play; it offers a supposed quick fix, a magical transformation that disguises the process—the labor—of risk and recovery inherent in all surgical procedures.

Conjoined neologisms such as *biomagical* are useful in conveying the disruption of modern conceptual dichotomies, such as rationality and magic, science and religion, and nature and culture. How could biomedicine be magical except though its promise of transformation and salvation? By juxtaposing the biological (the scientific) with the magical (the transformative), it can be shown that "what is at stake is *not* the complete disintegration or breakdown of categories, but rather the refiguring of boundaries and the visibility of new movements, mobilities or flows across them" (Roberts 2007, 198–9). Although cosmetic surgery involves risk, pain and recovery—decidedly unmagical qualities—it is both marketed and imagined (as are other rituals) as a magical solution to concerns with the flesh. Magic transforms, and the biomagical is full of promise. Cosmetic surgery then becomes what Taussig in *Beauty and the Beast* refers to as "cosmic surgery" because of its supernatural and transformative qualities. "The ancient arts of physiognomy (discerning insides from outsides, reading the soul in the face) may seem like hocus-pocus today, but when you stop to think about it, you realize it is imbedded in our everyday practice, such that you really have to wonder whether the fundamental reason for cosmic surgery is precisely to reverse this mechanism, to create a new inside by changing the outside. And once we have gotten a new inside, fate itself will change, making this cosmic tinkering akin to alchemy, and related magical practices. This is why cosmetic surgery is best considered cosmic surgery" (Taussig 2012, 44). Of course, the magic of cosmetic surgery is illusory, because there is no guarantee that one's fate will change with one's new exterior. However, in a culture in which appearance is paramount and still considered an indicator of personality and self-worth, the allure of such magic is often irresistible. Cosmetic surgery, in this paradigm, promises to change life itself, and although this is a spurious claim given life's unpredictability, enhancement can lead to happiness (at least temporarily) and the expectation of a better future, as demonstrated by the women's narratives shared in this book.

There has been much discussion, particularly in feminist literature, about women using cosmetic surgery to make themselves feel normal or to align how they feel inside with their outward appearance (Davis 1995; Davis 2003; Gimlin 2000; Heyes 2007a). Conversely, Taussig (2012, 44) suggests that the magic (or deceit) of cosmetic surgery lies in its supposed ability to "create a new inside by changing the outside." Perfectionists such as Kylie and Mia believe that their appearance, their outsides, reflect their personalities and that their perfect feminine bodies make them happy and therefore more socially engaging. These women have gained self-esteem and confidence through cosmetic surgery. Changing the outside has changed them inside, and they believe they are better able to contribute socially. Both Kylie and Mia are using their bodies to project a particular sort of feminine personality, one whose worth depends on care for appearance. In addition, a well-managed and overtly feminine body can accrue significant benefits, both in the workplace and socially: "Bodies have become increasingly commodified for the way they *look*," since bodily appearance "conveys status, authority, control, and success" (Holliday and Sanchez Taylor 2006, 191). For Kylie and Mia, a perfect body is a central component of their identity. Women who choose genital cosmetic surgery see surgery as productive in that it bolsters their social capital, making working on the self a worthwhile enterprise.

MAKEOVER CULTURE: "TECHNOLOGIES OF THE SELF"

Working on the self and aiming for improvement, even perfection, may not be a universal goal, but contemporary society rewards and values processes of self-regulation, what Michel Foucault (1988) terms "technologies of the self." These are ways in which people have come to express themselves individually within society, ways in which people are both enabled and constrained by contemporary discourse. Claire Tanner, JaneMaree Maher, and Suzanne Fraser (2013, 179) refer to technologies of the self as a form of "good vanity" in which "activities once considered vain—the pursuit of beauty, distinction and self-expression—are no longer seen as such." A certain amount of vanity is now "socially responsible self-care" (Tanner, Maher, and Fraser 2013, 179), demonstrating readiness for change, flexibility, and adaptability—valued attributes in the early twenty-first century.

We live in what Meredith Jones (2008) describes as a "makeover culture" in which we are expected to constantly improve ourselves, often through technological means. Makeover culture values and rewards the processes of working on the self. For Jones (2008, 120), "makeover culture is not about the creation of finished products—whether houses, psyches, bodies or gardens—rather it is about showing subjects, objects and environments being worked upon and improved. . . . Good citizens of makeover culture improve and transform themselves ceaselessly," which fits into the paradigm of what Taussig (2012, 9) refers to as "delirious consumption." Makeover culture consumes capital, time, and energy. Self-transformation involves a state where the process of transformation, or *becoming*, is more desirable than the end point. Becoming is fueled by desire (in Deleuzian terms) and involves not only policing in the Foucauldian sense, but also actively changing the body: "Bodies then can be thought not as *objects*, upon which culture writes meanings, but as *events* that are continually in the process of becoming—as multiplicities that are never just found but are made and remade. This is a fluid process of transformation" (Budgeon 2003, 50).

As Jones (2008, 1) suggests, "In makeover culture the process *of becoming something better* is more important than achieving a static point of completion. 'Good citizens' of makeover culture publicly enact urgent and never-ending renovations of themselves." This requires hard work, motivation, dedication, and willing partners, such as cosmetic surgeons who sit comfortably within, and benefit from, the self-improvement paradigm. Cosmetic surgery is "makeover culture's quintessential expression" (Jones 2008, 1).

The terms *self-enhancement* and *transformation* connote change for the better. The implication is that self-enhancement is both desirable and expected. The numerous terms describing the process of working on the self, what Foucault (1988) refers to as "care of the self" or "technologies of the self," include, but are not limited to, *self-improvement, self-discipline, self-regulation, self-policing, self-creation*, and *self-fashioning*. Whichever term is adopted, the notion involves movement and action within a limited framework of what is desirable. It also involves striving and discipline, traits that are admired within society and often materially rewarded through personal and professional relationships. Our bodies are particularly subject to self-improvement because our appearance is as important as what we say. In other words, our fleshy bodies speak volumes. Working on the self, aiming for improvement or some proximity to perfection, may not be a universal goal, but postmodern society rewards and values processes of self-regulation. These are the ways that people have come to express and police themselves individually within society, the ways in which they are both enabled and constrained by contemporary discourse. "'Technologies of the self' involve constant processes of self-monitoring and self-mastery, most of which operate on the mind and body through medical means. Biomedicine thus became the means by which the quality of collective and individual lives could be improved" (Hogle 2005, 701–2). Therefore, supposedly autonomous individuals have become the object of new forms of power that discipline them and result in "the individual pursuing aims of self-enhancement" (Crawford 1994, 1352).

Foucault (1988) explains four technologies, or "truth games," that people employ to develop knowledge about themselves. One such technology or technique is that of the self: "Technologies of the self permit individuals to effect by their own means or with the help of others a certain number of operations on their own bodies and souls, thoughts, conduct, and way of being, so as to transform themselves in order to attain a certain state of happiness, purity, wisdom, perfection, or immortality" (Foucault 1988, 18).

In late antiquity, Foucault argues, "to take care of yourself" was a central tenet of the art of life that has since been obscured by the Delphic principle of "knowing yourself" (Foucault 1988, 19). Morally, in Western society, it is considered inappropriate to care too much for yourself. Conversely, individuals are increasingly responsible for monitoring their own bodies from a medical perspective. Today, the central principle of taking care of the self has less to do with morality and the soul than with the body. Biomedicine has been harnessed in the care of the body because it involves the other three core meaning-making technologies of which Foucault (1988) speaks: production (the ability to transform things), power (of discourse to determine individual conduct), and signification (bodies are signs in themselves). Cosmetic surgery is implicated in identity formation, less the romantic notion of peeling away the layers to find the real or authentic self than care of the self through creative bodywork.

When care for the self meets the biomagical, it moves beyond necessity to enhancement. "Enhancement technologies aim to improve human characteristics, including appearance and mental or physical functioning, often beyond what is 'normal' or necessary for life and well-being" (Hogle 2005, 695). They are technologies of optimization (Rose 2007), and optimization implies being as perfect as possible, making the most of the available (biomedical) options to ensure we are "better than well" (Elliott 2003). Consequently, as Nikolas Rose (2007, 17) posits, medical technologies are no longer merely technologies of health; "they are technologies of life" and "the old lines between treatment, correction, and enhancement can no longer be sustained." As an enhancement technology, cosmetic surgery opens the human body to artifice and the biomagical because it does more than enhance—it changes what it is to be human. Enhancement technologies such as cosmetic surgery are concerned not with normalization but with what Adele Clarke et al. (2003, 181) refer to as "customization," whereby individuals decide for themselves which part of the body they wish to upgrade. "Previously expert medical interventions were utilized in order to cure pathologies, to rectify generally accepted deviations from desirable functioning or to promote biopolitical strategies through lifestyle modification. Now recipients of these interventions are consumers, making access choices on the basis of desires that can appear trivial, or narcissistic, or irrational, shaped not by medical necessity but by the market and consumer culture" (Rose 2007, 20).

Given the discourse (and activism) surrounding FGC, choosing female genital cosmetic surgery is frequently portrayed as narcissistic and irrational. Why would women choose a procedure that closely resembles one that the World Health Organization and the United Nations are endeavoring to eradicate? Despite this, the market and consumer culture appear to have worked their magic in creating a desire for female genital cosmetic surgery in women wanting to be perfect (or normal), and concerted efforts have been made to establish it as a legitimate medical intervention (see chap. 4).

Biomedicine is increasingly employed to optimize and enhance the self, leading to new ways of envisioning and achieving personhood (Rose 2007). Individuals are transformed through biomedicine at the level of personal identity—that is, who they conceive themselves to be. "We are increasingly coming to relate to ourselves as 'somatic' individuals, that is to say, as beings whose individuality is, in part at least, grounded within our fleshy, corporeal existence, and who experience, articulate, judge, and act upon ourselves in part in the language of biomedicine" (Rose 2007, 25–26). Through fitness regimens, body modifications, pharmaceuticals, and cosmetic surgery (along with many other biomedical interventions), "the corporeal existence and vitality of the self has become the privileged site of experiments with the self" (Rose 2007, 26). These experiments demonstrate that, as ontological security declines, individuals are increasingly reliant on the self (and the body) as a source of meaning and identity (Jones and Raisborough 2007).

Of course, working on the self, on the individual, is an entirely cultural and societal phenomenon, because we all act intersubjectively, despite protestations to the contrary by women claiming to be "doing it for themselves." In this context, cultural influences are so taken for granted, so subliminal, that they become thoroughly internalized. The biomagical melds biomedical technology with human life, resulting, as Rose (2007) argues, in more-biological bodies, not necessarily cyborgs in themselves but bodies touched by technological innovation. Edmonds (2007, 376) suggests that cosmetic surgery works "on the borders of proper medicine, it not only medicalizes the body but also in a sense 'de-medicalizes' itself." It becomes biomagical. In this paradigm, medicine has a new social purpose. When the salvational potential of medicine expands into "lifestyle treatments" that reconfigure the body and the mind for social reasons, new ways of imagining and experiencing selfhood are engendered (Petryna and Kleinman 2006, 3; Rose 2007).

BEFORE, AFTER, AND BECOMING

Working on the self has its roots not only in the before and after but also in becoming—the labor and process of self-enhancement. Cosmetic surgery has traditionally been represented not through process or becoming but through before and after photographs, which convey its biomagical and transformative properties. As confirmed in my interviews, these images, often found on the internet, lure prospective patients. Surgeons' websites depict vulvas before and after surgery with the before on the left and the after to the right, a kind of logical progression with the second image assumed to be unequivocally more aesthetically pleasing. The images in the left-hand column show vulvas of diverse shape, size, and color, whereas in the right-hand column they are uniform clean slits. Such representations give the impression of a magical transformation or, more correctly, transmogrification (Jones 2008.) The process of surgery—the pain, risk, labor, and recovery involved—are absent, making potentially harmful practices appear "trouble-free and inviting, on a par with putting on lipstick" (Jones 2008, 17). These images portray the transmogrification of cosmetic surgery as problem-free—a promise far removed from reality, as Kylie's story has demonstrated.

Although surgeons' websites predominantly display before and after images only, a number of television programs have aired over the past decade depicting graphic scenes of operations and recovery times—the actual transformative process. However, these depictions have served to normalize cosmetic surgery rather than deter prospective patients (Heyes 2007a; Heyes 2007b; Jones 2008). Along with television programs such as *Extreme Make-over*, *The Swan*, and *Doctor 90210*—which, although no longer produced, are still available for viewing—more-realistic documentary-style programs that offer medical advice also naturalize cosmetic surgery. Programs that purport to reduce the embarrassment that surrounds certain illnesses and conditions, such as the British Channel 4 program *Embarrassing Bodies*, frequently feature cosmetic surgery procedures (and labiaplasty), thereby normalizing aesthetic intervention. In *Extreme Makeover*, subjects are transformed through multiple surgical and nonsurgical interventions, which are portrayed as facilitating a new and better life. However, could the biomagical be deceptive? As Heyes (2007a, 105) comments in relation to *Extreme Makeover*, "The perfectability [*sic*] of subjects the show hopes for—this process of surgically facilitating becoming in which we all eventually manifest our essential goodness and live happily ever after—is ethically empty." The program is gripping because of its fairytale promise of a perfect body engendering a perfect life, something spurious but also compelling. However, the lure of changing the outside in order to become something new (happier, better) remains, and this promise is exploited by surgeons who stand to gain financially by promoting the transformative properties of cosmetic surgery. We live in a television-driven makeover culture, which extends to many aspects of life—our gardens and houses, our overweight bodies, our wardrobes and fashion, our relationships and cooking abilities—all of which promise contestants (and by association, viewers) happiness and personal success through "efficient" short-term projects of self-improvement.

"Makeover culture," argues Jones (2008, 55), "opens up the space between before and after and situates 'running' inside that space as the most productive and worthy activity for its citizens." Jones argues that this valorizes the process of what she calls "becoming," which is central to makeover culture: "Transformation becomes a temporal and spatial mode of being rather than a static end result. I use the word 'becoming' rather than 'transformation' because they are subtly different: transformation brings to mind a quick change, a definitive before and after, whereas becoming connotes growth and slower change. Becoming can be explained as a mode of living whereas transformation implies rupture and a stop-start action foreign to daily life. The cosmetic surgery recipient is not simply transformed: rather, she displays herself as a person manufacturing her own becoming" (Jones 2008, 55–56).

However, the difference between transformation (the biomagical) and becoming (labor) is more nuanced—there always exists the imagined end result, the "after" photograph, the perfect vulva, which makes the labor not only possible but also worthwhile. Both Kylie and Mia are continually becoming as they search for bodily perfection through logics of self-improvement. Lives then become liminal (Squier 2004), punctuated by a series of transformative events that the biomagical facilitates. Both Kylie and Mia downplayed the amount of labor expended on their body projects. Mia, particularly, recounted her experience lightheartedly, and even Kylie glossed over the pain and uncertainty of her recovery period despite enduring three consecutive operations. Instead, they focused on the end result, the transformation, the biomagical, because they have obtained their desired outcome. This is the *magic* of cosmetic surgery, its ability to persuade its subjects to take the risk and undertake the labor in order to achieve "more than I ever dreamed of" (Kylie). The "after" of cosmetic surgery, the result, appears as if by magic, and the perseverance, discomfort, cost, and labor are deemed worthwhile. As Kylie's comments about her final (perfect) result reveal, her expectations were surpassed through a blend of work and magic: "I think if it had never stuffed up in the first place, I would never have it as perfect as it is now, and I would never have expected it to be as perfect as it is now. I swear to God, now it is the best vagina I have ever seen." Mia described her labiaplasty as a quick and permanent fix, despite referring to her recovery as "full on" and expecting complete recovery to take a year. Jones argues that the difference between transformation and makeover lies in transformation's omission of the process of becoming, of working on the self, on which a makeover culture insists. With transformation, the labor, the brutality of surgery, is hidden. The magic of transformation is not lost, however, with the outing of process. Indeed, "the articulated makeover does not replace magical transformative discourse but works cleverly in conjunction with it: together, makeover and magic create a powerful set of rhetorics" (Jones 2008, 56–57) to which the perfectionist is beholden.

EXCESS

Michael Taussig (2012) views cosmetic surgery as excess, as consumption without production—in Georges Bataille's (1985, 117) terms, "nonproductive expenditure." Perhaps, then, cosmetic surgery involves extreme excess: excess vanity, excess bodily intervention, excess bodily anxiety, excess time, excess expenditure, even excess good fortune (which enables people to focus on vanity projects rather than survival) and, when it comes to female genitalia, excess skin. The notion of excess is parodied in *White Girl Problems*, where Babe is portrayed as emblematic of excess; her behavior is reprehensible, and her choice to have labiaplasty is as ridiculous as her excessive spending spree at Barneys, which results in her admission to a rehabilitation facility. However, to judge cosmetic surgery simply as excess fails to reconcile reality with opportunity—the hope for social inclusion and happiness that cosmetic surgery may offer. Although striving for bodily perfection can be seen as disciplining the body in the Foucauldian sense because women seek to conform to a narrow interpretation of beauty, Taussig suggests that cosmetic surgery is the ultimate expression of eroticized excess and therefore transgressive: "A boom in fashion and beautification not only absorbs male as well as female energies and fantasy but speaks more generally to the body as emblem and vehicle for a way of being that has displaced work and discipline in favor of style, transgression, and eroticized excess" (Taussig 2012, x).

Cosmetic surgery, particularly female genital cosmetic surgery, and fashion are closely linked. Vulvas need to look a certain way—hairless and nonprotruding. One plastic surgeon told me, "A few years ago a lot of boys were coming in wanting moles removed from their faces, and now they have stopped, and girls are coming. Cosmetic surgery is a trend, a fashion. It is the same with all body parts, boobs, waists, lip fullness, and fannies." Fashion drives consumer culture because it demands regular change to which women in particular are beholden, and cosmetic surgery has become its handmaiden. "The revealed—and—concealed female body," Taussig (2012, 152) explains, is "the center of desire around which consumerism revolves."

Cosmetic surgery lies somewhere between transgression and conformity. In the moral sense, it is a step too far because it crosses the boundary of the acceptable use of biomedicine. However, in the Foucauldian sense, cosmetic surgery facilitates an adherence to norms and care for the self. The controversial, intimate, and invisible nature of genital cosmetic surgery brings this tension into sharp relief. To set up an opposition between work and discipline on the one hand and style, transgression, and eroticized excess on the other is to overlook the fusion of eroticized excess with work and discipline encapsulated by the women's narratives presented in this chapter. Discipline is mediated through (excess) consumption, but it is also productive for the individual who imagines a better future. *White Girl Problems* and *Plastic Wives* portray cosmetic surgery as excessive consumption and vanity, yet perfectionists such as Mia and Kylie marry consumption with the biomagical in their quest for self-transformation. Technologies of the self have taken on new meaning as religious morality has waned; knowing oneself has been sublimated to taking care of oneself. Rather than revealing the inner self, the self can be created through cosmetic surgery. To not know oneself is to be inauthentic, but to take care of oneself allows for the biomagical. The question then becomes, can cosmetic surgery be taking care of oneself, or is it emblematic of excess? If the latter, where does the excess lie: with the women choosing these procedures or with the surgeons promoting them? Whether women are aiming for perfection or merely having genital cosmetic surgery to be normal seems immaterial. Fashion (and cosmetic surgery) may be frivolous, but it is part of the fabric of life, not always excessive but creative, and its magic can be difficult to resist.

THE INVISIBLE INTIMATE

Much that is to do with sexuality has been considered taboo and therefore invested with power and the possibility of transgression. Viewing or indeed talking about genitalia, except in intimate or medical situations, has generally been considered out of bounds. However, with the mainstreaming of pornography and the sexualization of society, this is no longer the case. As Dr. Marcos explained to me, "Female genital surgery is part of the culture of sexting and blowjob expertise. Girls just spread their legs and display their perfect fannies.[3]

The essence of female sexuality is just melting away, and women have lost the art of manipulation. It is all on the plate at a very young age. Women are less embarrassed to discuss their fannies these days. The fashion is dictating how women behave sexually and what they do with their fannies."

Dr. Marcos highlighted something of a paradox. According to her, the more explicit that sexuality becomes, the more it is overtly displayed and critiqued, the more the "essence of female sexuality is just melting away." Surely, however, when the biomagical is employed to fashion femininity, it is heavily implicated in this process of redefining femininity. Sexuality is now an exploitable commodity, and practitioners of female genital cosmetic surgery are as entangled in this process as are producers of pornography, manufacturers of sex toys, and fashion gurus. With multiple sexual partners over the course of one's lifetime becoming the acceptable norm (most women with whom I spoke had had several sexual partners), the popularity of Brazilian waxing, and the increased prevalence of participation in, or open discussion of, oral sex, unclad vulvas are seen by more people today (though perhaps not to the extent implied in Dr. Marcos's assessment). However, vulvas do retain an aura of mystery, and some boundaries cannot be crossed. The details of a woman's genitalia remain invisible to most. Despite this, a specific vulval ideal has emerged. "Could it be that as more attention is paid to the appearance of the body, to its aura and sex appeal, paradoxically the body becomes more of an object, a work of art, to be evaluated and discussed by everyone, acting like art critics or people discussing a soccer match, such that the older, sacred, tabooed qualities of the human body diminish or even disappear?" (Taussig 2012, 49). Aspects of the female body are visible, clothed or not—the female body is a public body in a manner that the male body is not (Braun and Kitzinger 2001a), and this is fueled by the fashion industry, the media, and pornography.

Body parts not on public display—for women, genitalia and nipples—constitute the invisible intimate. Their public exposure remains taboo; therefore, increased importance is placed on them. Taussig (2012, 143) speaks of the "tabooed cleft" (the crack exposed by low-slung jeans in certain positions) as something that is as much unseen as seen, the invisible intimate that is eroticized and, in our society, hints at transgression. "The beauty and the beastliness of beauty," its ability to create desire, "lies in its whiplash effect, which parallels the logic of taboo and transgression made manifest by the visible invisibility of the tabooed cleft" (Taussig 2012, 145). In this sense, the vulva is akin to the tabooed cleft or to a woman's cleavage. The invisible, intimate nature of the vulva invites transgression. As Taussig (2012, 144) asks, "How might one even begin to 'explain' this scotomic vision, this seeing and not seeing at the same time?" Given that a boundary is in place prohibiting the public display of vulvas, they enter the imagination, and their aesthetics become important as men and women internalize the images of perfect vulvas displayed in pornography and women's magazines. Thus, "'the taboo structure' no longer operates as it is meant to. . . . There is an extraordinarily interesting tension in this state of suspension of the norm. For it can unleash the creation of new desires, new fashions, and new ways of being human" (Taussig 2012, 146). There exists a certain fascination with what we cannot see (a blind spot), a cleavage, a cleft, a vulva—it is alluring, desirable, out of bounds (and now malleable).

Concern about appearance, generally considered by theorists to be a hallmark of the public realm, has emerged in the most private or intimate realm. Making the invisible and intimate public suggests an intrusion of stricter standards of bodily self-policing today, in the same way that genital policing has been considered normal in societies practicing circumcision. In such societies, the intimate has always been a matter of public concern for both social and aesthetic reasons. In the West, the public standard is an aesthetic one, but it is also one with moral implications, because only a certain aesthetic standard is allowed in the media. This standard is taken up by women who have internalized the public ideal of the perfect vulva. Vulvas are expected to look a certain (minimalist) way, and women who undergo genital cosmetic surgery are convinced they are doing it for themselves because of the very intimate nature of their genitalia. If circumcision for women and men is a marker of identity and belonging, so too are Western women's genitalia markers of their identity as women who strive for bodily perfection, who take care of themselves through self-enhancement, thereby reflecting desirable femininity.

As Suzanne Kessler explains in her work on intersexuality, "the fact that appearance is so important for a body part that is almost always hidden . . . is further evidence that more is at stake here than the body part itself" (Kessler 1998, 126). A great deal of symbolic power is invested in altering genitalia in any given context, whether to define femininity and masculinity as binary opposites or to produce a more perfect vulva. Since our genitalia are (sometimes problematically) assumed to define our sexuality, even clothed genitalia have symbolic significance, and "indeed an act of substitution is at play: the blank left by hidden genitals is typically supplied with mental images freighted with gender ideology" (Wall 2010, 81). When what constitutes normal or desirable female genitalia is defined in the media and endorsed by biomedicine, stricter codes of femininity are applied.

THE PURSUIT OF PERFECTION

Harnessing biomedicine, or the biomagical, to bring bodies and minds to perfection rather than to treat disease has drawn criticism from some quarters. Life is unpredictable and our bodies inherently vulnerable, making the possibility of bodily perfection an illusion. The pursuit of perfection is less about perfection than about the desire to improve or enhance a particular behavior, trait, or body part through the application of emerging medical knowledge or the use of existing technologies for new purposes. Detractors of enhancement technologies argue that the pursuit of perfection is frivolous and vain; not available to all, resulting in an uneven playing field; it goes against nature and could lead to sameness and conformity; driven by large corporate interests, particularly those of pharmaceutical companies; a sign of rampant consumerism in which individual shortcomings and inadequacies can be exploited for commercial profit; and accompanied by risks, which are frequently downplayed (Caplan and Elliott 2004; Elliott 2003; Taussig 2012). However, as Rose (2007) points out, we are already biological and technological creatures; as such, using biomedicine to enhance certain qualities seems inevitable. Science exerts a powerful hold on its practitioners and on the public (Rothman and Rothman 2003), and without medical innovation, improved and new cures for diseases and conditions would not be found. Neoliberal principles dictate that individuals have the right to do with their bodies whatever they choose. However, with enhancement technologies, argues Elliott (2003, xix), this could produce a more "homogenous cultural landscape, stripped of character and diversity, where everyone dreams and aspires to identical futures." Detractors of female genital cosmetic surgery contend that diversity is being replaced with conformity and that, regarding vulvas, a "cookie cutter" aesthetic has emerged—they all look the same (Braun 2005, 413). Malleable plastic bodies are akin to fashion in that a tension exists between fitting in and standing out as exceptional, between being different and not too different.

The philosopher Michael Sandel argues that advances in genetic engineering offer something of a conundrum; such breakthroughs offer the possibility of treating or preventing debilitating diseases, but this "newfound genetic knowledge may also enable us to manipulate our own nature—to enhance our muscles, memories, and moods . . . to make ourselves 'better than well'" (Sandel 2004, 1). As with cosmetic surgery, genetic enhancement "employs medical means for nonmedical ends" (2). Sandel considers genetic enhancement more problematic than surgical enhancement because it is more than skin-deep. However, the parallels are useful. He argues that excellence or giftedness (beauty, in cosmetic terms) is something to behold and admire and that these qualities should be appreciated over constantly striving for enhancement. For him, the moral significance of striving is inflated: "The deepest moral objection to enhancement lies less in the perfection it seeks than in the human disposition it expresses and promotes" (6)—that of individual willfulness, a trait Sandel finds distasteful. He argues that current enhancement technologies are "a way of answering a competitive society's demand to improve our performance and perfect our nature. This demand for performance and perfection animates the impulse to rail against the given. It is the deepest source of the moral trouble with enhancement" (8).

However, in makeover culture, striving *does* have a moral quality; it is both expected and rewarded. More pragmatically, Rose (2007, 104–5) predicts: "Freed from the portentous bioethical discourse that surrounds it, the distinction between normalization and enhancement will come to seem spurious, replaced by the more modest and pragmatic questions of what interventions are available to whom, at what cost, with what efficacy, and with what safeguards." Debates about female genital cosmetic surgery illustrate these pragmatic concerns. Issues of ethics revolve around unequal access. For instance, for women who come from circumcising societies, genital surgery would be considered illegal in Australia, and each Australian state has its own anti-FGM (female genital mutilation) legislation. In addition, the provision of female genital cosmetic surgery in public health-care systems and for adolescents is currently under debate in both Australia and Britain. Detractors cite a lack of medical evidence of safety and long-term outcomes and question whether surgeons have adequate medical training. Our enthusiasm for cosmetic surgery and other enhancement technologies exposes the fragility of the dividing line between consumer-driven (perhaps frivolous aesthetic procedures) and other medical interventions considered necessary for health and well-being. Rather than a dividing line separating enhancement and regular medicine, these interventions lie on a continuum, making it difficult to judge where treatment ends and enhancement begins.

The biomagical does not reside only in cosmetic surgery. Outside subsidized health care, it is generally agreed that individuals should be free to make an informed decision about how they spend their money, and enhancement technologies are just another consumer choice. However, the individual traits chosen for enhancement are particular to a certain culture. In Australia, as in much of the West, large breasts and minimal vulvas fit the Barbie-doll feminine ideal. Biomedicine, whether employed for cosmetic or therapeutic purposes, constantly sets its own agenda in ways that do not adhere to the supposedly strict scientific principles of the proven and the rational. As the boundaries of what biomedicine can fashion continually recede, its biomagical attributes flourish.

If cosmetic surgery becomes ubiquitous, women might feel they have to conform to narrower standards of beauty and femininity. Both Kylie's and Mia's pursuit of perfection is individual and culturally mediated. Rather than buying individual well-being at the expense of some larger social good, however, Kylie and Mia believe that cosmetic surgery has made them more-engaged members of society. Few women today do not enhance their bodies to some extent in order to conform to beauty standards. As Hogle (2005, 699) suggests, "Judgments about natural characteristics, particularly as they relate to merit, may also shift, providing an opportunity for enhancements to be seen as maintenance or needed self-improvements, rather than a luxury or a fantasy of perfection." Biomedicine and bodies are so firmly intertwined that the natural no longer exists, and some women increasingly envisage fantasies of perfection as necessary acts of self-improvement.

—m—

In contemporary Australian society, the pursuit of physical perfection has been normalized such that cosmetic surgery is marketed as a quick and permanent solution to fleshy failings. The actual process of surgery, its risks and brutality, is glossed over, both through before and after images on the internet and in patients' narratives, making the transformation appear magical. To be perfect is to optimize, to improve one's chances of happiness and success, and the invisible, intimate vulva has been co-opted into the self-enhancement paradigm. A perfect body is also an eroticized body. Cosmetic surgery uses the biomagical power of biomedicine to transform bodies (and, by association, minds) in a society that values technology itself (its salvational and magical properties) and technologies of the self—attributes that, in a makeover culture, are central tenets to living. Our bodies, even our vulvas, tell a story of who we are.

Through their narrative identity work, Mia and Kylie show that "their new appearance is both deserved and a better indicator of the self than the old appearance" (Gimlin 2000, 81). These two women use their narratives to explain their reasons for choosing genital cosmetic surgery as they simultaneously define their sense of self, their identity in relation to cosmetic surgery, and their wider transformative projects. Their perfect vulvas reflect their willingness to take care of themselves. In this sense, care, although corporeal, has a moral quality. In makeover culture, taking care of oneself is an individual's responsibility, and a certain amount of perfectionism is expected, even lauded. Too much perfectionism is, however, a psychological condition, and those showing traits of BDD are (theoretically) not suitable candidates for cosmetic surgery. Paradoxically, medicine defines excessive perfectionism as a disorder, while promoting a more perfect body through the medium of cosmetic surgery.

Makeover culture valorizes the process of becoming, of continually striving for self-improvement, which notions of perfection sustain. Cosmetic surgery may be excess, as Taussig posits (and *White Girl Problems* parodies)— that is, excess consumption—but it is also a disciplinary technology in the Foucauldian sense. A tension exists between excess and caring for the self, and this is mediated through consumption. The biomagical promise of cosmetic surgery is difficult to resist in a milieu in which working on the self is expected and enhancement technologies are available. To posit cosmetic surgery as excess is to suggest that a breach of the boundary of the acceptable use of biomedicine is immoral; however, Kylie and Mia situate their use of cosmetic surgery within a moral framework of self-improvement—a form of good vanity. This dynamic between discipline and excess is productive for the individual who imagines herself as a better person. The possibility of cosmetic surgery being conceived as morally defensible by its subjects is the *cunning* of cosmetic surgery, because it hides the fact that it is the medical professionals themselves who, through before and after images and promises of transformation, fuel the notion of surgery as magical—it is they who court excess. The magic of surgery for women is in the thrill of perfection, and both Kylie and Mia are grateful to their surgeons, who act as mediums for the biomagical. No longer do our imperfections make us fully human, as suggested in the past; instead, they must be erased as "we distance ourselves further and further from the flesh we inhabit" (Adams 2003, 1). The neologism *biomagical*, therefore, highlights how biomedicine has taken on new meaning with the rise of enhancement technologies, one that promises magical transformation to a better, more biological form of life. The boundaries between biomedicine and an imagined magical transformation, or transmogrification, are no longer as distinct.

NOTES

1. A hyaluronic-acid dermal filler.
2. A colloquial expression meaning to accept the facts of a situation.
3. A colloquial term used in Australia for female genitalia.

FOUR

—᠊ᚭᚭ᠊—

VULVA LAS VEGAS: SCIENCE, MAGIC (A GAMBLE), OR MORE OF THE SAME?

MY COLLEAGUE FRANCES D'ARCY-TEHAN AND I touched down in Las Vegas in late September 2011. We were to attend the World Congress on Female and Male Cosmetic Genital Surgery at the Venetian Hotel. The International Society of Cosmetogynecology (ISCG) organized the event, which they proudly announced as the first of its kind. The ISCG had held other congresses concentrating on female genital cosmetic surgery, but this was the first to include male genital cosmetic procedures. As the congress brochure stated, "The demand for cosmetic genital surgery in women and men is soaring. The Society has assembled the world leaders in aesthetic vaginal surgery, phalloplasty, and male/female, female/male transgender surgery to share their expertise and interact with the attendees. The Congress sets the standard for the new subspecialty and provides a complete overview of the field to gynecologists, urologists, uro-gynecologists, and cosmetic and plastic surgeons. The Congress will critically examine nomenclature, safety, effectiveness, complications, controversies, challenges, and innovations in this exciting new field." Despite the ISCG's intention to include male and transgender cosmetic procedures, only one session of the three-day congress was dedicated to this, and it was poorly attended. The focus was firmly on malleable, upgradable female genitalia and the controversies surrounding them.

Frances D'Arcy-Tehan, a psychologist researching female genital cosmetic surgery, was presenting a paper titled "Genital Image Perceptions amongst Australian Women and Attitudes towards FGCS [Female Genital Cosmetic Surgery]" at the congress, one of only three women to present (D'Arcy-Tehan 2011). She had been more excited than I about our impending trip to Las

Vegas. Despite the excellent research opportunities offered at the congress, I approached it with trepidation. I had spoken with many surgeons in Australia and had found them, with the odd exception, pleasant, reasonable, and even empathetic. However, the thought of suddenly being in a room full of surgeons promoting female genital cosmetic surgery as a new subspecialty made me feel vulnerable. As a woman, I felt uneasy that women's healthy genitalia were under the scrutiny of (mostly male) others who considered themselves experts in female genital form and function. Many of the presenters were undeniably leaders in the field of female cosmetic genital surgery. I had watched YouTube video clips of them performing surgery. I had read their articles, pored over their websites, and discussed their influence with surgeons in Australia.

The hotels in Las Vegas play host to masses of congresses and conferences. The complex where we initially stayed was enormous. Many of the people chatting in the elevators were attending a packaging conference, and they appeared animated by the whole experience. One eager young attendee said, "It's great, I'm talking to the bosses and I hope to make lots of money." I assumed he meant by furthering his contacts within the packaging company and by having success in the casino. There was an aura of excitement. Everyone was busy, focused on their specialties and hoping to further their various interests. Lady Gaga was coming to play that night.

Before the congress began, Frances and I attended the Crazy Horse Cabaret, a Parisienne burlesque show with a focus on breasts, perfectly rounded bottoms, and flat little vulvas hidden by black fabric triangles (which looked oddly like Charlie Chaplin mustaches). I was keen to discover whether this lack, this disappearance or blacking out, was the vulval ideal. We shared a table with an American couple during the performance, and they asked us what had brought us to Las Vegas. As we told them, I wondered whether they would be shocked or perhaps find nothing unusual or sinister about doctors congregating to teach others how they can help women rearrange their genitalia. "I love my vagina," the man said with a satisfied smile at his partner, affirming the oft-repeated rhetoric that men are "just happy to be there" when it comes to vulval aesthetics, yet perhaps they also feel some sort of ownership of this intimate part of their partner's body.

The next day was hot, sunny, and dry. The beautiful vermillion desert that I love so much can rarely be glimpsed from the Strip. Most activity takes place in an overly air-conditioned fantasy world of false skies and waterways and the often opulent and consumer-focused confines of the hotels where the pursuit of pleasure is paramount. The complex is filled with shops, bars, and restaurants; venturing outside is barely a consideration. In the Venetian complex

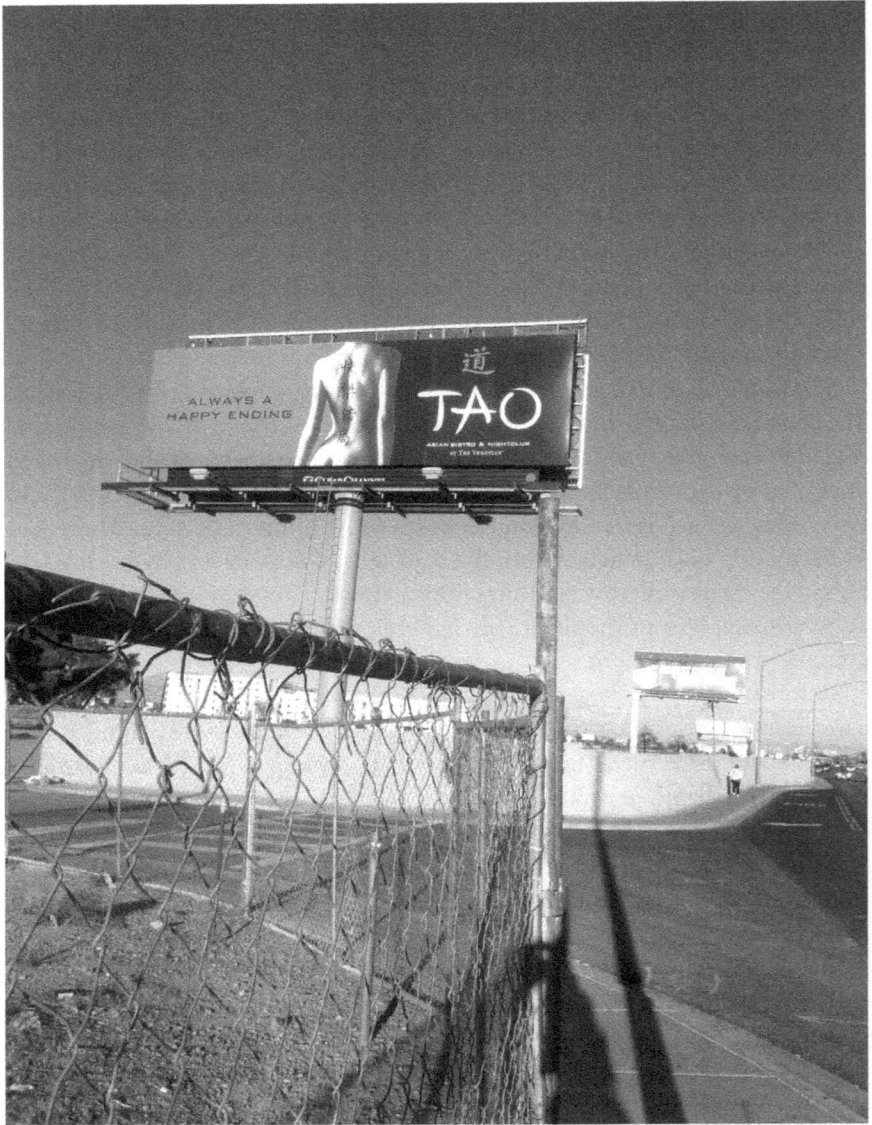

Figure 4.1. Tao nightclub billboard in Las Vegas, 2011. Photograph by author.

was the nightclub Tao, its aim and focus on female sexuality made explicit on its billboard outside, which shows the back of a naked woman with the words "Always a happy ending" emblazoned next to her (see fig. 4.1). The lines to enter the nightclub snaked through the complex as the sun dropped beneath the horizon. What better place to promote a nascent moneymaking scheme—cosmetogynecology! Feeling cold in the air-conditioning, I went out to buy a sweater and some long trousers.

As we walked up the stairs to the congress rooms in the morning, we passed a Victoria's Secret convention on the lower floor, promoting glamorous women's lingerie. The atmosphere was animated, colorful, and steeped in crimson, the enormous room populated by the young, beautiful, and enticingly clad. A cacophony of chattering and excitement emanated from the space. In comparison, the atmosphere of the rather plain rooms we entered upstairs was somber. The primarily middle-aged male attendees, dressed conservatively in dull suits, stood in small groups as they endeavored to eat their handheld breakfasts. For an outsider, it was difficult to break into these tight-knit clusters, and it was particularly challenging for a nonpractitioner like me. The room was adorned with cold, hard medical instruments, sophisticated machines for slicing flesh, pamphlets on G-spot amplification and courses in laser vaginal rejuvenation, and the odd medical journal: the face of science. Downstairs, female sexuality was being embellished with glamorous undergarments adorning breasts and genitalia. Here, however, the embellishment under discussion was not one of adornment but of subtraction: the removal of hair, the bleaching of external genitalia, the tightening of vaginas, and the paring away of unsightly, protruding labia—perhaps all the better to fit into the very items on display downstairs.

Female genital cosmetic surgery, at least in the United States, is increasingly being taught at profitable workshops and congresses such as the one I describe here. A similar congress was held just six weeks later in Tucson, Arizona—the Congress on Aesthetic Vaginal Surgery. The term *cosmetogynecology* has not been universally adopted to describe cosmetic genital surgeries, either within the United States or globally. According to its website, the ISCG was founded in 2004 by Dr. Marco Pelosi II and his son, Dr. Marco Pelosi III. The organization purports to have over one thousand members in more than thirty countries. Its stated aim is the advancement of surgical knowledge, skill, and excellence.

The Society was founded to fill an academic void in the field of women's healthcare in a milieu of changing societal opinions toward cosmetic surgery and medicine and a nontraditional shift in the practice patterns of many gynecologists. The founders experienced and observed that the traditional knowledge base and skill set of the practicing gynecologist formed an excellent foundation for the addition of new cosmetic surgical knowledge and skills. They also saw that the learning curve for most procedures was relatively short because of the broad transportability of pelvic surgical skills and experience to procedures outside this area. Furthermore, they understood that the gynecologist has a unique relationship with the female patient yielding the potential for more complete aesthetic management beyond the scalpel. (ISCG 2008)

Women's health care has primarily focused on reproductive health, along with mental health and domestic violence. Matters of aesthetics have traditionally not been considered essential to good health nor the province of the medical profession (except in the case of reconstructive plastic surgery). However, this has changed. Now, not only are body surfaces expected to conform to culturally defined beauty standards but the body must also function in prescribed ways. Medicine can now be harnessed in this endeavor. Women consult their gynecologists about intimate matters closely aligned to their sexuality, "yielding the potential for more complete aesthetic management beyond the scalpel" (ISCG 2008). The unique relationship women have with their gynecologists may give this group a competitive market advantage in the provision of genital (or other) cosmetic services. For instance, many obstetrics-gynecology clinics in the United States have expanded to offer liposuction, abdominoplasty, breast augmentation, and body contouring.

The specialist plastic surgeons with whom I spoke do not agree that the skills necessary for safe and successful cosmetic surgery are easily learned. Although women may visit their gynecologist more regularly than they do a plastic or cosmetic surgeon, they traditionally do so to seek reproductive and sexual health care rather than a judgmental aesthetic gaze that may find them wanting. While medical praxis is becoming increasingly specialized, when it comes to cosmetic procedures, doctors are expanding their area of expertise. Ear, nose, and throat surgeons; dermatologists; general surgeons; gynecologists; and general practitioners are increasingly providing cosmesis. Unlike in Australia, where female genital cosmetic surgery is primarily promoted by cosmetic and plastic surgeons (although it is also performed by gynecologists), in the United States, obstetrics-gynecology specialists are driving current practice. As was made explicit at the congress, this is because cosmetic procedures can add financial value to private practices. As one prominent doctor in the field, Dr. Michael Goodman, said, "Most of you are in independent practice, and these procedures provide a value-added service. It is tough. You receive no regular salary in an increasingly difficult market. We need something else if we are no longer practicing obstetrics, and it is the same for the plastic surgeons. This used to be the domain of plastic surgeons. Now it is becoming the domain of ob/gyn as well, so it is incumbent upon ourselves to be well trained and to know the pitfalls."[1]

To provide training so that pitfalls are avoided (and to make money), the ISCG runs frequent training sessions at the Pelosi Medical Center in Bayonne, New Jersey. This is consistent with the practice of other leaders in the field of female genital cosmetic surgery in their various locations. By appropriating the medical model of knowledge dissemination through scientific meetings and fellowships, ISCG members hope to deflect criticism that, to date, no medical board certifies their subspecialty. According to one journalist (Bates 2010), training courses are expensive, often in the tens of thousands of dollars (over US$50,000, according to some reports), but those who consider themselves experts in genital cosmetic surgery believe they should be compensated for sharing their specialized knowledge with surgeons who stand to profit from including these new cosmetic procedures in their practice armory.

From my research in Australia, it appears that surgeons' attitudes toward knowledge sharing vary. Most board-certified plastic surgeons learn to do la-biaplasties (to a limited extent) as part of their surgical training, so competition between plastic surgeons is not intense. Cosmetic surgeons, on the other hand, are not board certified and have no specific surgical training, and because they are self-taught, some are reluctant to share the techniques they have learned or developed. One female cosmetic surgeon with a busy labiaplasty practice told me she was planning to publish her technique in the Australasian College of Cosmetic Surgery (ACCS) journal.[2]

> Dr. Silver: I am about to publish it [my technique] so, once it is published, I'll talk all over the world at conferences, yeah. I plan to train a surgeon from Sydney and one from Melbourne.
> Lindy: Do you charge for training?
> Dr. Silver: I don't. I think that is unethical, but would I share it with the plastic surgeon around the corner? No. He'll have to read my journal article, and he'll have to—if he feels uncomfortable doing it just from my text—then, um, I might ... [laughs softly, and pulls a face].
> Lindy: Is that because of competition?
> Dr. Silver: I would think so.

According to the ACCS, "Cosmetic surgery and medicine has emerged as a new specialty and thus has not been a significant part of the training of any of the established colleges. Indeed, any doctor wishing to specialise in this field had no option but to acquire privately organized training on an apprentice-ship basis. This training was not subject to any quality controls and varied greatly in its quality. Some doctors obtained adequate and appropriate training and others did not. To fill this vacuum, the Australasian College of Cosmetic Surgery was established in 1999 as a multidisciplinary body for those already practicing cosmetic surgery" (Australasian College of Cosmetic Surgery 2012). Although the ACCS was established to ensure that cosmetic surgery performed by those other than trained plastic surgeons is more regulated, scrutinized, and therefore legitimate, as with the ISCG, any qualifications gained through the college are not board certified.[3] However, this does not deter ACCS members from disseminating their so-called expertise.

The distinction between plastic and cosmetic surgeons (and the paucity of the latter's training) is often referred to on plastic surgeons' websites, and plastic surgeons were keen to highlight this disparity during interviews. As one plastic surgeon, Dr. Luke Stradwick, states on his website:

> Becoming a surgeon in Australia requires years of additional training and examinations—no shortcuts. The only way you can be sure your surgeon has completed this rigorous process is by looking for the letters FRACS. This denotes fellowship of the Royal Australasian College of Surgeons—the only recognised body for training surgeons. Not everyone can be accepted into surgical training and not everyone makes it through....
>
> Unfortunately, some doctors need a shortcut. They may have not met the entry criteria to gain a place on an Australian surgical training program. Maybe they couldn't make it through. Instead, they seek training outside the accepted pathways. Some spend time "observing" overseas. Maybe they watch a few DVDs when they get back. (Stradwick 2009)

Dr. Stradwick is based in Queensland, the only state in Australia where it is prohibited for cosmetic practitioners to call themselves surgeons unless they are board certified. He points out that membership to a college such as the ACCS does not guarantee a level of surgical training above a basic medical degree. Although intense competition exists between plastic and cosmetic surgeons in Australia because of the commercial nature of cosmetic surgery, women are often unclear about the distinction between the two categories. Some of the women I spoke with who had undergone labiaplasty specifically chose a cosmetic sur-geon believing they would have more experience with cosmesis, and cosmetic surgeons themselves deem that because they specialize in cosmetic procedures, they have a better understanding of aesthetics than do plastic surgeons.

CONGRESS PROCEEDINGS

The first day of the Las Vegas congress was a postgraduate training day with an emphasis on the treatment of pelvic floor defects, pelvic anatomy, and other vaginal and vulval repairs requiring surgical correction. According to the gynecologists present, such training is necessary because often, patients presenting for cosmetic procedures also have underlying functional problems, such as uterine prolapse and stress urinary incontinence.

Dr. Pelosi III, who along with his father was the prime organizer of the congress, greeted the seated group of about sixty attendees, who were predominantly but not exclusively male. The following day, for the congress proper, participant numbers increased to more than one hundred. On registration, name tags were distributed, as is usual at such an event. However, many of the speakers sported more substantial badges festooned with ribbons identifying them as faculty, fellowship, attendee, and more. In an article describing another congress in Tucson, Arizona, one journalist compared the participants to "generals returning from battle with a chest full of medals" (Lee 2011, 2). Some presenters were identified as recipients of awards for teaching excellence, conferred by the ISCG (of which they were members). The anthropologist Thomas Strong has suggested—rather tongue in cheek—that conferences are not about ideas; rather, they are status rituals. Conferences and congresses are performances; the content of what anyone says matters less than the way they deliver it. Paramount is the physical appearance of the attendees and presenters—the clothes they wear and how they comport themselves. The most important item attendees can wear, Strong (2007) says, is their name tag.

The organizing committee displayed an obvious hierarchy and sense of pride. Early on, Dr. Pelosi II made a dramatic entrance, flamboyantly dressed, sporting oversized dark glasses and a mane of longish graying hair, an imposing, heavily accented Marlon Brandoesque figure, well pleased with himself and his creation—the ISCG. Although his son, Dr. Pelosi III, was clad in a smart gray buttoned-up suit, he was a dull figure in comparison with his father. Showing a grainy 1972 film on female genital surgeries as the congress began, Dr. Pelosi II stated, "See, even then they spoke of sexual satisfaction and cosmesis, and this is increasingly important now because most women are shaving." As a defensive stance on genital cosmetic surgery began to emerge, I started to wonder whether more than medical science and the welfare of women were at play here. Perhaps it was a carnival, a performance—or the affirmation of a brotherhood with strategic goals (Cohen 1995; Gawande 2003). As two prominent American physicians opined:

> The genie is out of the bottle, and she's not going back and that's a fact! (Dr. David Matlock)

> The question really becomes, is there any science behind vaginal rejuvenation and sexual gratification? It certainly hasn't been answered yet but we are making moves in that direction. It is refreshing and rewarding to be involved in another new aspect of vaginal surgery, but now we are trying to put some science behind it as well. We have talked about all the media hype, the news, the magazines and recent TV shows behind this. Is this the final frontier? Is all this just marketing hype; is there any really true scientific evidence behind what we are doing in this field? So, have we found paradise; have we found the hallowed ground; have we opened the heavens and are we here, or are we opening the gates of hell and getting some of the wrath of God? There are plenty of critics out there when it comes to vaginal surgery. You see, Matlock, he is an innovator, and he is the guy who stepped outside the box. He said way back when, "If you can exist in Beverly Hills doing this type of surgery, you must be doing something right" (Dr. Robert Moore).[4]

Tension is evident in the above statements. There is pride and an assertive belief in the benefits of female genital cosmetic surgery as an innovative practice, but also an acknowledgement by Dr. Robert Moore that female genital cosmetic surgery is controversial and for the practice to burgeon, it needs to be safeguarded.

Many of the presenters were from Central and South America, reflecting the popularity of cosmetic surgery in those countries (as well as their geographical proximity). Others came from Turkey, Korea, Egypt, England, and Greece. It has been suggested that Brazilian surgeons are often pioneers in aesthetic surgery because it is performed there in the public hospital setting, where women's bodies are "a resource both to teach medical students about plastic surgery, and to develop surgical techniques that are marketable in private clinics and abroad" (Jarrin 2012, 6). Also, the fact that Brazil has fewer institutional and legal barriers to technological innovation than many countries increases the likelihood of novel procedures emanating from there (Edmonds 2010; Jarrin 2012).

Topics discussed over the two days included the evolution of the subspecialty, recommended training for practitioners, patient selection, and the G-spot (with the emphasis on authenticating its existence rather than techniques for its augmentation). Other discussions described new technologies and instruments, vaginal rejuvenation and issues of sexual satisfaction, liposculpting, bleaching of the external genitalia, and even advanced surgical bodybuilding (a procedure one of the surgeons himself had undergone) whereby fat is transferred into muscle groups under the guidance of ultrasound. Various surgical techniques were briefly demonstrated using slides, videos, and stylized diagrams—methods of learning about new procedures similar to those described to me by some Australian surgeons who said they developed new techniques by reading articles or watching videos. Many presenters emphasized the less technical, more social aspects of their medical field. As proceedings got underway, tensions arose around topics such as nomenclature and ways to respond to critics and defend the practice of female genital cosmetic surgery. The congress's goals were strategic as well as medical, with the focus as much on countering bad press and establishing the subspecialty as on sharing medical expertise.

One female Brazilian doctor, a pioneer in the field, chatted with me in the bathroom as we were washing our hands. She was about to give her presentation and was immaculately dressed in a figure-hugging outfit. She confided in me that when she had started practicing female genital cosmetic surgery, everyone had thought she was crazy and would avoid her. Now, as she observed, there were entire congresses dedicated to the discipline, and more female practitioners. "We women need to stick together," she said, smiling broadly and handing me her business card. Over the two days, I asked attendees why they had decided to attend the congress. Some said their practice had sent them because they were receiving requests for cosmetic procedures from their patients; others said they were simply curious or were trying to decide on a specialty to focus on. Others mentioned wanting to make more money to compensate for rising malpractice insurance costs or abandoning obstetrics for a specialty with more acceptable working hours.

A GENEROUS OFFER OF PEARLS

One of the most vocal and articulate doctors to speak at the congress was Dr. Goodman, an older surgeon who admits to being self-taught when it comes to female genital cosmetic surgery. As he said, "I am a much better surgeon now than I was at the beginning." He was warmly welcomed to the podium with an anticipatory "Michael, let's see what you've got this time." Dr. Goodman promised to present a "generous offer of pearls"—a sharing of his female genital cosmetic surgery techniques. Dr. Goodman began, "I have known Marco [Dr. Pelosi II] for about thirty-five years. We fought the laparoscopy wars together—now we are fighting these wars." He continued:

> This is a clinical presentation; it is going to be totally different to anything
> I have presented before because I am going to be showing you techniques.

We all hold these things close but why [else] are you guys here? Firstly, you should be a member of the International Society of Cosmetogynecology.

Experience is a hard teacher; she gives the tests first and the lessons after. If you haven't had complications, you probably haven't been doing this type of surgery for long. . . . With all due respect to some of the presenters, you are not just going to cut it off straight; you are going to sculpt it, because if you cut it off straight you get a Barbie-doll look. Now that may be something [some of] your patients want, but all your patients want something different.

All you folks are clinicians and independent practitioners. You would like to keep people coming into your office. The reason people come into my office is that they have seen the forty photos that I have on my website—you can take a look at it to see how you can build a good site. They come in because all my afterwards look different and, if you want to build a successful practice, as I said before, if all you have is a hammer, everything looks like a nail. So, there are different techniques.

Despite, or maybe because of, the availability of different techniques that can be tailored to vulval morphology, the vulvas in the after photographs on Dr. Goodman's website vary only marginally, especially compared with the before photographs (Goodman 2014). All the postsurgery vulvas approximate a clean slit, a look that ensures a successful (i.e., lucrative) practice. Dr. Goodman's introduction to his conference presentation highlights the tension between sharing knowledge and maintaining a competitive edge in the field. Surgeons are somewhat reluctant to share new surgical techniques yet want acknowledgment for their expertise and innovation. New surgical techniques are experimental, and satisfactory results are not guaranteed.

Dr. Goodman spoke of the "evolution of the new subspecialty" and offered the audience what he termed *pearls*: "How to decide on the right procedure for the right patient for the right reasons, so you can stay out of trouble." The war analogy he invoked when he was welcomed to the podium reveals not only the degree to which proponents of female genital cosmetic surgery feel unduly victimized but also their determination to defend their practices by asserting their power. As Michel Foucault (1980, 123) wrote in *Truth and Power*, "Isn't power simply a form of warlike domination? Shouldn't one therefore conceive all problems of power in terms of relations of war?" Whether the genital cosmetic surgery wars are for the benefit of women's health, are driven by commercial imperatives, or are the resolve of surgeons to maintain the power to reshape women's bodies according to their own interpretation of desirable genitalia is questionable. One of the few female speakers at the congress, an obstetrician-gynecologist interested in cosmetic procedures, Dr. Mona Alqulali, said:

So, we have had some pioneers in this field who felt that they were empowered because they decided that to really make a difference in women's lives, and when you choose to do this, you are actually becoming an advocate for women. People may say, "No, you are taking advantage of women, because women with diseases or deformities need attention but this [genital anxiety] is all in a woman's head, and you are taking advantage of them because you take money off them but you are not supposed to be doing this; that's bad, this, that, and the other." The thing is this: it is because they can't do it!

As with Dr. Alqulali, congress presenters frequently mentioned that their involvement with female genital cosmetic surgery was in response to women's unmet needs. They spoke of themselves as pioneers who possess skills that other surgeons, often their critics, do not. Thus, parallel discourses of empowerment are engendered. Surgeons become empowered through the acquisition of new skills from which their patients supposedly benefit, and according to surgeons' websites, women themselves are similarly empowered because "our mission is to empower women with knowledge, choice and alternatives" (Laser Vaginal Rejuvenation Institute 2013). However, degrees of power are relative when women rely on surgeons to execute their desires because, to achieve their goals, women must abdicate their bodies to surgeons (Gilman 1999), who appear to have their own ideas of genital beauty.

At the congress, Dr. Pelosi II proudly spoke of the new tools they had developed to make surgery easier (quicker and cheaper) to perform. There were balloons to insert into the rectum, retractors to hold open the introitus (the opening of the vagina), and the implement of which he was proudest (invented by a Chilean presenter), the Aguilera vaginal tonometer. This device is a dildolike instrument with a mercury pressure gauge, which is used for measuring vaginal tone pre- and post-vaginal tightening, the purpose being to prove that surgery has done something, thereby legitimizing the procedure, even when the patient feels little difference. "With labiaplasty, before it was ugly, now it is pretty. But with vaginal tightening, it is more difficult to prove what you have done and, if the patient is not happy, then the tonometer is useful," Dr. Pelosi II said blandly. Over tea and coffee, surgical implement representatives demonstrated their wares. The precision of one high-frequency radio-wave scalpel was demonstrated by cutting slices of raw steak. Dr. Ralph Zipper gave a presentation about his patent-pending method of labiaplasty using his GyneShape Diamond Laser, which promises to preserve the vaginal nerves and tissues. At the end of the congress, a man in a sharp suit was permitted to explain his product, Luscious Lips, to the dwindling audience. He then presented all attendees with a glossy hardcover book, *Luscious Lips*. Apparently, full, pouty, more kissable lips can be attained with a suction-pump device rather than injectables (Cynthia Rowland Beauty Systems 2014).

Much time was given to extolling the virtues of tumescent anesthesia, the subcutaneous infiltration of a large volume of highly diluted local anesthetic and adrenaline, which causes the targeted tissue to become swollen and firm, or tumescent. This "holy water," as it was described, allows procedures to be performed in the surgeon's medical offices rather than in a hospital. "Ninety percent of all cosmetic surgery will be done on an outpatient basis within five years. I don't go to the hospital anymore," Dr. Pelosi II said. Performing surgery in one's offices reduces time and costs, allowing surgeons to perform more pro-cedures, but it is an unregulated arena and can make these operations appear less invasive and less risky than they are (Bartholomeusz 2012). Furthermore, it allows surgeons whose qualifications are not recognized by hospitals to per-form procedures for which they have little training. As one non-board-certified doctor in Australia confided to me:

> Dr. Doron: They didn't accept me in the public system, they didn't allow me
>   to become a consultant, and I didn't get a job the way I would like to, or
>   to have operating rights here and there. So, I sophisticated my surgical
>   practice with minimally invasive procedures, all done strictly under local
>   anesthetic. I have not used sedation since 2000.
> Lindy: Why?
> Dr. Doron: Firstly, I am very experienced academically and clinically. I am
>   one of the most experienced doctors in the world.
> Lindy: Is it difficult sometimes in Australia?
> Dr. Doron: Not really. They didn't like me because I am a foreigner. It's very
>   simple, and then I didn't like them either because they didn't like me.
>   I told them to piss off, and now I have the best and largest clinic in the
>   country, one of the best and largest in the world.

Not only was this doctor's statement a flagrant exaggeration, but it also high-lights how a lack of regulation can be dangerous for women, who are often at-tracted to doctors offering surgery in their offices because the costs are lower, doctors' premises offer more privacy than hospitals, and without a general anesthetic, the patients' surgical experience is briefer.

The increasing number of cosmetic procedures being performed in doctors' offices ("rooms," as they are called in Australia) has drawn criticism locally. In an article published in the *Medical Journal of Australia*, Dr. Hugh Bartholomeusz (2012, 493) declared, "An urgent need exists for Australian regulatory authori-ties to rectify the lack of regulation in this burgeoning area of medical practice and provide a nationwide system of accreditation for office-based surgical facilities." Bartholomeusz argued that the procedures performed in doctors' offices and the practitioners themselves should be subjected to regulation, and this has begun in New South Wales. The Australian Medical Council does not recognize the qualifications of cosmetic surgeons; as such, cosmetic surgeons find it difficult to obtain operating privileges in private hospitals and licensed day surgeries. Therefore, they are more likely to operate in their offices than are plastic surgeons or gynecologists. Similarly, not all US states require the premises where doctors perform surgery to be accredited or licensed. Some states are starting to address the growing issue of practice drift—doctors working outside the areas in which they are trained and board certified. Insurance companies and hospitals typically prohibit doctors from practicing outside their specialties, but office surgery facilities are often unregulated (O'Donnell 2011). This lack of regulation works to the economic advantage of doctors who perform cosmetic procedures.

THE NOTION OF VULVAL BEAUTY

Genital beauty (and vaginal tightness) ran like an undercurrent throughout congress proceedings: "Does genital beauty really exist—the perfect vulva?" was asked by more than one presenter. The answer was a resounding, "Yes, it really exists. Some vulvas are more beautiful than others . . . a beautiful vulva is tight and closed." It is also, apparently, recognizable: "Is that one of yours, Robert?" asked one surgeon when a particular image of a vulva appeared on the screen. It seems images of vulvas circulate at congresses and workshops or as before and after images on surgeons' websites to the extent that they become recognizable within the fraternity. The certainty of the existence of genital beauty was demonstrated through before and after photos of women's vulvas. "The after photos look much better," was the emphatic response.

Female genital cosmetic surgery relies on women believing that their genitalia are less than adequate in their natural state, and the medical gaze validates these beliefs. Although surgeons agree that vulvas vary widely and that most fall within the normal range, patients come in with expectations to look a certain way. As Dr. Oscar Aguirre explained, "I had a thirteen-year-old come in with her mum, and I asked her, 'How do you want to look?' She is a virgin as far as I could tell, she has not looked at porn, she doesn't know what girls look like, and her description was, 'I want my labia to be inside the hamburger buns,' and that is the kind of look that they want. Even a thirteen-year-old knows what is attractive and what really is not attractive. I think that's the message."

By stressing (perhaps incorrectly) that the girl had not compared her genitalia with others, Dr. Aguirre implies that ideals of vulval beauty are natural rather than learned. For him, genital beauty exists, and both the teenager and the doctor recognize it.

Although ideals of genital beauty are generated outside medicine—in the media, in pornography, and on the internet—the ubiquitousness of before and after photographs on surgeons' websites reinforces a certain limited aesthetic as more appealing. The fact that many surgeons subscribe to the notion of genital beauty increases the likelihood that women will undergo surgery. Even if surgeons do not divulge their preferences to patients, it is difficult to imagine that their preferences do not influence their actions. When explaining why he believes a small rim of labia minora should be left to protrude below the labia majora, Dr. Jack Prado said, "It is important for the sexuality, but also I think it looks more beautiful." Furthermore, women who do have their own preference for vulval aesthetics are unable to achieve their desires without medical assistance. As Rhian Parker (2010, 57) says, "If women are trying to recreate their identity through cosmetic surgery, they do so through offering themselves to surgeons who reflect and transpose their own understandings of culture through their scalpels." Clearly, surgeons are in a powerful position vis-à-vis their patients in that they make the incisions.

Although adamant that vulval aesthetics are important and that the G-spot truly exists, Dr. Goodman, a fellow of the International Society for the Study of Women's Sexual Health, espoused a conservative approach to surgery with an emphasis on *listening* to women. Although this is a trope oft used by surgeons, his sympathetic approach was disarmingly convincing. Despite some dissent, Dr. Goodman was adamant: "I've seen women come to my office. They have huge labia, much larger than women that I have operated on. I don't tell them, 'Oh my goodness, you need work done.' If it ain't broke, don't fix it. And if the patient says, 'What do you think I need?' [I] don't answer that." Conversely, Dr. Aguirre argued:

> I kind of disagree with what Dr. Goodman said, [that] if they don't complain about it, don't address it. They are looking to you for expert advice and opinion, and if they want to look youthful, ask them to hold a mirror. Have them look as you examine them; ask what bothers them and point out all the things you identify, and they will tell you, "No, that doesn't bother me, I really don't care about that," or "Yes I do." You have to point it out or else she is going to come back and say, "Well, I did get what I asked for but that is not what I wanted." There is really a lack of understanding of what's going on down there. Sometimes women come in requesting a labiaplasty when

what they really need is a repair of their prolapse. Some women need vaginal rejuvenation, but they don't know what that is.

Women are often portrayed as ignorant of their own genital anatomy and, consequently, as reliant on the (mostly male) medical gaze. One wonders why a woman would need vaginal tightening or rejuvenation if she has no complaints. The approach taught at the congress entails an all-encompassing medical and aesthetic gaze, where genital structures are individually examined and found to be in need of surgery. As Carole Spitzack (1988, 39) says, "The female patient is promised beauty and re-form in exchange for confession, which is predicated on an admission of a diseased appearance that points to a diseased (powerless) character. A failure to confess, in the clinical setting, is equated with a refusal of health; a preference for disease." Cosmetic surgery works by having women confess, in Spitzack's terms, to bodily shortcomings and the doctor then explaining how they can assist them. Certain aesthetic preferences are so ubiquitous that they are assumed to be natural.

Some of the cosmetic surgeons I interviewed in Australia employ an all-encompassing eye, one that is focused on female genital detail. When describing female genitalia, one cosmetic surgeon pronounced, "It's a piece of architecture—it is not a two-dimensional thing—it's very three dimensional, and so is the clitoris and the labia minora—right down to the bottom of the perineum. You have to look at the whole thing and I think work out what you're going to do with the whole thing rather than just trim off the edges that are sticking out."

Doctors approaching female genitalia as a "piece of architecture" ensure that procedures offered to women are more extensive than they may be if doctors were to attend solely to a woman's specific aesthetic concerns. Unlike the cosmetic surgeons I interviewed, most plastic surgeons said that they learned their skills during their specialist training in Australia rather than at congresses or on short courses such as those offered by the ISCG. Many said they would not operate on any genital structure other than the labia.

The media (and pornography) are assumed to be driving a certain vulval aesthetic to which doctors and patients are exposed, even if unwittingly. In 2009, a study in the Netherlands set out to discover whether doctors held aesthetic preferences similar to those of the public and whether this might influence their willingness to perform labiaplasty. General practitioners, gynecologists, and plastic surgeons were shown four photographs of vulvas (two preoperative and two six months postoperative) and asked whether they would refer the women in the photographs for surgery or perform surgery. Male doctors in all specialties were more likely to agree to a labial reduction than were their female colleagues, and plastic surgeons were significantly more open to surgery than were gynecologists. According to the study, "Ninety percent of all physicians believed that the most minimalist of the two postoperative vulvas most closely matched the societal ideal, and the male doctors found this vulva closest to their private ideal in contrast to their female colleagues" (Reitsma et al. 2011, 4). In this study, the male ideal was firmly in line with the public ideal of a contained vulva. The plastic surgeons I interviewed did not view operating on labia differently from other cosmetic procedures, as altering bodies for aesthetic purposes is their specialty.

In contrast with the gynecologists at the congress, several female Australian gynecologists with whom I spoke expressed a lack of concern for vulval aesthetics. One explained, "As gynecologists, we are trained to identify and deal with specific organic or anatomical problems. Where the female external genitalia are concerned, we all have a good idea of what constitutes normality, and if the presenting problem involves the area, we know what to look for—there are infections, rashes, cancers, and so on. Otherwise, we pay little attention to the appearance of the vulva and perineum in a routine gynecological examination." Unlike in the United States, few gynecologists in Australia specialize in female genital cosmetic surgery. With one exception, the gynecologists I spoke with in Australia stressed that they perform cosmetic work as part of their regular practice only when there is significant labial asymmetry, discomfort, or damage as a result of childbirth.

Women's bodies are prone to reductionism. Women are more likely to be described (mostly by men) as a sum of their features—breasts, bottoms, and legs, for instance—in a way that male bodies are not, and this renders women more vulnerable than men to cosmetic intervention (Culbertson 1998). Medicine uses fragmentation as a diagnostic and teaching tool; the body is seen not as a whole but as a sum of its constituent parts, each subjected to the medical gaze, one of "seeing and knowing" (Foucault 1973, 55; Good 1994). By viewing female body parts as separate entities rather than as constitutive of a whole, they are more easily subject to evaluation and intervention.

This fragmentation of the body is used to particular effect in cosmetic surgery, where body parts are aesthetically critiqued, fetishized, and subjected to market forces and the possibility of being serially upgraded (Frank 2002; Martin 2001). Women's genitalia are further fragmented and categorized into their component parts, each category a site for medical intervention. Figure 4.2 shows the complexity of female genitalia—each of these structures has become the target of cosmesis.

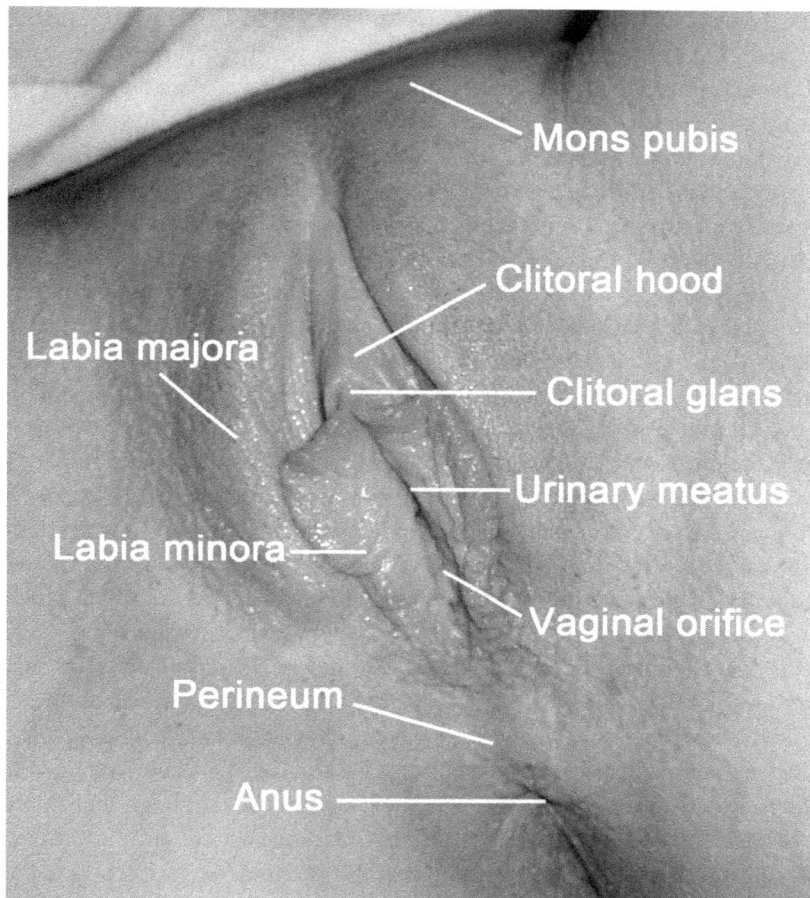

Figure 4.2. Female genitalia (Wikimedia Commons 2013).

At the congress, labia majora were described as "deflated" or "flaccid," as "hamburger buns" or "flat tires," while labia minora were "redundant," clitoral hoods "excessive," and vaginas "wide," "gaping," and "loose." While such fragmentation is an essential tool in the practice of clinical medicine, the medical gaze risks rendering the subject disembodied, as a graphic image shown during one presentation highlighted. A photograph of a prone woman, in the necessary position for genital surgery, was projected onto the screen, her legs spread, vulva exposed, and the remnants of her two labia minora and two folds of clitoral skin placed in an arc around her groin. This powerful imagery exceeded that of naming body parts pejoratively, judging them, and describing suitable intervention. To me, it screamed, "Look what we can do—look what we can pare away, so much excess!" As Byron Good (1994, 73) suggests, "It is not that anatomy is a 'dehumanizing' experience, rather cultural 'work' is required to reconstitute the person who is the object of medical attention." What cultural work can we offer to reconstitute the woman in such an image? A focus on female genitalia in isolation is to be expected at a congress dedicated to them, but such a powerful image makes it difficult to see female genital cosmetic surgery as a rational practice totally distanced from female circumcision (see fig. 4.3, from the exhibition *Love Me* by Zed Nelson).

Discussions among male surgeons about the existence of the notion of vulval beauty, despite ambivalence about how the necessity for certain procedures should be conveyed, conflates common tropes to which female bodies are subjected—the medical gaze, the male gaze, and the aesthetic gaze. The medical gaze, as conceived by Foucault, confirms that "visual culture and contemporary medicine are intertwined" (Jones 2008, 71), and nowhere is this more apparent than with cosmetic surgery. The judges of genital beauty described here are almost exclusively male doctors, whose evaluative gaze functions in a disciplinary manner (Foucault 1977): "According to Spitzack, the physician's clinical eye functions like Foucault's medical gaze; it is a disciplinary gaze, situated within apparatuses of power and knowledge that constructs the female figure as pathological, excessive, unruly, and potentially threatening" (Balsamo 1992, 208).

Such excess and unruliness is made explicit in the language that doctors use to describe women's genitalia and to validate the use of "rational" medical intervention to restore order to the chaos. To gaze implies more than to look. It is a judgmental, potentially active exercise constituted in uneven power relations given that female patients rely on surgeons to fulfill their desires to have their genitalia altered. "Mistrust works to encourage confession and consumption because the male physician, the 'other,' is both knowledgeable and 'centered.' He, unlike the fragmented female patient, is in a position to render an a priori judgement" (Spitzack 1988, 44).

According to surgeons, women today are likely to be demanding patients with their own aesthetic ideals, medical knowledge, and expectations (often gleaned from the internet). Surgeons are wary of demanding patients, not because they are concerned about body dysmorphic disorder (BDD) but because demanding patients are difficult to please. Despite this, few surgeons I spoke with refuse to operate on patients. Describing the ethical dilemmas that surround genital cosmetic surgery, one surgeon at the congress proudly explained that she had operated on a patient who had been refused surgery by another doctor who requested the patient have a psychological assessment. The patient was offended because she felt the doctor was rude and was intimating that she was mentally unstable. The surgeon said, "She wasn't crazy; that is just how she is, so I did the surgery." Although she stressed the need to obtain informed consent and to be vigilant with documentation, this surgeon sympathized with the patient and agreed to operate.

Given that the presenters at the congress appeared to be familiar with each other's handiwork and agreed that such a thing as a beautiful vulva exists, the gaze they employ surpasses that of medicine; it is also an aesthetic and erotic gaze. As Welmoed Reitsma et al. (2011, 2383) suggest in their study of doctors' aesthetic preferences and female genital cosmetic surgery, "Male physicians, especially considering the esthetic aspects of the vulva, may attach erotic values to its appearance." In *Ways of Seeing*, John Berger (1972, 8) states, "The way we see things is affected by what we know and what we believe." This cultural aspect of the gaze, of ways of looking at others, is particularly pertinent when medicine, sexuality, and aesthetics collide, as is the case with female genital cosmetic surgery. Women rely on the presumed capability of doctors (who are predominantly male) to not only alter their genitalia but to also interpret what is desirable aesthetically.

Although there is nothing inherently sexist in medicine's use of "seeing and knowing" (Foucault 1973, 55), the medical gaze cannot be untangled from the male gaze. The male gaze, as a second-wave feminist concept, turns a subject into an object, and when the male gaze is turned onto a woman, it is also one of desire. Patricia Gagne and Deanna McGaughey (2002, 815–6) state, "The notion that men exercise power over women through socially constructed standards is known as the 'male gaze,' a concept developed by Laura Mulvey (1998) to explain how feminine subjectivity is constructed as women judge and create themselves on the basis of their perception of men's desires." As feminist philosopher Kathryn Morgan (1991, 36) articulates, the male gaze comprises actual men, "male beauty experts"—or, in this case, male surgeons—and "hypothetical men" who live in the "aesthetic imaginations of women." Therefore, given that media images are assumed to depict forms that are desirable to men as well as to women, women may judge themselves through male eyes. The hegemony of the male gaze posits women as devoid of agency in problematic ways. At the congress there did appear to be what Alexander Edmonds (2010, 185) describes in his analysis of the interactions between plastic surgeons and mothers seeking plastic surgery in Brazil as "a certain amount of misogyny in the medical gaze." Surgeons *do* imagine women in terms of surface appearance and individual body parts ripe for intervention. However, at the congress, any suggestion of misogyny was disguised within a discourse of empowerment for women.

Philip Culbertson (1998) suggests that the male gaze is important to "homosociality," a term coined by Eve Kosofsky Sedgwick (1985) to describe the basic structure of patriarchy: men pleasing other men through the medium of women. In *The Elementary Structures of Kinship*, Claude Lévi-Strauss (1969) describes exchange in marriage as a relationship between two groups of men, not a partnership between a man and a woman. Women are conduits for affiliations between men. Today, "it appears that men exercise power interpersonally, by virtue of the visual attentions they devote to women deemed physically attractive," and they "exercise power institutionally, through medicine, the fashion industry, the media, and in the workplace" (Gagne and McGaughey 2002, 835). The power to judge vulval aesthetics forms bonds between surgeons, and these bonds are reinforced at forums such as the medical congress I describe in this chapter. Even if, contrary to what some women think, most men are not concerned about vulval aesthetics, the construction of vulval beauty by the doctors at the congress (and communicated on their websites) reinforces genital anxiety in vulnerable women. As described elsewhere in this book, women interested in genital cosmetic surgery develop their ideas about genital aesthetics as much from surgeons' websites as they do from pornography or other media sources.

EVOLUTION: HINTING AT HISTORY

At the congress, the practice of female genital cosmetic surgery was also validated through an oblique allusion to its place in history. In her presentation, Dr. Alqulali offered some sound advice for surgeons who perform female genital cosmetic surgery. Although claiming that such surgery was nothing new, she acknowledged that the practice, as promoted and performed contemporarily, had met with some harsh criticism, and she stressed that training (rather than evidence) was imperative to deflect it:

> I thank all of those who are choosing to understand and learn a little bit about this developing, evolving, um, the revolution, or whatever you want to call it, because ah, in reality, what we are doing is actually not new. This is as ancient as humanity, since the creation of this race, and it will continue. The issues that deal with sex were always important, and have been talked about—maybe in closed rooms—but now we can talk about them in public meetings and discuss it more openly. This is a very infective process—you

start with something and then you end up doing more and more and then you don't become comfortable with what you are doing, maybe you should have started down and then you find yourself slowly progressing up, up, up, so it is a process, an evolution when you choose to become a part of this unique, eclectic group of providers for women. Maybe it's a good time to be in this field, but maybe it's a curse; it's a double-edged sword and you need to know that [there is all] this hype and everybody is talking about it. There are pros and cons and critics, and people who are going to support you. You just need to decide where you want to be.

Whether Dr. Alqulali was suggesting that female genital cosmetic surgery has evolved from female circumcision (which she did not mention directly) is not entirely clear. Perhaps what is "as ancient as humanity" is body modification or embellishment, or even moral concerns about sex and sexuality. Although it was not explicit, in her efforts to validate the practice, she did hint at an historical precedent for female genital cosmetic surgery. Comparisons with female genital cutting (FGC) fuel the ethical concerns about the "infective process" of female genital cosmetic surgery and using history to validate contemporary practices is probably disingenuous given that female circumcision is illegal in most Western countries and vigorously opposed by the World Health Organization.

Dr. Alqulali exposed surgery as an inexact science, an organic process that changes as surgeons innovate with new techniques and aesthetic ideals change. One female surgeon I interviewed in Australia drew an analogy between perfecting her labiaplasty technique and baking a cake. She said, "Usually when you develop a technique, it's a work in progress. It's just like, um, you know, if you make a particularly difficult cake. Every time you make it, you go, 'That didn't quite work. Maybe I should try something else. Maybe I should soak the fruit in wine this time before I add it, or maybe I should whisk the egg whites and fold them in afterwards so that it is lighter.' So, that is essentially what you do. I did not like the look of the old techniques—the original technique was just an amputation."

The idea of surgical practice as evolutionary assumes that techniques are always improving, which fits seamlessly with the scientific paradigm of linear progress. In his presentation, Dr. Goodman compared the evolution of female genital cosmetic surgery as a subspecialty to the move from women wearing bloomers in the eighteenth century to G-strings today—perhaps the evolution from genital surgery suppressing pleasure to (supposedly) enhancing it and from FGC to the G-shot—mirroring the neoliberal imperative toward the pursuit of individual pleasure.[5] Genital cosmetic surgery, as described by its practitioners, is a dangerous field to be in but one well worth the risk. Dr. Alqulali went on to say:

> Why is there this big interest in female genital cosmetic surgeries? People are asking for it, the magazines are talking about it, everybody is talking about this, it's hip and a good thing, and it is not just people in the sex industry or the porn industry who are obsessed with it—it is now becoming mainstream. In reality, it is a very contested field, everybody is trying to get a piece of it, which is common because when you do anything with women and their sexuality it's a problem; when you do anything with women and their reproduction it's a problem.

Although it may be true that "when you do anything with women and their sexuality, it's a problem," female sexuality has long been viewed as not only problematic but also a site of social control, particularly through medical intervention.

Women's bodies in the eighteenth century were imbued with problematic sexuality; the feminine body was analyzed, qualified, disqualified, and described "as being thoroughly saturated with sexuality" (Foucault 1978, 104) and intrinsically pathological, thereby demanding medical attention. Female sexuality and reproduction have a long history of being scrutinized and controlled, and therefore, although this may be problematic, it is nothing new. Novel cosmetic procedures such as genital cosmetic surgery exist within a long trajectory of medical incursions into female bodies and sexuality, and these are bound up (mirroring many reproductive practices) in a language of increased choices for women, but choice is not necessarily empowering for women. Female genital cosmetic surgery may be an evolution of sorts, but perhaps not to the benefit of women. It may not be the "up, up, up" progression that Dr. Alqulali suggested. Rather than being a linear progression offering women more choice regarding their sexual bodies, the rise of genital cosmetic surgery demonstrates a cyclical historical transformation, where the techniques of intervention change but the problematizing of and interference in women's sexuality remains the same.

Early in the congress proceedings, Dr. Pelosi III also referred to historical precedents. He rather churlishly stated, "A lot of people focus on the negative things we do. They focus on our procedures as a branch of genital mutilation." With this statement in mind, I was curious when an Egyptian doctor delivered a presentation on female circumcision. Only a few attendees remained for the presentation, and I wondered why it had been accepted given that at the congress—and in my interviews with surgeons in Australia—analogies between the two procedures were met with derision by surgeons, notwithstanding Dr. Alqulali's allusion to female genital cosmetic surgery's historical underpinnings. The presentation did not spark much interest, despite the presenter, Dr. Amr Seifeldin, stating that both labiaplasty and clitoral hood reduction would come under the World Health Organization classification for female genital mutilation. Dr. Seifeldin described how, despite it being illegal, FGC is still requested in Egypt. He performs clitoral surgery for pain alleviation (rather than for sexual enhancement) on women who have undergone FGC, as well as reinfibulations—the resuturing of the vulva after childbirth for infibulated women. Describing how women in Africa, as elsewhere, use the insertion of herbs to tighten their vaginas after delivery, Dr. Seifeldin commented, "So, that beats Matlock!" intimating that women have always attended to the tightness of their vaginas and that methods to effect this vary across cultures. In an earlier presentation on vaginal tightening, Dr. Seifeldin had begun by saying, "A tight vagina is very important. How tight is still an area for discussion, but all cultures describe a normal woman as one with a tight vagina." He also stated that clitoral hypertrophy is common in hot regions.

I found Dr. Seifeldin's presentation on FGC ambiguous, and I was unable to discern his position on genital alterations until I visited his website and discovered that he specializes in genital cosmetic surgeries in Cairo. Describing how female Egyptian mummies show signs of circumcision, Dr. Seifeldin highlighted that female circumcision is an ancient practice. Surgeons alluded to traditional practices—even those condemned by global medical bodies—and genital surgeries as being "as old as humanity itself" to validate female genital cosmetic surgery and thereby naturalize the premise that women's genitalia are in need of surgical intervention. I am not suggesting that women do not have aesthetic and functional concerns, but we must acknowledge that expert medical discourse and allusions to historical precedents perpetuate the idea that women's genitalia are not good enough for sex in their natural state. Performing surgery on women to ensure that they conform to an idealized and primarily male-generated version of femininity leaves gender stereotypes intact.

RESPONDING TO CRITICISM

A key theme at the congress was a rebuttal of the 2007 American College of Obstetricians and Gynecologists (ACOG) statement cautioning against female genital cosmetic surgery: "It is deceptive to give the impression that vaginal rejuvenation, designer vaginoplasty, revirgination, G-spot amplification, or any such procedures are accepted and routine surgical practices. Absence of data supporting the safety and efficacy of these procedures makes their recommendation untenable. Patients who are anxious or insecure about their genital appearance or sexual function may be further traumatized by undergoing an unproven surgical procedure with obvious risks. Women should be informed about the lack of data supporting the efficacy of these procedures and their potential complications, including infection, altered sensation, dyspareunia, adhesions, and scarring" (ACOG 2007). ACOG members at the congress displayed pride in their opposition to the statement. By broadening their base to include cosmetic, plastic, and other surgeons in an effort to forge a subspecialty, the ISCG has become a counterforce to more institutionalized opinion.

The Royal Australian and New Zealand College of Obstetricians and Gynaecologists (RANZCOG 2015) issued similar statements in 2008, 2011, 2015, and 2016. Although doctors who perform these surgeries have responded to the ACOG statement by publishing articles in peer-reviewed academic journals demonstrating patient satisfaction with genital cosmetic surgery, there remains no credible body of evidence to support either the efficacy or safety of these procedures. Few prospective studies have been conducted. One pilot study published by Goodman et al. (2011) found that, in their small study of thirty-three women who underwent various forms of genital cosmetic surgery, most experienced a lessening of their BDD symptoms six to nine months after surgery. However, since BDD tends to be a lifelong condition, Goodman et al. (2011, 224) noted that "it is unlikely that bodily dissatisfaction will abate completely" with surgery. Even though the authors concluded that BDD is a significant issue with female genital cosmetic surgery, researchers do not appear to be deterred. Currently, several pilot studies are underway, which, by using validated psychological scales, aim to prove the efficacy of surgery in relieving genital anxiety.

Although any new subspecialty in medicine may be met with resistance, the ACOG's statement cautioning against female genital cosmetic surgery has placed extra pressure on practitioners of these procedures to legitimize their actions. In their presentations, the physicians wasted no time in suggesting that the ACOG issued its statement not only to warn but also to punish, and this irritated them. Dr. Goodman explained:

> In the mid- to late 2000s, along comes Dr. Trouble who is a gynecologist and a good surgeon, an innovator and unashamedly a marketer. You know we don't like that. Our doctors are not supposed to market themselves; everyone else can, but we are above that. Well, because we [the medical profession] have put ourselves above that, that is why we are in the bag that we are today with insurance companies running the whole system and using patients and us as a means to make their money. When David [Matlock] came out and basically marketed it, that got everyone in the establishment really pissed off, and what did we see? A backlash. OK. Why, why was there a backlash? This is the first time I have ever seen an opinion from ACOG that was based on one

person. ACOG was pissed at David Matlock because he came up and said, "Here I am; here are these procedures; let's do them."

Most of the North American doctors presenting at the congress mentioned the ACOG statement. The ISCG was founded before the statement was issued, but as Dr. David Matlock reveals below, the proponents of female genital cosmetic surgery saw the ACOG response coming. That your professional institution disapproves of your practices may be upsetting or infuriating, but the ACOG's response has not resulted in a decline in demand for surgery.

The Los Angeles-based Dr. Matlock, whose statement "The genie is out of the bottle" was quoted earlier in this chapter, is referred to as the father of female genital cosmetic surgery. He founded the Laser Vaginal Rejuvenation Institute of America, an institution that has trained a number of surgeons in Australia, one of whom I interviewed. Dr. Matlock is well known to the media and appears comfortable with his image as the so-called bad boy (and innovator) of female genital cosmetic surgery, blatantly exploiting it as a commercial enterprise. As he said, "This is a lucrative business and you need to remember, medicine is a business." In his congress presentation, Dr. Matlock discussed the ACOG's opinion:

> Another thing is that we brought up ACOG a couple of times, and I would say that I have been in the public eye for, you know, the last fourteen years, and I noticed maybe about four years prior to the ACOG opinion letter coming out, I would see in some of the media response that I had in interviews with national magazines [regarding these procedures], they would then ask ACOG, "What is your opinion?" For four years, ACOG said, "We have no opinion." I do believe they got tired of saying "We have no opinion," but I saw that coming. For a good ten years, it was just a lot of fluff pieces; it was just "Give me the information." The other thing too on that—they had a task force commissioned by the president [of ACOG] to review cosmetic surgery GYN and they came up with the statement prior to them ever meeting.

Dr. Matlock was intimating that the ACOG statement was as much about satisfying the media (who were interviewing him about female genital cosmetic surgery) as about producing a thorough investigation into the safety of genital cosmetic surgeries. According to many practicing doctors, the ACOG statement was directed firmly at Dr. Matlock and his aggressive marketing style, which made him and his ilk appear unprofessional and overtly materialistic. Adam Ostrzenski, a former university professor and gynecologist specializing in female genital cosmetic surgery, after reviewing the scientific literature on it, concluded that "practicing cosmetic gynecology within ACOG

recommendations is desirable and possible" (Ostrzenski 2011, 617). Ostrzenski does not consider cosmetic procedures as outside the range of traditional
gynecological practice; however, he is critical of "creating medical terminology trademarks and establishing a business model that tries to control clin-
ical-scientific knowledge dissemination" (Ostrzenski 2011, 617). The ACOG
statement appears to have had the unintended effect of strengthening practitioners' resolve, indignation, and sense of purpose. Similarly, in Australia, the
RANZCOG statement has had little impact on practice, because plastic and
cosmetic surgeons, who do not come under the purview of RANZCOG, carry
out most procedures. For gynecologists, vaginal tightening for multiparous
women is considered reconstructive surgery, and labiaplasties to correct obstetric trauma are deemed appropriate by RANZCOG (2016).

The review that Dr. Goodman was referring to appeared in *The Journal of
Sexual Medicine* in 2011. The article gives an overview of female genital cosmetic
surgery but provides only anecdotal evidence of patient satisfaction. "Every
study relating to outcome in the peer-reviewed English literature reports subjective success rates well in excess of 80–90%. However, all of these studies are
retrospective; all have relatively short-term follow-up of sexual satisfaction,
none delve more than superficially into body image issues, and all lack a control
group" (Goodman 2011, 1823). Perhaps this exposes these procedures as just as
much a pseudoscience as the pseudofeminism that Dr. Goodman critiqued.

Along with the criticism from the ACOG, there has been growing debate
about female genital cosmetic surgery in the popular press, which also irritates
surgeons specializing in these procedures. As Dr. Goodman commented in his
presentation, "Freelance journalists write shock pieces on this subspecialty.
The people who are writing against it have their own agendas. What they say
is not based on fact." He described how one journalist conducted an in-depth
interview with him at the last ISCG meeting, but "she chose to write a totally
fictional shock piece to sell; these are freelance journalists, and excitement sells.
Negative stuff sells; sober information doesn't sell." Dr. Goodman explained
how he had attempted without success to open a dialogue with certain academics who have written about female genital cosmetic surgery in peer-reviewed
journals.[6] He said, "These are authors with preconceived prejudicial positions
based either on financial goals of selling sensational chat pieces or academics
pushing their personal concepts of sexuality for paternalistic or pseudo- or
retro-feminist purposes, and where does their data come from? They don't have
any—no data. This is why I have written a review of these procedures. If you
want to answer your critics, you should look at it."

However, as he rightly notes, "The field of female genital cosmetic revision is in flux. As it evolves, it is anticipated that unanswered questions will be addressed by means of well-designed studies evaluating both sexual and body-image issues, and evaluating long-term satisfaction, benefit, and risk" (Goodman 2011, 1823). To answer some of these questions, in 2016, Goodman et al. published the results of a prospective study of 120 women undergoing female genital cosmetic surgery, which indicated that surgery alleviates sexual dissatisfaction and negative genital self-image.

Criticism of female genital cosmetic surgery published in the popular press threatens not only doctors' reputations but also their profits, resulting in the defensive stance at the congress and previous ISCG meetings. In 2010, after the inaugural Global Symposium on Cosmetic Vaginal Surgery held in Orlando, at least two relevant articles appeared in the mainstream press in the United States. One appeared in the *Huffington Post* (Bonavoglia 2010) and one in *Cosmopolitan* magazine (Triffin 2010), with the titles "Cosmetic Vaginal Surgeons Clueless about Female Sexuality" and "Warning: These Doctors May Be Dangerous to Your Vagina," respectively. Criticism of these procedures was brought to the public's attention for the first time. Prior to the publication of these two articles, female genital cosmetic surgery had been portrayed in women's magazines and the popular press as a novelty and as yet another opportunity for women to alter their bodies. All media had been considered good media. However, surgeons today are warier of the press, and although they still use the media to promote their practices, articles such as those described above are considered biased by doctors who practice genital cosmetic surgery. Surgeons now portray themselves as unfairly under attack. Yet any media attention or discussion of female genital cosmetic surgery serves to normalize it in some way—to make it a possibility.

One focus of the congress as outlined in its glossy brochure was to "critically examine" nomenclature for genital cosmetic surgery procedures. Dr. Goodman explained:

> You guys do very great work, but I must respectfully disagree with you on nomenclature. If I give a postmenopausal woman who is maybe sixty-five—she isn't on hormones, hasn't had sex in ten years, and has a vagina I can barely get my finger into—if I give her estrogens and dilators and slowly her vagina is able to accommodate a penis, I am doing vaginal reconstruction. You will not get anything into any journal using the term "vaginal rejuvenation." So, I would say let's use "reconstruction" rather than "rejuvenation"—that means to "make new."

Adopting correct nomenclature is deemed necessary to facilitate the acceptance of papers for publication in peer-reviewed journals, because publication can prove difficult when unscientific terms such as "designer vagina" and "vaginal rejuvenation" are used. Also, as one doctor said, "If we use names like 'designer vagina,' our position is made worse, as the terms are taken up and splashed around in the press," reducing the likelihood that female genital cosmetic surgery will be considered proper medicine, something vital to congress participants.

THE CONGRESS: CELEBRATION OR STRATEGY?

What is the purpose of a medical congress or conference today? Is it a tribal event, as Gawande (2003) proposes, a space to be among your peers—to network and belong—or is it a site for significant (and impactful) knowledge sharing?

Carnival

It has become popular to use the concept of carnival as a prism through which to critique society and its symbolic order through an analysis of transgression and boundary crossing (Jenks 2003). Carnival involves a temporary reversal of the perceived natural order of things; participants cross the line, go beyond the limits that mark off the dualisms that ontologically and symbolically structure society. Applying the carnival model more broadly, "Every social moment is like a carnival in the sense that it is an occasion for artifice in which multiple levels of power and resistance are operative, each responding to different forces at the same time that they accommodate themselves to one another" (Washabaugh 2005, 1). For Mikhail Bakhtin (1984), the social is carnivalesque in the sense that all social moments involve renegotiations of power: "Carnival, after all, is a *licensed* affair in every sense, a permissible rupture of hegemony, a contained popular blow-off as disturbing and relatively ineffectual as a revolutionary work of art" (Eagleton 1981, 148). Carnival is an instrument of social control, even as it allows for minor and temporary transgressions (Eco 1984). In the carnivals of professional academic conferences, scientific authority is not ruptured, only reaffirmed.

I began this chapter with a description of Las Vegas as a conference location that invoked a carnival atmosphere, one of glitz, excitement, and perhaps deception. Anthropologist Lawrence Cohen (1995, 320) referred to a medical conference he attended as an "epistemological carnival," a site of both knowledge production and contestation—a celebration of knowledge to an extent but one that hides as much as it reveals. As with inversion at carnival, the status quo, the structure underpinning medical knowledge production, remains largely untouched. "Large conferences are often carnivals, colossal events where academic proceedings are overshadowed by professional politics, ritual enactments of disciplinary boundaries, sexual liminality, tourism and trade, personal and native rivalries, the care and feeding of professional kinship, and the sheer enormity of discourse" (Cohen 1995, 323).

Ostensibly, most doctors attend medical conferences to gain further knowledge and skills in what is a rapidly changing scientific field, but frequently, more is at stake. Who benefits from this "enormity of discourse"? Although the ISCG congress was not large enough to exude a vivacious carnival atmosphere, unlike the Victoria's Secret gathering below, there was much self-congratulation and bravado. Professional politics and kinship were at play, and disciplinary boundaries were being established in an effort to legitimize this nascent subspecialty through the power of discourse. Notions of brotherhood and solidarity emerged as forms of defense against criticism from both within and outside the medical realm—a form of social capital.

Rather than treating carnival as transgression across boundaries, Cohen's use of the carnival metaphor exposes the artifice of the conference, the posturing and flamboyant display; things are not entirely what they seem. The ISCG congress was as much about self-congratulation, professional kinship, and the construction of an academic edifice with which to refute critics of female genital cosmetic surgery and further its acceptance in the medical realm as about the dissemination of knowledge and the relief of women's supposed suffering. An effort was made to lay epistemological anxiety to rest through discourse, but if carnival is a time for celebrating antistructure and opening up liminal realms for flouting norms (Cohen 1995), that is not what transpired in Las Vegas. The ISCG congress did not offer a post-carnival utopia for women: there was no flouting of norms; rather, their affirmation, and no celebration of female flesh; rather, strategies to remove and control it. The future envisioned was one in which the hierarchical structures (Bakhtin 1984; Parker 1997) and authority of biomedicine were reinforced. What is acceptable regarding the intrusion of medicine into the lives of women remains the province of those who orchestrate power, and power rests with those who stipulate which surgeries are or are not in the best interests of women.

At carnivals, particularly Brazilian carnivals, an ideal and frequently cosmetically enhanced body is foregrounded. Edmonds (2012) describes how, at one carnival parade, homage was paid to a famous plastic surgeon, Dr. Ivo Pitanguy, who "led the procession surrounded by samba dancers in feathers and bikinis," not unlike Victoria's Secret models. The female body was central to both the ISCG congress and the Victoria's Secret convention. However, while the latter displayed a certain playfulness and *jouissance*—a carnivalesque celebration of the female form—the mood upstairs held a different effervescence in the Durkheimian sense; professional reputations (and money) were at stake. As has been the case historically, discourse was being invoked to legitimize medical intervention into women's problematic bodies. The troubling disjuncture at the ISCG congress, the carnivalesque, was the relationship between the medical knowledge espoused there and its practice. The presenters described themselves as responding to women's requests, but they completely glossed over why women feel their genitalia are inadequate in the first place.

Nancy Scheper-Hughes and Margaret Lock (1987) theorize how individual bodies exist in relationship to the social body and the body politic; medical knowledge dwells within the latter category, the most powerful. "For as the body and its afflictions are rooted in and between these multiple frames, the meaning of bodily knowledge is slippery" (Cohen 1995, 321), and this slipperiness ensures that there cannot be one totalizing (expert) knowledge of women's bodies—medical or otherwise. As doctors spoke of women as having gaping, protuberant, redundant, and deflated genitalia, the discursive bodies that emerged served to produce real women defined by these attributes. As Richard Parker (1997, 376), referring to carnival, aptly says, "It is impossible to ignore the extent to which the symbolic structures of the festival exaggerate the most oppressive structures of the real world—male fantasies and desires continue to define a particular vision of female sexuality," a vision increasingly vulnerable to aesthetic ideals.

Cohen (1995, 330) uses the term *air-conditioned knowledge* to emphasize the distance between the knowledge produced in the sanitized rooms of an international hotel in Bombay and the real India outside. The boundary separating the Venetian Hotel from Las Vegas was far more porous. In fact, each reflected the other, even as the reality of Nevada's sunbaked desert and the social world outside the casinos and hotels were rendered distant and irrelevant. The focus on showgirl bodies, consumption, money, and pleasure seeped into the discursive terrain of the congress. Unlike in Bombay, five-star space was not confined to the lobby in Las Vegas. Instead, it permeated discourse, making it seem inevitable rather than transgressive that surgeons spoke freely of addressing the final frontier of the female form with their aesthetic gaze, capable hands, and scalpels.

The idea of a unitary knowledge of the body, in this case what is best for women as far as genital aesthetics and function is concerned, is problematic if the social and political forces impinging on female autonomy are not interrogated. There is no scientific evidence that suggests medically altering women's genitalia for cosmetic purposes improves women's lives. Women's individual bodies and their genitalia exist in a particular social and political milieu that the air-conditioned knowledge produced at conferences fails to acknowledge. Although there was some attempt to address the social body—the environment in which women make decisions about their genitalia—it was presented as immutable and inevitable, whereas corporeal bodies were portrayed as malleable, allowing doctors to profit from women's genital anxieties.

Using carnival as a metaphor for sites of medical knowledge production alerts us to the questionable utopian nature of the medical quest. This remains so whether it is a cure for the lack of agency of India's poor or the search for a perfect vulva and a satisfying sex life as if they are somehow crucially important to twenty-first-century femininity. As with Cohen's Āyurvedic medical conference, where knowledge production and reproduction was articulated more through an oppositional dialogue of legitimacy by using biomedicine as a straw man—a "dialogic third," in Bakhtin's sense—rather than addressing the suffering of the patient, so too there arose at the ISCG congress a contest for the female body, the dialogic third being the detractors of female genital cosmetic surgery. Surgery was legitimated through a dialogue of female empowerment, knowledge, and choice—an appropriation of feminist discourse that disguised the lack of scientific rigor supporting the surgical procedures. Rather than providing empirical evidence, presenters attacked their detractors (ACOG, the popular press, and feminist academics) as a distraction. The carnival of the congress was less about the object of the search, in this case helping women to be comfortable with their genitalia, than about other powerful "projects of mastery," such as institutional recognition, wealth, status, and brotherhood (Cohen 1995, 341).

Brotherhood

Reflecting on a large surgical conference he attended in Chicago, Atul Gawande (2003) concluded that medical conventions offer more than the carnivalesque. They facilitate a sense of being among your tribe, networking and belonging, because to be a doctor is often an isolating experience. "Doctors belong to an insular world—one of hemorrhages and lab tests and bodies sliced open" (Gawande 2003, 85–86), and this world is made more insular if your professional body and peers doubt your motivations and practices. For this reason, the sense of being among your tribe took precedence over the carnivalesque at the ISCG congress, whose mission statement in part reads as follows:

> The Society seeks to cultivate and fortify relationships with surgeons around the globe from all specialties which participate in the cosmetic and aesthetic management of women.
> We will increase our visibility in the fields of Medicine and Surgery by acquainting other organizations having regional, national and international significance with our activities. This visibility will be supported through an open technical milieu to encourage member participation.
> The International Society of Cosmetogynecology is dedicated to serving the needs of the cosmetic gynecologic surgeon, to enrich the member's life both personally and professionally. By delivering superior educational programs on a regular basis, the members of the ISCG have the opportunity to grow and evolve professionally with the sense of brotherhood the Society imparts. (ISCG 2008)

This mission statement places a strong emphasis on relationships and support for practicing members, something that Paul Rabinow suggests is typical in scientific communities: "Today the daily life of the sciences is saturated with personal ties that serve diverse functions. It is sometimes forgotten that mutual advantage needs to be identified and negotiated as much as anything else. . . . Scholarly and scientific conventions play a significant role in the American economy; the face-to-face encounters they foster, while hard to justify in quantifiable economic terms, clearly continue to be valued" (Rabinow 1997, 200–1). According to Rabinow, friendship is "an ethical and epistemological *practice*"; it serves a purpose in the circulation of knowledge (Rabinow 1997, 201). Brotherhoods have strategic purposes and consist of like-minded people with a common goal. Colleagueship, or a sense of brotherhood, may be one of the most sensitive indicators of what Rue Bucher and Anselm Strauss (1961) refer to as segmentation, or subspecialization, within a profession. Whom someone considers a colleague is linked to their own place within their profession, and what ties someone more closely to one member of their profession may alienate them from other members. If a group develops a unique mission, they may become alienated from others in the same profession (Bucher and Strauss 1961). This is certainly the case with female genital cosmetic surgery, which is not recognized as a legitimate subspecialty by the certifying body, the American Board of Obstetrics and Gynecology, or by the overarching body, the American Board of Medical Specialties. Potentially, this has serious implications for patients. Doctors who profess to be experts in the area are not required to pass select examinations, making their claims to expertise perhaps deceptive and certainly unverifiable by patients.

The ISCG was established to fill a perceived academic void in women's health care, one that gynecologists are well suited to fill because of their unique relationship with women. By establishing a mission to forge new relationships with patients, surgeons can develop subspecialties that distinguish them from other medical groupings. Often, these relationships, and the services the doctors provide, are referred to in idealized ways (Bucher and Strauss 1961). Although Cohen refers to the "enormity of discourse," the language of conferences and mission statements can take on a more rhetorical form when the endeavor is to establish a new area of expertise, "probably because it arises in the context of a battle for recognition and institutional status" (Bucher and Strauss 1961, 326). Returning to the war analogy (as in the "laparoscopy wars" referred to by Dr. Goodman), "It's astounding to see how easily and self-evidently people talk of *war-like* relations of power" (Foucault 1980, 123) when devising strategies to establish epistemological truths. By isolating a given anatomical area for the purpose of cosmetic improvement and creating a society around that purpose, ISCG members hope to gain legitimacy and, by including doctors other than obstetrician-gynecologists, they aim to build a defense against ACOG.

In *Cyborgs and Citadels*, Gary Downey and Joseph Dumit (1997) describe how medical knowledge is constructed, enacted, and protected for strategic purposes through the maintenance of boundaries: "The Citadel Problem is a problem of cultural boundaries: it calls attention to the centering effects of science, technology, and medicine within discourses of objectivity and practices of both legitimation and sovereignty. The word 'citadel' denotes a small fortified city or a fortress at the center of a larger city that protects and oversees it. We use the term to highlight the ways in which prevailing modes of popular theorizing about science, technology, and medicine displace societal issues and concerns into expert and often expensive technical problems, thereby isolating participation and discussion while transforming the stakes involved" (Downey and Dumit 1997, 6).

Boundaries are set up to protect expert medical knowledge, and they are vigorously defended. For those choosing to practice female genital cosmetic surgery, the "larger city," ACOG, not only offers no protection but also is openly hostile. Maintaining this analogy, the citadel, the ISCG (and similar bodies promoting female genital cosmetic surgery, such as the American Academy of Cosmetic Gynecologists), must adopt strategies of self-defense to ensure impenetrability to criticism. These strategies include creating a sense of brotherhood and accepting nongynecologists into the society.

Knowledge about new procedures and technologies is normally controlled and reproduced through training and accreditation (and at congresses), and practitioners "build up social capital around such technologies" (Manderson 2012, 4) by creating a professional space for themselves. As a scientific practice, cosmetic surgery, like other sciences, relies on boundary-work for legitimacy: "Because expansion, monopolization and protection of autonomy are generic features of 'professionalization,' it is not surprising to find the boundary-work style in ideologies of artists and craftsmen (Becker 1978) and doctors (Friedson 1970; Starr 1982)" (Gieryn 1983, 792). However, for a medical specialty to evolve from an area of interest into a recognized subspecialty requires more than boundary-work; it needs a critical mass of doctors to decide to carve out a unique clinical role and to develop the education and research programs to support it, as is the case with the ISCG. Although subspecialization can be useful when new knowledge and techniques develop in a discrete area of practice, it is a cause for concern when the narrow scope of some fields of specialization is the product of overt medicalization (Sinclair 2005). In addition, the term *subspecialty* can convey legitimacy where none may lie.

The medicalization of health "problems" often follows a well-trodden trajectory. The advent of Viagra as a cure for erectile dysfunction is one example. The road to Viagra involved the nomenclatural morphing from impotence into erectile dysfunction, a concerted medical effort to explain the phenomenon in physiological rather than psychological terms, thereby medicalizing it and, lastly, proffering a pharmaceutical solution: Viagra (Fishman 2006). Similarly, female genital cosmetic surgery offers a surgical solution to protruding labia, wide vaginas, and female sexual dysfunction. The pharmaceutical industry is also intent on creating and capitalizing on female sexual dysfunction as a condition (now listed in the *DSM-5*) in need of a cure. Providing a cure for a new illness category is anything but accidental, as Jennifer Fishman suggests: "Relying on 'serendipity' is a way of maintaining a notion that technologies, scientific facts, and scientific knowledge developments, more generally, are simply out there in the world, waiting to be discovered, rather than social and cultural productions in their own right" (Fishman 2006, 245). Serendipity in this case involves an orchestrated and strategic enterprise from those seeking to expand into new medical arenas. Strategies involve the creation of a supporting society, journal publications, the uptake of persuasive terminology, medical conferences, the strident discourse of "experts," and more than a modicum of determination. In this case, serendipity (women have a problem and surgeons have the skills to solve it) involves a great deal of cultural work.

Global Flows

In Australia, I had a conversation with Dr. Johnson (a pseudonym), one of the few gynecologists (as opposed to cosmetic or plastic surgeons) in the country who advertises female genital cosmetic surgery. Our conversation highlights how congresses such as the one just described, their players, and their content can have a global reach. Although various genital cosmetic surgery procedures have been adopted unevenly globally (for instance, labiaplasty is more popular in Australia than is vaginal tightening or hymenoplasty), American surgeons have been innovators and key educators in the field. More importantly, they see female genital cosmetic surgery as a viable niche profession in its own right, one that requires the validation of a "whole area" approach to genital aesthetics, as described previously. Consequently, the past few years have seen a proliferation of surgeons in Australia offering a greater variety of procedures. Dr. Johnson, who has trained with Dr. Matlock, described how he came to do so in a conversation with me over lunch one day.

> Lindy: Have you been doing the surgery for a long time?
> Dr. Johnson: I've been doing sort of sexual function type surgery for the last ten years. But I did David Matlock's training. In fact, the thing is, when I was in the UK, I was doing, I was doing some and looking at what other people were doing. Trying to work it out. And then I heard about David Matlock. For a while, he wasn't training people in the UK; a lot of his customers came from the UK before he trained any UK doctors. What happened was, at a meeting in Paris, a combined meeting between the International Urogynecology [*sic*] Association and the Incontinence Society, fabulous meeting, one of the best opening ceremonies, in fact the best opening ceremony I've been to for a conference. It was good. But on one of the evenings, um, I for some reason went to a bar, because I had a couple of friends there. I thought, "Oh, I'll just go out for a bit." Anyhow, in that bar, I met a chap for the first time. I'd heard about him, John Miklos, and I met also at the same time, what's his name, from Chile?
> Lindy: Prado?
> Dr. Johnson: Anyway, it was one of those evenings when you're just chatting, nice bunch of guys, started talking about our interests, and I said to them, "Oh yeah, I was interested in all this kind of stuff [female genital cosmetic surgery]." "Oh, have you done," the Chilean guy asked, "have you done Matlock's course?" And I said "No, because I thought he wasn't going to train people from the UK." So, John Miklos, who is very interesting, very American, very big, you know. One of the best laparoscopic surgeons you'll ever come across. Brilliant. Very, very fast. Just, precise. Really

good—watched him operate one day. Fantastic. He just flipped open his phone at the bar and said, "Hold on David, I've got my friend with me. He's based in the UK but you're going to train him." When I got to Australia, I communicated with him [Dr. Matlock] and said I wanted to do his course.

He's in Hollywood, the center of, you know, money and complaint, and you know, if people don't like it, they tell you about it. He's doing well, and for all the criticism he has taken he's actually taught a lot of people, a lot of people, some very, very good surgical techniques. The reason why he gets a lot of flak is there is a lot of professional jealousy. People don't like to give their secrets out to everybody. People don't like to pay him. As far as I'm concerned, I spend a lot of time traveling to surgeons all over the world to teach and also to observe because I want to . . . if I go somewhere and pick up one little thing that makes my practice a bit better, it's money well spent, but a lot of people won't get the money out of their wallet. The same people who have criticized me for not telling them about lasers, it's not a hidden secret, the more people who get trained in this sort of work, the better for women generally, I think, but they sort of want to somehow sit in their office and get the information from me. Without me knowing about it, without me even knowing that they want the information. I'm much more likely to get someone from Taiwan visiting me, or India or somewhere like that, to say, "Can you teach me your techniques?" which happens all the time.

Lindy: Training is a question I always ask surgeons about, where have they trained.

Dr. Johnson: Well, generally the ones who want to be trained in Australia want to use the term "LVR [laser vaginal rejuvenation]," so I say to them, "If you want to use the term 'LVR,' you need to go and do Matlock's course. I will support you in that. I'll even mail them and tell them that you're a good guy or whatever, good girl, you know." Sometimes when they get people from around the world, they're not sure and they'll email me and say, "Do you know this person?" So, I say, "But you need to go and do it, the course."

Despite his small concession to political correctness in acknowledging there may be "good girls" as well as "good guys" seeking training, Dr. Johnson was describing a brotherhood moment. Doctors travel worldwide to share knowledge at conferences, which reinforces a global network of female genital cosmetic surgery providers. Those who seek training in these practices gain admission to the global network through some form of personal recommendation—along with a payment, of course. Therefore, although female genital cosmetic surgery is a global phenomenon, practitioners are at the same time consolidating tight personal networks, and the sense of (homosocial) brotherhood is strengthened.

Specialist doctors have always traveled abroad to congresses, conferences, and workshops, especially from Australia, which, due to its geographical isolation, recognizes that much medical knowledge emanates from elsewhere. Furthermore, many Australian specialists complete their qualifications overseas. However, current social networking technologies, the ease of international travel, and the flow of medical information through congresses and workshops make it increasingly easy to acquire new skills. What happens in one geographical and medical space soon moves to another. This has led to a marked increase in female genital cosmetic surgery, with more novel and invasive procedures becoming the norm. Such surgery is now performed almost universally: in Asia, Europe, Mexico, South America, North America, the Middle East, Australia, and South Africa. In Brazil, Dorneles de Andrade (2010, 79) refers to genital cosmetic surgery as "very common," perhaps indicating the emergence of a "global aesthetic norm" for female genitalia. Learning new techniques for body parts previously left untouched by cosmetic procedures may be "money well spent" for surgeons, but whether it is true that "the more people who get trained in this sort of work, the better it will be for women generally," as Dr. Johnson suggests, is less certain.

Describing how female genital cosmetic surgery is becoming more acceptable, one prominent Australian surgeon I interviewed said, "There are now chapters in American textbooks describing cosmetic genital surgeries. There, it is a subspecialty, but because of the numbers and volume, it is not a subspecialty here in Australia yet. There is not enough of it, but we always follow the Americans." Although female genital cosmetic surgery is not yet officially recognized as a subspecialty within medicine, it seems increasingly likely that this might eventuate as doctors continue to network across the globe. Goodman et al. published the edited volume *Female Genital Plastic and Cosmetic Surgery* in 2016 in order to bring medical legitimacy to the practice. When money can be made through training doctors in new techniques, professional jealousy is laid to rest, and the ideas of a small number of surgeons, a select club (all the surgeons mentioned in the conversation above are key members of ISCG), can have a worldwide impact.

—∽—

Medical congresses are performative, in Judith Butler's (1990) terms. They embody the quintessential speech act because, cloaked in scientific discourse and often taking on a rhetorical air, they have the ability to *do* something, to set in motion the possibility of acting on bodies rather than merely representing them. Although congresses such as the one described here are integral to the process of medical knowledge production, they are also political in that they work to legitimatize new medical practices that have social implications. They also align the knowledge economy with medical economics in these moments of exchange. While "the genie may be out of the bottle" regarding female genital cosmetic surgery, her whereabouts requires monitoring until other than anecdotal evidence is available to support the validity of altering women's genitalia for cosmetic reasons. Without rigorous scientific evidence and without attention to the social world in which women choose to have genital surgery, these procedures appear, from a health perspective, to be as much of a gamble as FGC and one just as imbued with the "magic" of culture as its historical precedent. Cosmetic surgery relies on the desire for "more of the same" as growing numbers of women are persuaded to surgically alter their bodies to comply with increasingly exacting beauty and functional standards. In this case, what happens in Vegas does not stay in Vegas. Although we may all be cyborgs in that medical technologies "routinely contribute to the fashioning of selves," as Downey and Dumit posit (1997, 7), the citadel also needs to be challenged and its purposes made visible.

A carnival suggests a coming together of bodies and minds in a moment of spectacle, one that results in little permanent change to the status quo. In a sense, this is applicable to the ISCG congress; medical science retained the power to judge a healthy body, and gender hierarchies remained intact. However, the carnival metaphor also highlights the strong sense of brotherhood or *communitas* displayed at the congress, as boundaries to found and protect a novel area of expertise were established. Congresses have strategic aims. The carnivalesque atmosphere of the congress, the feeling of belonging, passed, but the power of discourse, the epistemological residue of the congress, remained to impinge on female bodies and on how women experience their sexuality through new medical imaginaries. The efficacy or relevance of new medical technologies and surgical techniques is dictated by culturally constructed expectations. The not-yet-proven aspects of new areas of medical intervention and the imagined benefits they offer are fields ripe for investigation and critique to ensure that medicine is used to the benefit of its subjects, not merely its practitioners. Without scientific evidence, the promise of a more beautiful vulva and increased sexual satisfaction is elusive. Nevertheless, this ambiguity is what gives doctors and their technologies both social meaning and power (Dumit, cited in Karim 2012). The remark by one congress presenter, "If you can exist in Beverly Hills doing this type of surgery, you must be doing something right," is scarcely a convincing argument for these invasive procedures.

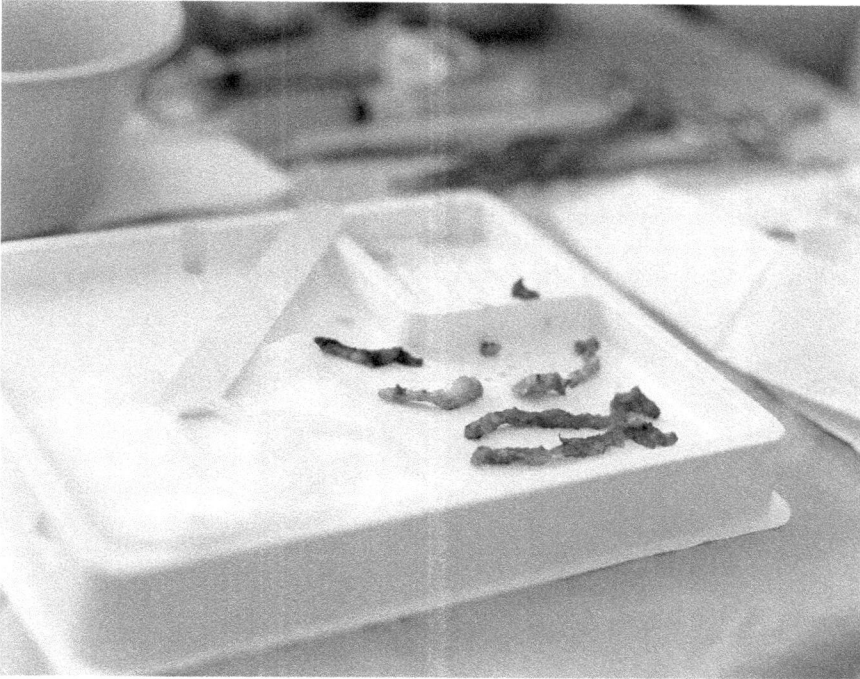

Figure 4.3. "Vaginal tissue removed during 'designer vaginal rejuvenation' surgery to 'tighten and neaten appearance'" by Zed Nelson, 2009, from the photographic series *Love Me*. Reproduced with permission from Zed Nelson.

NOTES

1. I personally took field notes at all the presentations I attended at the conference, and I draw on these in this chapter. A DVD of congress proceedings was produced, and I purchased a copy from the ISCG. Dr. Goodman's presentations are not included on the DVD, so where I quote him, it is from my own field notes.

2. In this chapter, I have provided full names for those presenting at the congress but pseudonyms for physicians I interviewed in Australia.

3. In Australia, board certification is gained through the Australian Medical Council for recognized medical specialties. Similar recognition applies in the United States and Europe. In the United States, a new subspecialty was approved by the American Board of Medical Specialties in 2013: female pelvic medicine and reconstructive surgery.

4. Drs. Matlock and Moore are at the forefront of the growing field of female genital cosmetic surgery in the United States. They are key educators in these procedures, and they featured prominently at the congress.

5. A G-shot is a technique that involves augmenting the G-spot with fillers to purportedly increase sexual responsiveness in women.

6. For instance, Virginia Braun, an academic who has written extensively on female genital cosmetic surgery, was asked to present at the equivalent ISCG congress in 2010. A presentation she gave to the New View Campaign on this experience can be found at http://www.newviewcampaign.org/video.asp#2010.

FIVE

—ɷ—

AUTONOMY, RISK, DESIRE, AND MAGIC

TO WRITE THIS CONCLUDING CHAPTER, I escaped to the country for some peace and quiet. I also wanted to spend time with my beautiful but slightly unpredictable horse. Unfortunately, I had a bad fall and broke some bones. Doctors are often risk-averse; for them, exposing oneself to risk is a bad choice, and some see horse-riding as a dangerous activity. I know there are dangers, yet I choose to ride. I choose risk and the happiness I derive from threading through the countryside on the back of a magnificent and physically adept beast. I see so much more of nature: being higher, I gain a new perspective. I see and hear the birds more clearly. I have company—we talk, we lapse into long silences, my horse and I. In riding, I choose to take a calculated risk with my body. Although I acknowledge that the risks involved with activities such as horse-riding are different from those inherent in cosmetic surgery, they both involve issues of choice and desire. People take bodily risks for different reasons, seeking various pleasures, and they judge risks accordingly. What *is* interesting is that medical praxis is often deemed less risky than many recreational pursuits (and less risky than it actually is) because of the faith people place in biomedicine.

My accident brought to my attention something of a paradox. On the one hand, the authority of medical knowledge can be censuring, prompting us to feel guilty for choosing certain activities deemed risky, self-indulgent, or vain; on the other hand, it declares certain conditions worthy of medical attention and sympathy. Medical knowledge is particularly authoritative. My general practitioner, my specialist, and the hospital staff mildly censured me for putting myself at risk on a horse whose habits I was unfamiliar with. One suggested I should get rid of the horse altogether; another asked me how I was planning to control him in the future—both social, not medical, opinions. Nevertheless, they were sympathetic to my medical condition. "You should not have put yourself at risk, but we are willing to help" was their attitude.

My experience led me to reflect on the topic of this book, female genital cosmetic surgery, and its relationship to risk, autonomy, desire, and the intersection of social values and the medical profession. Should women be free to take risks with their bodies by choosing genital cosmetic surgery, and if so, who should decide this? Who is delegated the power to judge: practicing surgeons, women, the public? Risk-taking activities are always ethically fraught, whether they are medically induced risks for cosmetic purposes or recreational risks. The themes that arose in my research highlight both the influential and contested nature of biomedicine. The practice of medicine is a fine balance now that it no longer focuses solely on health but is increasingly bound up with beauty and issues of happiness and self-esteem.

My accident also reinforced for me the malleability and restorative properties of the body. The injuries and swelling were painful initially, as was the recovery from the bones of my nose being pushed back into position and my wrist bound, but the pain subsided more quickly than the ugly bruising. I soon recovered and came to appreciate the amazing healing properties of the body, making the concept of damaging it temporarily in the quest for beauty (or recreation) seem less irrational than it might at first appear.

For the medical profession, there is money to be made when aesthetics are foregrounded, as my surgeon explained: "There are some shady doctors out there who tell their patients not to do anything at first with their [facial] injuries. They advise them to come in for a rhinoplasty or facial reconstruction at a later date rather than attempting to fix things up before the broken bones set, which is less invasive. They prefer to do more major and expensive surgery, usually for cosmetic purposes. Women, particularly, want their faces to be perfect, but often men don't bother."

Listening to these comments, I thought to myself, rather disappointedly, that there would be no opportunity for a smaller, neater nose at this stage. Having to surrender my body to medical authority because of my accident afforded me fresh insights into the practice of female genital cosmetic surgery, from both a social and medical perspective. Whether medicine is employed traditionally—to restore an injured or diseased body—or more innovatively, as in the case of genital cosmetic surgery, aesthetics are an important consideration. Mirroring my informants, I too am driven by an internalized cultural compulsion dictating that the body should look, as well as feel, good.

—ᴍ—

My goal with this book has been to impart a sense of the "problem" of female genitalia in the West in the early twenty-first century and explore how they are increasingly subject to authoritative forms of medical knowledge and public scrutiny. Although female genital cosmetic surgery is a minority practice, female genitalia are tightly policed. They are represented verbally and visually in very specific ways. Women who are anxious about their genital aesthetics seek out medical knowledge (and intervention) as they embark on their identity projects. I have drawn attention to the cultural landscape in which women decide to undergo genital cosmetic surgery and surgeons choose to perform these procedures. A vulval ideal, the clean slit, is promulgated in the media, and the medical profession increasingly facilitates the attainment of this aesthetic for those women concerned about their genital appearance. Some women experience their vulvas as not normal, embarrassing, uncomfortable, or simply not ideal, and a biomagical solution is at hand. When health and beauty are as firmly entwined as they are today, a body that is less than ideal or perfect is readily pathologized.

The phenomenon of cosmetic surgery is a complex one that raises the following questions: What should be the purpose of medical science? Should the magic of biomedicine be harnessed for pleasure or beauty as legitimately as it is for survival or health? Female genital cosmetic surgery brings this last question into sharp relief. Richard Shweder (2015) suggests broadening the meaning of medicine to include what he terms "social medicine," a recognition that medical science can be used to "shape the body in socially functional ways," thereby enhancing it in order to "have a positive effect on a person's sense of well-being" (Schweder 2015, 179). However, it must be cautioned that medicine is also a largely commercial enterprise in the West, which encourages physicians to seek out new ways to capitalize on people's bodily insecurities. This is occurring at the same time as the internet is bringing new knowledge and opportunities into the homes and palms of most people, ensuring that novel opportunities for bodily alterations can be materialized. Cosmetic surgery has a biomagical quality; it is, as Michael Taussig (2012, 44) suggests, "akin to alchemy, and related magical practices" because, by changing the outside of the body, it promises to alter how people feel about themselves. For women harboring perfectionist traits, caring for the self is a significant aspect of daily living. However, most women with whom I spoke were not perfectionists. Their concerns were more prosaic—they wanted to relieve their genital anxiety. Nevertheless, perfecting or improving the body, its functions, and its form is ultimately the goal of biomedicine. As such, biomedicine's foray into the biomagical appears less

an aberration and more a natural progression in a consumer-driven environment in which the body reveals inner truths. Biomedicine can dictate what is
normal and what is desirable, and women respond to the authority of cosmetic
surgeons, who imprint their personal preferences onto women's bodies.

The clean-slit ideal is a simulacrum, a hyperreality that has become attainable through surgery and depilation; the map, the representation, precedes
the territory, in Jean Baudrillard's (1994) terms. The simulation, the clean slit,
only has its original version or prototype in prepubescent girls. Although nonprotruding labia *do* occur in nature, hairlessness for adult women does not.
The clean-slit ideal is modeled on an imagined female sexuality devoid of hair
and external genitalia. The privacy of female genitalia, their invisible, intimate
quality, makes the hyperreality of the airbrushed clean slit (as seen in soft-
core pornography and women's magazines) particularly compelling, because
there is no clear social reality with which it competes. Baudrillard (1994) argues
that in a postmodern world, individual experience is increasingly influenced by
the media, technology, and the hyperreal. The full spectrum of female genital
morphology is not portrayed in the mainstream media, and what is deemed
normal, ideal, or perfect is constructed by medicine in dialogue with cultural
aesthetics. The corporeal, therefore, is replaced by the hyperreal, and the reality
of genital diversity seems, for some women, to be inauthentic and inadequate
for happiness. The biomagical, then, brings the corporeal and the hyperreal
closer together. In an increasingly uncertain biomedical age, the body "provides
the metaphor of metaphors so to speak, as both stability and flux, order and
transgression" (Williams 1997, 1048). Bodies are at once concrete and malleable,
and when biomedicine is harnessed to the production of the hyperreal,
stricter codes of femininity can be imposed on the body. Despite women's awareness that much genital imagery is manufactured, hyperreality creates desire.

Cultural influence operates not only through symbols or models but also
through erasure or omission, through disappearing part of the range of what
is possible for bodies, resulting in some women feeling not only unfeminine
but also undesirable. Censorship and the regulation of visual imagery in mainstream media does not merely conceal the true range of genital variation; it
actively attempts to erase it, making the absence appear to be the normal state
of things—what female genitalia actually look like. Body image, therefore, is
influenced as much by what is *not* represented as by what is represented. With
regard to female genitalia, bodily erasure shapes individuals' expectations, and
the resultant pressure makes some women feel they need to eradicate what
makes them feel incomplete, different, or stigmatized. Culture, therefore, is
not merely what is positive or present; it is also conveyed through absences,

silences, and censure—the gaps in the symbolic system's account of reality. This visible evidence of lack often goes unacknowledged, especially in the case of the body. The fact that bigger women and women from different ethnic backgrounds are underrepresented in the mainstream media in Australia affects how women perceive their bodies and how they form their ideas of what is desirable, as does the ubiquitousness of the clean-slit image for genitalia.

This absence of female genitalia is eroticized and presented as desirable. Cosmetic surgery is predicated on the belief that it can turn the "unerotic into the erotic" (Gilman 1999, 207). At the same time as secondary sexual characteristics are eroticized, so too is genital absence. The clean-slit ideal is a paradox. It involves the eroticization of a desexualized but clearly feminized image: a woman with markers of her secondary sexual status—breasts, buttocks, and curves—heightened and exaggerated (with the exclusion of body hair) but with primary sexual markers—the vulva and vagina—reduced to absence. This paradox reinforces a concept of femininity as opposite to masculinity, contained and desirable but not desiring.

From an anthropological perspective, female genital cosmetic surgery can be understood as the ritual excision of a body part that has symbolically become the somaticized repository of a woman's psychic distress about her body and her sexuality. Genital cosmetic surgery is represented by some (academics, medics, laypersons) as excess, as irrational behavior. However, Susan Bordo (2003, 139) suggests that psychopathology also represents "the crystallization of culture." Mental health disorders (such as body dysmorphic disorder or anorexia) are not "aberrant and idiosyncratic features of pathological individuals" but instead offer "a window into a culture's pressures, incitements, history and structures of power" (Heyes 2009, 73), all of which have traditionally disadvantaged women. What we worry about, what we consider abnormal, is a window into our culture, into what we expect and consider appropriate. If, for instance, women such as Kylie and Mia are portrayed as almost pathological in their search for bodily perfection, then we shift our unease about cosmetic surgery from the practice itself and unfairly place it on its recipients. In this way, the overall cultural structure—its pressures and incitements—is left intact, ensuring that cosmetic surgery remains a desirable option for some women.

The effects of surgery are more than physiological; they demonstrate a concretization of bodily anxiety, which surgery (temporarily) expunges. Portions of the vulva are considered ugly or, following Mary Douglas (1966), polluted, and their excision allows a sense of control and relief, because bodily anxieties have been condensed onto the vulva as a source of unhappiness. I suggest that the so-called excess tissue of the vulva is not merely an issue of aesthetics; it has become a scapegoat for greater social anxieties, echoing other powerful techniques employed for mitigating suffering, fear, or pollution. The surgeons I interviewed acknowledged that female genital cosmetic surgery has symbolic qualities but only for women who have experienced sexual abuse. However, I believe that the symbolic nature of the invisible, intimate vulva extends beyond this to women who (perhaps because of comments they have received, language they have heard, or images they have seen) consider their genitalia unattractive or abnormal. There is a cultural insistence in the West on maintaining binary sex and gender categories, which female genital cosmetic surgery plays into— any protrusions are considered inappropriate and masculine. For women who choose genital cosmetic surgery, bodily concerns are projected onto the genitalia, and their genital anxiety personifies cultural pathology writ large.

Cosmetic surgery involves sacrifice; there is the risk of a loss of sensation, a poor result, embarrassment, and pain. However, sacrifices connote meaning. The rise of female genital cosmetic surgery as a treatment for a new anxiety and its inclusion into the "symptom pool" of culture (Shorter 1992, 5) exposes new forms of suffering. Articulating concerns about having a suboptimal vulva is a form of cultural communication. Bodily anxiety is not a new phenomenon; however, the availability of new medical technologies, such as female genital cosmetic surgery, and anxieties arise hand in hand. Anxiety is free-floating and turns back upon the self in a society where constant self-invention and transformation are valorized as indicating "a personal readiness for change, flexibility and adaptability" (Elliott 2008, 46), traits that mirror the wider economy. The medical profession is implicated in the rise of female genital cosmetic surgery as a solution to new symptoms of bodily distress because it determines which symptoms are declared valid and treatable (Watters 2010). Although many medical institutions consider female genital cosmetic surgery a worrying practice, it is a growing specialty avidly defended by its practitioners, reaffirming genital anxiety as a genuine concern for some women.

Janice Boddy describes female circumcision in Northern Sudan as a ritual experience that sacrifices sensation for heightened femininity: "The girl lies docile. . . . Her hands and feet are stained with henna applied the night before. Several kinswomen support her torso; two others hold her legs apart. Miriam [the midwife] thrice injects her genitals with local anesthetic, then, in the silence of the next few moments, takes a pair of scissors and quickly cuts away her clitoris and labia minora; the rejected tissue is caught in a bowl below the bed" (Boddy 1989, 50). I include Boddy's description of female circumcision not to be provocative but to draw an analogy between the ritual characteristics of female genital cutting (FGC) and female genital cosmetic surgery.

As with FGC, cosmetic surgery "provides a culturally meaningful ritual setting in which self-transformation can be enacted" (Huss-Ashmore 2000, 32).
Cosmetic surgery is often employed to mark significant life transitions, and
genital cosmetic surgery allows women to embark on their sexual lives with
increased confidence. Traditional rituals often enhance the body, making it
more (culturally) beautiful and endowing it with "erotic allure" (Edmonds
2010, 29). Employing the rhetoric of ritual enables a view of cosmetic surgery
as a practice that, despite its increasing naturalization and acceptance, is no
less exotic than FGC. I propose that cosmetic surgery be theorized as a form
of *ritualization*, a term proposed by Ronald Grimes to describe more prosaic
contemporary rituals as "activity that is not culturally defined as ritual but that
someone could interpret as if it were" (Grimes 2000, 28).

Critics of female genital cosmetic surgery see it as a nontraditional and
improper use of biomedical technology, too innovative, commercial, and
dangerously creative to be considered akin to traditional, socially inscribed
ritual. However, interpreting cosmetic surgery as ritual facilitates an understanding of why even the invisible, intimate vulva has been co-opted into
beauty regimens. Cosmetic surgery is a contemporary ritual undertaken at
the individual level. Ritual does not only involve tradition. For instance,
in Chad, FGC has been adopted as an innovative practice in a traditionally noncircumcising society—as a fashion and an expression of modernity
(Leonard, 2000). Ritual requires imagination and innovation. Contemporary
rituals (including cosmetic surgery) are performative practices that recom-
bine "traditional actions [or technologies] in new ways" (Schechner 1993, 228).
When biomedicine is used for ritualizing purposes, it becomes biomagical;
it is imbued with "mystical beings and powers" (Turner 1967, 19), and its
meaning therefore outstrips its corporeal potential. Looking at cosmetic
surgery as ritual highlights the sacred potential of medical authority in the
West, because medical opinions are generally considered sacrosanct, ensuring that the biomedical imaginary, that part of biomedicine that may be
fictitious but fuels desire (Walby 2000), is infused with possibility.

For women who choose female genital cosmetic surgery as part of their
individual projects of "care of the self", the practice has symbolic meaning. If
cosmetic surgery is a biomagical practice, should we then consider it deceptive, or does it gain legitimacy by promising transformation despite the dearth
of scientific evidence that it results in enduring satisfaction? I acknowledge
that there are multiple and contested realities that posit female genital cosmetic surgery as not merely a product of hegemonic medical practice but also
a consequence of consumerism producing desire and perhaps genuine medical

empathy concerning the plight of women and their wayward vulvas. However, the magic of cosmetic surgery is its ability to persuade its subjects to take the risks and endure the pain of surgery in their search for happiness, no matter how fleeting that happiness may be. Faith *is* placed in ritual practices, and a belief in change has enormous power to motivate women and persuade them to endure the pain and uncertainty of surgery. Rituals are often rites of passage. Some women choose genital cosmetic surgery in order to reclaim their bodies after negative comments, sexual abuse, childbirth, or failed relationships, or before reentering the sexual market. For others, it is an aspect of routine bodily maintenance. Ritual behaviors help make meaning out of life's exigencies; they facilitate a process of wresting back bodily control through transformation, the achievement of a new (more desirable) identity. Seeing female genital cosmetic surgery as a ritualizing experience focuses attention on the surgery itself, something that women often glossed over when they spoke of their surgery as a "quick" or "permanent" fix. Such language mirrors the before and after images that promote cosmetic procedures rather than emphasizing the pain and recovery that surgery entails.

As a practice, female genital cosmetic surgery crystallizes public concerns around the role of biomedicine in contemporary lives. As my observations of the cosmetogynecology congress reveal, powerful and authoritative voices are at play within the field of genital cosmetic surgery, and they have direct consequences for women concerned about their genital aesthetics and function. While the cosmetogynecology congress and other professional proceedings draw attention to the erection of boundaries and notions of brotherhood within the medical field, they also illustrate how the walls of the citadel are porous. Physicians must garner support for their practices if the subspecialty is to thrive. They accomplish this by publishing articles in academic journals, a practice that validates female genital cosmetic surgery as a legitimate form of medical intervention despite a paucity of data to substantiate this claim. Practitioners also generate support by being visible in the media and at medical congresses, as well as by lobbying professional bodies to recognize these new procedures (Martin 1998), often employing a rhetoric of listening to women and responding to women's needs. To survive, scientists must gather allies and create networks both within and outside the field of medicine, ensuring that the boundaries between science and culture are permeable. Surgeons respond to women and women respond to their surgeons in a shared social space. Therefore, physicians, patients, and the public are forever "forging ways of acting, being, and thinking in the world, or in other words, forging what anthropologists call culture" (Martin 1988, 28). Women's stories and representations found in the media, be they real or hyperreal, meld with science in the production of female genital cosmetic surgery as an emergent medical practice, ensuring that it is science responding to culture as much as its antithesis.

Emily Martin (1998, 29) has argued that "many powerful collectives and interested groups dot the landscape all around the citadel of science." Consequently, I propose that rather than being merely a citadel—an analogy appropriate to much of biomedicine—cosmetic surgery resembles a *rhizome*, in Gilles Deleuze and Félix Guattari's (1987) terms. There is no single identifiable cause and effect or beginning and end when biomedicine is entwined with beauty, which itself is a potent cultural construct. Female genital cosmetic surgery involves a multitude of players, and within this assemblage, power and influence operate on different levels (Deleuze and Guattari 1987). Interweaving women's narratives with medical perspectives and media representations exposes the always complex and changing cultural and social field in which concepts of the gendered body materialize in the early twenty-first century. "As a machinic assemblage, cosmetic surgery combines discourses, people (both as recipients and as professionals, such as doctors, lawyers, psychologists, advertising agents and scientists), equipment and locations (hospitals, clinics, courtrooms, etc.)" (Fraser 2003, 27).

Deleuze explains how cultural milieus are "worlds at once social, symbolic, and material, infused with the 'affects' and 'intensities' of their own subjectivities—and *trajectories*—or the journeys people take through milieus to pursue needs, desires, and curiosities or to simply try to find room to breathe beneath social constraints" (1997, cited in Biehl and Locke 2010, 323). Female genital cosmetic surgery provides some women with this "room to breathe beneath social constraints," and it provides a window into the social and cultural milieu in which women make meaning of their material bodies, their anxieties, and desires in relation to biomedical opportunities (magics), media influences, and social pressures at this particular time in history.

Female genital cosmetic surgery raises some ethical dilemmas. In countries such as Australia (and elsewhere in the West), the increased prevalence of the practice highlights an unevenness, where some (predominantly white) women are permitted to alter their genitalia for cultural reasons whereas women from circumcising societies now residing in Australia are not. Although there is no suggestion that adult women who seek cosmetic surgery need to be protected from themselves through legislation, women who choose to undergo FGC are seen as particularly vulnerable to culture from which they require legal protection and medical exclusion (Allotey, Manderson, and Grover 2001). If we consider female genital cosmetic surgery and FGC as being on a continuum of genital alterations—all of which involve ritual and sacrifice, cultural aesthetics, and therefore meaning—it becomes obvious that cultural coercion is implicated in both practices. The most obvious (and troubling) differences between these practices are those of age and consent, with FGC in practicing countries mostly performed on minors without their consent. However, an increasing number of Western mothers are now expressing concern about their daughters' genital aesthetics and taking them to see physicians (as was the case with Tara and Nell from chap. 2), and some adult women from circumcising backgrounds but living in the West seek FGC or reinfibulation in their countries of origin.

In the West, cosmetic surgery is viewed within a liberal humanist conception of the autonomous subject, where the individual is granted the right to make almost any choice regarding their bodily integrity. Seen through this prism, cosmetic surgery is the ultimate individual choice that reflects "a contemporary preoccupation with the self that is portrayed as entirely independent and internally located, rather than being a product of culture" (Fraser 2003, 86). However, the culture of the individual that underpins consumer-driven choice and into which cosmetic surgery taps is as culturally embedded as that of a community-based society practicing FGC whose members (also) operate in relational terms. Peer pressure works as forcefully in Western society as it does in non-Western settings, particularly in a makeover culture where working on the self, a certain amount of "good vanity," is expected.

Conforming to social ideals of acceptable or desirable femininity restricts other ways of being. Although some minorities may resist gender identity rules, "in all social settings, gender identity rules do not leave much room for 'choice,' whatever the dominant narrative says in the West" (Grande 2004, 7). For those who are anxious about their bodies, cosmetic surgery makes a more ideal body (and more ideal genitalia) attainable, and this puts pressure on women to conform to the ideal. In this sense, having more options paradoxically leads to women feeling they have less choice. If a more perfect body is possible in a makeover and consumer culture in which "care of the self" is valorized, pursuing this ideal becomes more likely. Not unlike FGC, female genital cosmetic surgery functions to produce a particular type of constrained female sexuality. Contradictorily, genital cosmetic surgery is promoted as increasing sexual confidence for Western women, which is assumed to be liberating, while at the same time, the media perpetuates a narrow version of female sexuality (and genital aesthetics) so that this version of femininity can reach a wide audience. Confining acceptable female sexuality to such a narrow range constrains and misrepresents women. Although female genital cosmetic surgery promises more, it delivers less by defining how women's genitalia should look and how women should respond sexually. There is no space for unbridled female sexuality, given that all sexuality is constrained by cultural gendered expectations.

Consequent to these impositions on female sexuality, female genital cosmetic surgery has become the focus of increasing but limited activism. The New View Campaign, established by Leonore Tiefer and based in New York, is particularly active in opposing the medicalization of sexuality, including unnecessary genital cosmetic surgery. *Centrefold*, an animated documentary about labiaplasty, was designed and directed by Ellie Land in the United Kingdom in 2012. It features the narratives of three women who have undergone labiaplasty. The documentary was funded by the Wellcome Trust to counter the rise in these procedures and includes interviews with Sarah Creighton and Lih-Mei Liao from University College London Hospitals.[1] In Australia, Women's Health Victoria has developed an issues paper with recommendations for further action and established the Labia Library, a website that confirms female genital diversity. Various medical bodies globally have produced guidelines and recommendations, but there has been no direct nonadvisory action (of which I am aware) dealing with the legal disparity between female genital cosmetic surgery and FGC. The consensus is that adult (Western) women should be able to choose what they do with their bodies, providing they have undergone psychological assessment, been made aware of genital diversity, been told of the risks of surgery, and ensured that the surgeons they consult have been properly trained. I have not been able to verify that any of these recommendations are guaranteed.

An examination of cosmetic surgery, particularly female genital cosmetic surgery, reveals that the role of medicine is constantly changing. Although biomedicine has historically exerted a strong influence on female sexuality in the West, the newer model of medicine with which women engage extends beyond management or healing to personal quality-of-life issues and the pursuit of beauty and happiness—concepts that are more subjective and difficult to define. This allows medicine to enter new spaces and find new opportunities for intervention. Female genitalia have provided such an opportunity. Breast augmentation, which started from a small base in the late nineteenth century, is one of the most prevalent forms of cosmetic surgery in the United States, Great Britain, and Australia today, and it has seen an exponential rise in the last fifty years. It is impossible to predict the future of female genital cosmetic surgery, but labiaplasty procedures in the United States increased by 23.2 percent in 2016 (ASAPS 2016), although figures vary, and an increasing number of physicians (36 percent of plastic surgeons in the United States, according to the 2016 American Society for Aesthetic Plastic Surgery report) offer these procedures globally. The International Society of Aesthetic Plastic Surgery reported a global increase in labiaplasties of 45 percent in 2016 (ASAPS 2016). Certainly, there appears to be a desire for an erotized female body today, one with an emphasis on breasts and buttocks. However, as Sander Gilman (1999, 206) posits, "Once the 'visible' body is seen to be mutable, and the patient is seen to be able to 'pass' 'in public,' then the 'hidden' aspects of the body become materials of the surgeon." This observation suggests that the invisible, intimate vulva may be a target for ongoing cosmetic attention.

When happiness can be attained through medical intervention, as is the case with cosmetic surgery, a consumer medical model emerges, and this creates incentives for finding new problems with body parts and bodily functions while simultaneously providing solutions to these problems. Offering procedures alleged to improve self-esteem can prey on the insecurities of vulnerable women, and using medicine to produce normal or ideal body parts undermines the range of acceptable difference. In this realm, medical ethics are colliding with commercial interests, new technologies, and cultural expectations of desirable femininity in complex ways that demand attention. The new biomedical model releases medicine from its rigid scientific underpinnings and exposes the practice of medicine as an increasingly cultural and commercial pursuit, one with important implications for women, and for men.

Although freedom from aesthetic ideals may theoretically be liberating, it is difficult to imagine a world without aesthetics, even though aesthetics are value judgments. In the West, new medical technologies combined with an increasingly persuasive media and a consumer-driven milieu *do* impinge on women's lives and increase the likelihood of more radical body alterations. Indeed, in the same manner as non-Western women's bodies are subject to their own cultural imperatives, it seems impossible to imagine a Western female body untouched by medicine, technology, consumerism, and specific regimens of femininity. Perhaps, as Deborah Covino (2004, 107) suggests, "resistance to social beauty norms should be one of the options that the industry sells; interpellation by the aesthetic surgical imaginary might then consist of a 'Hey, you there' accompanied by a menu of options that does not include body loathing." Unlike horse-riding, body loathing is not something women intentionally choose. Rather, it is subtly acquired. However, medicine (and aesthetics) can become entangled in both. I believe an informed woman should be free to decide for herself what she chooses to do with her body, but information today is both the solution and the problem. The "Hey, you there," the interpellation of the aesthetic surgical imaginary, is a loud shout, and the symbiosis between risk and pleasure is a potent aspect of human experience that is often played out through the body. The biomagical promise of female genital cosmetic surgery is seductive for some women and lucrative for physicians, and intimately bound up with gendered expectations and makeover culture. As such, it appears unlikely that the allure or magic of genital cosmetic surgery will fade away. Fashioning desirable femininity has a long history across cultures, and the rise of female genital cosmetic surgery fits perfectly within this paradigm.

NOTE

1. Creighton and Liao recently published the edited volume Female Genital Cosmetic Surgery: Solution to What Problem? (2019). Also in 2019, Camille Nurka published Female Genital Cosmetic Surgery: Deviance, Desire and the Pursuit of Perfection. Both these books provide valuable insights into the practice of female genital cosmetic surgery and highlight the increasing concern regarding these procedures.

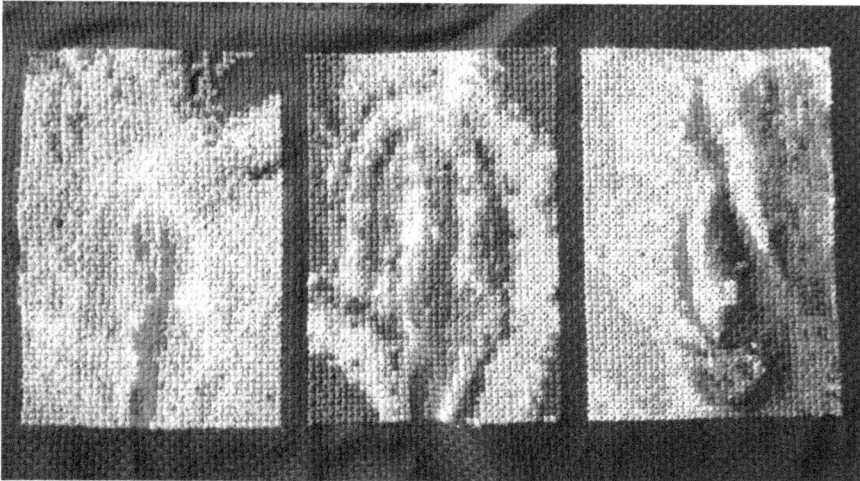

Figure 5.1. "The vulva is under increasing aesthetic scrutiny," closeup of *Bitches Get Stitches* by Jessy Jetpacks, 2016. Reproduced with permission from J. E. Challenger.

APPENDIX 1

Details of Women Interviewees Who Had Undergone or Were Contemplating Female Genital Cosmetic Surgery

Table 1. Age, marital status, and parity of women informants

Name	Age	Marital status	Number of children
Mandy	29	Married	3
Tara	22	Single	0
Nell	18	Single	0
Jane	59	Single	1
Kylie	30	Single	0
Mia	34	Married	2
Bella	26	De facto	0
Ann	52	Single	4
Hilda	41	Single	1
Parintin	40	Married	3
Cassie	26	De facto	0
A	46	Partner	0
B	26	Married	1
C	26	Married	2
D	21	Single	0
E	54	Partner	2
F	30	Married	3

(Continued)

Table 1. Age, marital status, and parity of women informants (*Continued*)

Name	Age	Marital status	Number of children
G	44	Single	0
H	44	In relationship	4
I	27	Married	0
J	24	Single	0
K	22	Single	0
L	49	Single	0
M	25	Partner	2
N	17	Single	0
O	23	Single	0
P	31	Dating	2
Q	79	Married	2
R	31	Partner	0
S	36	Married	1
T	24	Single	0
U	52	Single	0
V	29	Partner	0
X	41	Single	1
Y	25	Partner	2
Z	18	Single	0
a	20	Boyfriend	0
b	16	Single	0
c	19	Single	0
d	42	Single	0

Table 2. Summary of women interviewees by age, marital status, parity, and occupation.

Characteristic	Number of women
Age (years)	
17–24	12
25–34	14
35–44	7
45–54	5
55+	3
Marital status	
Married	9
Partner/de facto/boyfriend	10
Single	20
Number of children	
>2	6
2	7
1	5
0	23
Occupation*	
Student	9
Psychologist	5
Administrator	
Human resources manager	2
Business/development manager	2
Sales manager	2
Nurse/Health worker	2
Retired	2
Homemaker	2
Air traffic controller	1
Health foods and supplements salesperson	1
Personal trainer/life coach	1
Barrister	1
Veterinary surgeon	1
Civil servant	1
Travel industry salesperson	1

* Not all noninterviewed women gave their occupation.

APPENDIX 2

Questionnaire for Women Undergoing or Contemplating Female Genital Cosmetic Surgery

To complete the questionnaire, please place an X in the appropriate box for each question or write in the space provided. If you feel comfortable contacting me, I would love to speak with you, anonymously of course, so that I can better gain an idea of why some women think female genital cosmetic surgery is a good choice for them. If you would rather speak with me than fill out this questionnaire, please contact me at lindy.mcdougall@mq.edu.au and I will call you back. If you would rather complete this questionnaire online, please go to http://www.surveymonkey.com/s/genitalcosmeticsurgery. All information I receive from you will be treated as strictly confidential. There is no need to give your name.

1. Your details:

How old are you? _____

What is your occupation/profession? _____

What is your ethnic background? _____

Are you single or do you have a partner? Single [ ] Partner [ ]

Do you have children, and if so, how many? Yes [ ] No [ ] _____

---

2. What type of surgery have you had or are you considering?

_____

3. How did you find out about genital cosmetic surgery?
   Magazines [　] 　 Television programs (please specify)

   _____

   Friend(s)　[　]　Partner　[　]　Doctor　[　]　Other

   _____

4. Were you concerned about the risks of surgery?

   _____

   Has there been any pain (beyond what you expected from surgery) or any loss of sensitivity?

   _____

   How was the healing process?

   _____

5. Were alternatives to surgery suggested for your problem?
   　　　　　　　　　　　　　　　　　　Yes　[　]　No [　]
6. Did you discuss your surgery with your partner or family before deciding to undergo the procedure?
   　　　　　　　　　　　　　　　　　　Yes　[　]　No [　]
   Details:

   _____

   _____

7. Have you had previous cosmetic surgery?
   　　　　　　　　　　　　　　　　　　Yes　[　]　No [　]
8. Have you wanted to have genital surgery for a long time?
   　　　　　　　　　　　　　　　　　　Yes　[　]　No [　]
9. Are you happy with the results of your surgery?
   　　　　　　　　　　　　　　　　　　Yes　[　]　No [　]

   ┌───┐
   │ **I am interested in the _reasons_ why women are prepared to have** │
   │ **cosmetic surgery, particularly on their genitals.** │
   └───┘

10. Why did you decide to have surgery?

    _____

    _____

    _____

11. Would you say the decision to have this type of surgery was essentially a private one? Was it to please you alone or also, perhaps, to please your partner?

_____

_____

_____

12. If you have a regular partner, have they noticed/commented on your new look? Please describe.

_____

_____

_____

13. Did you have surgery to return to the look you had when you were younger?

Yes [ ] No [ ]

14. Did you have surgery because of the effects of childbirth on your body?

Yes [ ] No [ ]

15. Do you think that having a caesarian section may have led to less stress on your vulva and vagina and, therefore, fewer problems in this area?

_____

_____

_____

> **As women, we spend a lot of time working on our bodies. It seems women have become more _worried_ about the appearance of their genitals recently and are more prepared to discuss this and take action.**

16. Have you ever felt ashamed or embarrassed about the appearance of your body, particularly your genitals?

Yes [ ] No [ ]

Comments:

_____

_____

_____

17. Did you have surgery to make your genitals look more **normal**?

_____

_____

_____

18. If so, where did you get your idea of what normal genitals look like?

_____

_____

19. How do you look different in the genital area since you have had surgery?

_____

_____

_____

20. Have you ever had a Brazilian wax?

                          Yes [ ] No [ ]

21. Do you think there is a link between images in pornographic material and the desire for women to alter the appearance of their genitals?

                          Yes [ ] No [ ]

Comments:

_____

_____

_____

22. Have you seen many advertisements for genital cosmetic surgery or read articles about the available procedures, and if so, where?

_____

_____

_____

_____

> **I am interested in how we, as women, view ourselves as _sexual beings_ and how we might use genital surgery to fashion our sexuality.**

23. Did you have surgery to enhance the appearance of your genitals, to make you feel more feminine, or so that you look more like other women?

_____

_____

_____

24. Were you persuaded to have surgery in order to be more attractive to men (or, if you are homosexual, to be more attractive to women)?

_____
_____
_____

25. Have you experienced increased sexual satisfaction since your surgery? If so, why do you think that is?

_____
_____
_____

26. Thank you for completing this survey. Any further comments about your personal experience or views of genital surgery would be much appreciated. Please add them here.

_____
_____
_____
_____
_____
_____
_____
_____
_____
_____
_____
_____

If you are happy for me to contact you so that I can better understand your point of view, please leave your details here and I will get back to you.

_____
_____

Many thanks,
Lindy

REFERENCES

Abbie, K. 2009. "My Vagina Stinks." Yahoo! Answers. Yahoo.com. Accessed June 3, 2013. https://answers.yahoo.com/question/index?qid= 20090223222424AA7J40Q.

Adams, Alice. 1997. "Molding Women's Bodies: The Surgeon as Sculptor." In *Bodily Discursions: Gender, Representations, Technologies*, edited by Deborah Wilson and Christine Laennec, 59–80. Albany: State University of New York Press.

Adams, Tim. 2003. "The Skin We Are In." *The Observer*, October 26, 2003. Accessed June 6, 2016. https://observer.guardian.co.uk/bodyuncovered/story /0,,1067744,00.html.

Aesthetica. 2012. Aesthetica Image Centre. Accessed May 20, 2013. https:// aesthetica.com.au/.

Albury, Katherine, Catharine Lumby, and Alan McKee. 2008. *The Porn Report*. Melbourne: Melbourne University Press.

Alinsod, Red. 2013. "Labiaplasty Photo Gallery." South Coast Urogynecology. Accessed November 29, 2013. https://urogyn.org/avs_minora/.

Allotey, Pascale, Lenore Manderson, and Sonia Grover. 2001. "The Politics of Female Genital Surgery in Displaced Communities." *Critical Public Health* 11 (3): 189–201.

Alter, Gary. 2008. "Home Page." Gary J Alter, MD, Beverly Hills, California. Accessed August 7, 2008. https://www.altermd.com/services/.

American College of Obstetricians and Gynecologists. 2007. "Vaginal 'Rejuvenation' and Cosmetic Vaginal Procedures." ACOG Committee Opinion No. 378. ACOG. Washington, DC. Accessed September 6, 2009. https://www .acog.org/Resources_And_Publications/Committee_Opinions/Committee _on_Gynecologic_Practice/Vaginal_Rejuvenation_and_Cosmetic_Vaginal _Procedures.

American Psychiatric Association. 2013. *Diagnostic and Statistical Manual of Mental Disorders,* 5th ed. Washington, DC: American Psychiatric Association.

American Society for Aesthetic Plastic Surgery. 2016. "Cosmetic Surgery National Data Bank Statistics." ASAPS. Accessed September 20, 2017. https://www.surgery.org/sites/default/files/ASAPS-Stats2016.pdf.

American Society of Plastic Surgeons. 2020. "Vaginal Rejuvenation: Surgical Options." Accessed August 25, 2020. https://www.plasticsurgery.org/cosmetic-procedures/vaginal-rejuvenation/labiaplasty.

Angier, Natalie. 1999. *Woman: An Intimate Geography.* New York: Anchor Books.

Armstrong, Jennifer. 2008. "Vagina Anxiety: The Rise of the Labiaplasty." *Sirens,* June 24, AlterNet. Accessed May 1, 2013. https://www.alternet.org/.

Ashong, Ashong, and Herbert Batta. 2013. "Sensationalising the Female Pudenda: An Examination of Public Communication of Aesthetic Genital Surgery." *Global Journal of Health Science* 5 (2): 153–65.

Attorney-General's Department. 2005. Office of Legislative Drafting and Publishing. *Guidelines for the Classification of Publications 2005* (consolidated March 19, 2008, Canberra, Australia). Accessed December 3, 2012. https://www.comlaw.gov.au/Series/F2005L01285.

Australasian College of Cosmetic Surgery. 2012. "About ACCS." Australasian College of Cosmetic Surgery. Accessed May 12, 2012. https://www.accs.org.au/about/the-college.

Australian Bureau of Statistics. 2012. 4364.0.55.001—Australian Health Survey: First Results, 2011–12. Accessed September 5, 2013. https://www.abs.gov.au/ausstats/abs@.nsf/Lookup/4364.0.55.001Chapter1002011–12.

Australian Government, Department of Communications and the Arts. 2015. "Classifications for Publications Including Magazines." Accessed July 20, 2018. http://www.classification.gov.au/Guidelines/Pages/Guidelines.aspx.

Australian Health Ministers' Advisory Council. 2011. "Cosmetic Medical and Surgical Procedures: A National Framework Final Report." Australian Health Ministers' Conference, 2011. Accessed June 6, 2013. https://www.health.nsw.gov.au/publications/Documents/cosmetic-surgery.pdf.

Baker, Katie. 2013. "Popular Cosmetic Procedure Called 'The Barbie' Hacks Off Women's Labia So She's Smooth Like a Doll." *Jezebel,* January 28. Accessed February 8, 2013. https://www.alternet.org/culture/popular-cosmetic-procedure-called-barbie-hacks-womens-labia-so-shes-smooth-doll.

Baker Brown, Isaac. 1866. *On the Curability of Certain Forms of Insanity, Epilepsy, Catalepsy and Hysteria in Females.* London: Robert Hardwick.

Bakhtin, Mikhail. 1984. *Rabelais and His World.* Translated by Hélène Iswolsky. Bloomington: Indiana University Press.

Balsamo, Anne. 1992. "On the Cutting Edge: Cosmetic Surgery and the Technological Production of the Gendered Body." *Camera Obscura* 28:206–37.

Barnes, Andrew, and Yvonne Lumsden. 2010. *Heart of the Flower: The Book of Yonis*. Brisbane: Pangia.

Bartholomeusz, Hugh. 2012. "The Need for Regulation of Office-Based Procedures: Closing a Regulatory Gap to Ensure Patient Safety in All Surgical Procedures." *Medical Journal of Australia* 196 (8): 492–93.

Bataille, Georges. 1985. *Visions of Excess: Selected Writings, 1927–1939*. Translated by Allan Stoekl. Minneapolis: University of Minnesota Press.

Bates, Betsy. 2010. "Controversy Rages over Female Genital Cosmetic Surgery." *Ob.Gyn. News*, 45 (3). Accessed June 9, 2012. http://www.lvratlanta.com/pdf /OB%20Gyn%20News%20Cosmetic%20Controversy%20March%202010%5B2 %5D-2-1.pdf.

Battaglia, Cesare, Bruno Battaglia, Paolo Busacchi, Roberto Paradisi, Maria Meriggiola, and Stefano Venturoli. 2013. "2D and 3D Ultrasound Examination of Labia Minora." *Archives of Sexual Behaviour* 42:153–60.

Baudrillard, Jean. 1994. *Simulacra and Simulation*. Translated by Sheila Glaser. Ann Arbor: University of Michigan Press.

Bell, Kirsten. 2005. "Genital Cutting and Western Discourses on Sexuality." *Medical Anthropology Quarterly* 19 (2): 125–48.

Belt, Paul. 2013. *Taboo Tuesday: Labiaplasty*. Radio 612 ABC, Brisbane, October 1. Accessed November 11, 2013. http://blogs.abc.net.au/queensland/2013/10/taboo -tuesday-labiaplasty.html.

Berger, John. 1972. *Ways of Seeing*. London: Penguin Books.

Better Health Channel. 2012. "Body Dysmorphic Disorder (BDD)." State Government of Victoria. Accessed December 10, 2012. http://www.better health.vic.gov.au/bhcv2/bhcarticles.nsf/pages/Body_dysmorphic_disorder _(BDD).

Biehl, João, and Peter Locke. 2010. "Deleuze and the Anthropology of Becoming." *Current Anthropology* 51 (3): 317–51.

Blackledge, Catherine. 2003. *The Story of V: Opening Pandora's Box*. London: Weidenfeld and Nicolson.

Blank, Joani. 2011. *Femalia*. San Francisco: Last Gasp.

Blum, Virginia. 2003. *Flesh Wounds: The Culture of Cosmetic Surgery*. Berkeley: University of California Press.

Boddy, Janice. 1989. *Wombs and Alien Spirits: Women, Men, and the Zār Cult in Northern Sudan*. Madison: University of Wisconsin Press.

———. 2007. "Gender Crusades: The Female Circumcision Controversy in Cultural Perspective." In *Transcultural Bodies: Female Genital Cutting in Global Context*, edited by Y. Hernland and B. Shell-Duncan, 46–66. New Brunswick, NJ: Rutgers University Press.

———. 2016. "The Normal and the Aberrant in Female Genital Cutting." *Hau: Journal of Ethnographic Theory* 6 (2): 41–69.

Boellstorff, Tom. 2008. *Coming of Age in Second Life: An Anthropologist Explores the Virtually Human*. Princeton, NJ: Princeton University Press.

Bonavoglia, Angela. 2010. "Cosmetic Vaginal Surgeons Clueless about Female Sexuality." *Huffington Post*, February 24. Accessed May 24, 2011. http://www.huffingtonpost.com/angela-bonavoglia/cosmetic-vaginal-surgeons_b_475929.html.

Bordo, Susan. 2003. *Unbearable Weight: Feminism, Western Culture and the Body*. Berkeley: University of California Press.

Bramwell, Ros. 2002. "Invisible Labia: The Representation of Female External Genitals in Women's Magazines." *Sexual and Relationship Therapy* 17 (2): 187–90.

Bramwell, Ros, and Claire Morland. 2009. "Genital Appearance Satisfaction in Women: The Development of a Questionnaire and Exploration of Correlates." *Journal of Reproductive and Infant Psychology* 27 (1): 15–27.

Bramwell, Ros, Claire Morland, and Anne Garden. 2007. "Expectations and Experience of Labial Reduction: A Qualitative Study." *BJOG: An International Journal of Obstetrics and Gynaecology* 114 (12): 1493–9.

Braun, Virginia. 2005. "In Search of (Better) Sexual Pleasure: Female Genital 'Cosmetic' Surgery." *Sexualities* 8 (4): 407–24.

———. 2008. "Making Sense of Female Genital Alteration Practices." Women's Health Action, Auckland. Accessed October 10, 2013. https://www.womens-health.org.nz/.

———. 2009a. "'The Women Are Doing It for Themselves': The Rhetoric of Choice and Agency around Female Genital 'Cosmetic Surgery.'" *Australian Feminist Studies* 24 (60): 233–49.

———. 2009b. "Selling the 'Perfect' Vulva." In *Cosmetic Surgery: A Feminist Primer*, edited by Meredith Jones and Cressida Heyes, 133–49. Farnham, UK: Ashgate.

———. 2010. "Female Genital Cosmetic Surgery: A Critical Review of Current Knowledge and Contemporary Debates." *Journal of Women's Health* 19 (7): 1393–407.

———. 2012. "Female Genital Cutting around the Globe: A Matter of Reproductive Justice?" In *Reproductive Justice: A Global Concern*, edited by Joan Chrisler, 29–55. Santa Barbara, CA: Praeger.

Braun, Virginia, and Celia Kitzinger. 2001a. "The Perfectible Vagina: Size Matters," *Culture, Health and Sexuality* 3 (3): 263–77.

———. 2001b. "'Snatch,' 'Hole,' or 'Honey-Pot'? Semantic Categories and the Problem of Nonspecificity in Female Genital Slang." *The Journal of Sex Research* 38 (2): 146–58.

Braun, Virginia, and Leonore Tiefer. 2010. "The 'Designer Vagina' and the Pathologisation of Female Genital Diversity: Interventions for Change." *Radical Psychology* 8 (1): 1–19.

Braun, Virginia, and Sue Wilkinson. 2001. "Socio-cultural Representations of the Vagina." *Journal of Reproduction and Infant Psychology* 19 (1): 17–32.

Brookman, Nicole. 2011. "My Problem with #whitegirlproblems." *Huffington Post*, December 1. Accessed December 3, 2012. https://www.huffing tonpost.com/nicole-brookman/my-problem-with-whitegirl _b_1121382.html.

Bucher, Rue, and Anselm Strauss. 1961. "Professions in Process." *American Journal of Sociology* 66 (4): 325–34.

Budgeon, Shelley. 2003, "Identity as an Embodied Event." *Body and Society* 9 (1): 35–55.

Buhlmann, Ulrike, Nancy Etcoff, and Sabine Wilhelm. 2008. "Facial Attractiveness Ratings and Perfectionism in Body Dysmorphic Disorder and Obsessive-Compulsive Disorder." *Journal of Anxiety Disorders* 22:540–7.

Buni, Catherine. 2013. "The Case for Teaching Kids 'Vagina,' 'Penis,' and 'Vulva,'" *The Atlantic*, April 15. Accessed June 4, 2013. https://www.theatlantic.com/health/archive/2013/04/the-case-for-teaching-kids-vagina-penis-and-vulva/274969/.

Butler, Judith. 1990. "Performative Acts and Gender Constitution: An Essay in Phenomenology and Feminist Theory." In *Performing Feminisms: Feminist Critical Theory and Theatre*, edited by Sue-Ellen Case, 270–82. Baltimore, MD: Johns Hopkins University Press.

Canguilhem, Georges. 1978. *On the Normal and the Pathological.* Translated by Carolyn Fawcett. Dordrecht, NL: Reidel.

Caplan, Arthur, and Carl Elliott. 2004. "Is It Ethical to Use Enhancement Technologies to Make Us Better than Well?" *PLoS Medicine* 1 (3): 172–5.

Chang, Peter, Mark Salisbury, Thomas Narsete, Randy Buckspan, Dustin Derrick, and Robert Ersek. 2013. "Vaginal Labiaplasty: Defense of the Simple 'Clip and Snip' and a New Classification System." *Aesthetic Plastic Surgery* 37 (5): 887–91.

Clarke, Adele, Janet Shim, Laura Mamo, Jennifer Fosket, and Jennifer Fishman. 2003. "Biomedicalization: Technoscientific Transformations of Health, Illness, and U.S. Biomedicine." *American Sociological Review* 68 (2): 161–94.

Cleo. 2008. "Cleo Sex: The Hottest Bedside Guide Ever." *Cleo*, April, 104–9. Australia: ACP Magazines.

Cohen, Lawrence. 1995. "The Epistemological Carnival: Meditations on Disciplinary Intentionality and Āyurveda." In *Knowledge and the Scholarly Medical Traditions*, edited by Don Bates, 320–43. Cambridge, UK: Cambridge University Press.

Coman, Mihai. 2013. "Media Anthropology: An Overview." Working paper. Accessed June 24, 2013. http://www.philbu.net/media-anthropology/coman _maoverview.pdf.

Conrad, Peter. 2005. "The Shifting Engines of Medicalization." *Journal of Health and Social Behavior* 46:3–14.

Conroy, Ronán. 2006. "Female Genital Mutilation: Whose Problem, Whose Solution?" *British Medical Journal* 333:106–7.

Corrina, Heather. 2008. "Give 'Em Some Lip: Labia That Clearly Ain't Minor." Scarleteen. Accessed August 26, 2013. http://www.scarleteen.com/article/advice/giveem_some_lip_labia_that_clearly_aint_minor.

Cosmopolitan. 2012a. "What Do You Like to Find When You Head Down There?" Issue 463, February. Sydney: Hearst/Bauer Media.

———. 2012b. "The Last Taboo: Your Body Map." Issue 464, March. Sydney: Hearst/Bauer Media.

———. 2013. "Hooray for a Fresh Hoo-ha." Issue 479, June. Sydney: Hearst/Bauer Media.

Cosmos Clinic. 2013. "Vaginal Cosmetic Surgery—Labiaplasty." Cosmos Clinic. Accessed June 6, 2013. https://www.cosmosclinic.com.au/body/vaginal-cosmetic-surgery/.

Coventry, Martha. 2000. "Making the Cut." *Ms. Magazine*, Oct./Nov. Arlington: Liberty Media for Women. Accessed January 1, 2013. https://www.msmagazine.com/octoo/makingthecut.html.

Covino, Deborah. 2004. *Amending the Abject Body: Aesthetic Makeovers in Medicine and Culture.* Albany: State University of New York Press.

Crawford, Robert. 1994. "The Boundaries of the Self and the Unhealthy Other: Reflections on Health, Culture and AIDS." *Social Science and Medicine* 38 (10): 1347–65.

Creighton, Sarah M., and Lih-Mei Liao, eds. 2019. *Female Genital Cosmetic Surgery: Solution to What Problem?* Cambridge, UK: Cambridge University Press.

Crerand, Canice, Martin Franklin, and David Sarwer. 2006. "Body Dysmorphic Disorder and Cosmetic Surgery." *Plastic and Reconstructive Surgery* 118 (7): 167–80.

Crouch, Naomi, Rebecca Deans, Lina Michala, Lih-Mei Liao, and Sarah Creighton. 2011. "Clinical Characteristics of Well Women Seeking Labial Reduction Surgery: A Prospective Study." *BJOG* 118 (12): 1507–10.

Culbertson, Philip. 1998. "Designing Men: Reading the Male Body as Text." *The Journal of Textual Reasoning* 7. Accessed May 10, 2012. https://jtr.shanti.virginia.edu/designing-men-reading-the-male-body-as-text/.

Cynthia Rowland Beauty Systems. 2014. "Luscious Lips: Naturally Gorgeous Lips at Your Fingertips." Accessed February 15, 2014. https://www.cynthiarowland.com/luscious-lips/.

D'Arcy-Tehan, Frances. 2011. "Genital Image Perceptions amongst Australian Women and Attitudes towards FGCS." International Society of Cosmetic

Gynecology. *World Congress on Female and Male Cosmetic Genital Surgery,* September 29 and 30, and October 1 [DVD]. United States: ISCG.

Davis, Kathy. 1991. "Remaking the She-Devil: A Critical Look at Feminist Approaches to Beauty." *Hypatia* 6:21–43.

———. 1995. *Reshaping the Female Body: The Dilemma of Cosmetic Surgery.* New York: Routledge.

———. 2003. *Dubious Equalities and Embodied Differences: Cultural Studies on Cosmetic Surgery.* Lanham, MD: Rowman and Littlefield.

Davis, Lennard. 1995. *Enforcing Normalcy: Disability, Deafness, and the Body.* London: Verso.

Davis-Floyd, Robbie. 1994. "The Rituals of American Hospital Birth." In *Conformity and Conflict: Readings in Cultural Anthropology,* 8th ed., edited by David McCurdy, 323–40. New York: Harper Collins. Accessed November 19, 2013. http://davis-floyd.com/the-rituals-of-american-hospital-birth/.

Davison, Steven, and Jorge de la Torre. 2011. "Labiaplasty and Labia Minora Reduction." Medscape Reference, WebMD. Accessed July 19, 2013. https://emedicine.medscape.com/article/1372175-overview#showall.

de Waal Malefyt, Timothy. 2017. "Enchanting Technology." *Anthropology Today* 33 (2): 1–2.

Deleuze, Gilles, and Félix Guattari. 1987. *A Thousand Plateaus.* Translated by Brian Massumi. Minneapolis: University of Minnesota Press.

Dickinson, Robert Latou. 1949. *Atlas of Human Sex Anatomy,* 2nd ed. Baltimore, MD: Williams and Wilkins.

Dictionary.com. 2014. *The American Heritage® Stedman's Medical Dictionary.* Houghton Mifflin Company. Accessed December 1, 2013. https://dictionary.reference.com/browse/pudenda.

Dines, Gail. 2010. *Pornland: How Porn Has Hijacked Our Sexuality.* Boston: Beacon.

Dissident X. 2010. "Is There a Beautiful Vulva and Ugly Vulva. What Does a Perfect Vulva Look Like?" [post to online forum], Yahoo! Answers, Yahoo. com. Accessed June 28, 2012. https://answers.yahoo.com/question/index?qid=20100720032729AASRoex.

Dobbeleir, Julie, Koenraad van Landuyt, and Stan Monstrey. 2011. "Aesthetic Surgery of the Female Genitalia." *Seminars in Plastic Surgery* 25:130–41.

Dodson, Betty. 1974. *Sex for One: The Joy of Selfloving.* New York: Three Rivers.

Dorneles de Andrade, Daniela. 2010. "On Norms and Bodies: Findings from Field Research on Cosmetic Surgery in Rio de Janeiro, Brazil." *Reproductive Health Matters* 18 (35): 74–83.

Douglas, Mary. 1966. *Purity and Danger: An Analysis of Concepts of Pollution and Taboo.* London: Routledge and Kegan Paul.

Downey, Gary, and Joseph Dumit. 1997. "Locating and Intervening: An Introduction." In *Cyborgs and Citadels: Anthropological Interventions in Emerging Sciences and Technologies*, edited by Gary Downey and Joseph Dumit, 5–29. Santa Fe, NM: School of American Research Press.

Drysdale, Kirsten. 2010. "Healing It to a Single Crease." *Hungry Beast* blog. Accessed July 21, 2010. http://hungrybeast.abc.net.au/blog/kdrysdale/healing -it-single-crease (site discontinued).

Eagleton, Terry. 1981. *Walter Benjamin or Towards a Revolutionary Criticism.* London: Verso Books.

Eaves III, Felmont, Rod Rohrich, and Jonathan Sykes. 2013. "Taking Evidence-Based Plastic Surgery to the Next Level: Report of the Second Summit on Evidence-Based Plastic Surgery." *Aesthetic Surgery Journal* 33 (5): 735–43.

Eco, Umberto. 1984. "The Frames of Comic 'Freedom.'" In *Carnival!* edited by Thomas Sebeok, 1–9. Berlin: Mouton.

Edmonds, Alexander. 2007. "'The Poor Have the Right to Be Beautiful': Cosmetic Surgery in Neoliberal Brazil." *Journal of the Royal Anthropological Institute* 13:363–81.

———. 2009. "'Engineering the Erotic': Aesthetic Medicine and Modernization in Brazil." In *Cosmetic Surgery: A Feminist Primer*, edited by Meredith Jones and Cressida Heyes, 153–69. Farnham, UK: Ashgate.

———. 2010. *Pretty Modern: Beauty, Sex, and Plastic Surgery in Brazil.* Durham, NC: Duke University Press.

———. 2012. "A Right to Beauty." Anthrownow.com. Accessed December 30, 2013. http://anthronow.com/print/alex-edmonds-a-right-to-beauty.

———. 2013a. "Can Medicine Be Aesthetic? Disentangling Beauty and Health in Elective Surgeries." *Medicine Anthropology Quarterly* 27 (2): 233–52.

———. 2013b. "The Biological Subject of Aesthetic Medicine." *Feminist Theory* 14 (1): 65–82.

Elliott, Anthony. 2008. *Making the Cut: How Cosmetic Surgery Is Transforming Our Lives.* London: Reaktion Books.

Elliott, Carl. 2003. *Better than Well: American Medicine Meets the American Dream.* New York: W. W. Norton and Company.

Ellis, Havelock. 1900. *Studies in the Psychology of Sex.* Vol. 2, *Sexual Inversion.* London: Watford University Press.

Ensler, Eve. 2001. *The Vagina Monologues: The V-Day Edition.* New York: Villard.

Esteem Cosmetic Studio. 2013. "Labiaplasty." Esteem Cosmetic Studio. Accessed August 30, 2013. http://www.esteemstudio.com.au/body/labiaplasty.

Fausto-Sterling, Anne. 2000. *Sexing the Body: Gender Politics and the Construction of Sexuality.* New York: Basic Books.

Fishman, Jennifer. 2006. "Making Viagra: From Impotence to Erectile Dysfunction." In *Medicating Modern America*, edited by Andrea Tone and Elizabeth Siegel Watkins, 229–52. New York: New York University Press.

Foucault, Michel. 1973. *The Birth of the Clinic: An Archaeology of Medical Perception*. Translated by Alan Sheridan Smith. London: Tavistock.

———. 1977. *Discipline and Punish: The Birth of the Prison*. Translated by Alan Sheridan. New York: Vintage Books.

———. 1978. *The Will to Knowledge*. Vol. 1, *The History of Sexuality*. Translated by Robert Hurley. London: Penguin Books.

———. 1980. *Power/Knowledge: Selected Interviews and Other Writings 1972–1977*, Brighton, UK: The Harvester.

———. 1988. "Technologies of the Self." In *Technologies of the Self: A Seminar with Michel Foucault*, edited by Luther Martin, Huck Gutman, and Patrick Hutton, 16–49. Amherst: University of Massachusetts Press.

Franco, T., and Franco, D. 1993. "Hipertrofia de Ninfas." *Jornal Brasileiro de Ginecologia* 103 (5): 163–5.

Frank, Arthur. 2002. "What's Wrong with Medical Consumerism?" In *Consuming Health: The Commodification of Health Care*, edited by Saras Henderson and Alan Petersen, 13–30. London: Routledge.

Fraser, Suzanne. 2003. *Cosmetic Surgery, Gender and Culture*. Basingstoke, UK: Palgrave Macmillan.

Freedman, Mia. 2009. "Genital Surgery: Two Words You Don't Want to Read in the Same Sentence," Mamamia, November 30. Accessed December 3, 2012. https://www.mamamia.com.au/news/genital-surgery-two-words-you-dont -want-to-read-in-the-same-sentence/.

Freud, Sigmund. 1905. *Three Essays on the Theory of Sexuality*. Vol. 7 of *The Standard Edition of the Complete Psychological Works of Sigmund Freud*. Translated and edited by James Strachey. London: Hogarth.

Gagne, Patricia, and Deanna McGaughey. 2002. "Designing Women: Cultural Hegemony and the Exercise of Power among Women Who Have Undergone Elective Mammoplasty." *Gender and Society* 16 (6): 814–38.

Gawande, Atul. 2003. *Complications: A Surgeon's Notes on an Imperfect Science*. New York: Picador.

Geest, Sjaak van der, and Susan Whyte. 1989. "The Charm of Medicines: Metaphors and Metonyms." *Medical Anthropology Quarterly* 3 (4): 345–67.

Gell, Alfred. 1988. "Technology and Magic." *Anthropology Today* 4 (2): 6–9.

Giddens, Anthony. 1991. *Modernity and Self-Identity: Self and Society in the Late Modern Age*. Cambridge, UK: Polity.

Gieryn, Thomas. 1983. "Boundary-Work and the Demarcation of Science from Non-science: Strains and Interests in Professional Ideologies of Scientists." *American Sociological Review* 48 (6): 781–95.

Gillespie, Rosemary. 1997. "Women, the Body and Brand Extension in Medicine." *Women and Health* 24 (4): 69–85.

Gilman, Sander. 1999. *Making the Body Beautiful: A Cultural History of Aesthetic Surgery*. Princeton, NJ: Princeton University Press.

Gimlin, Debra. 2000. "Cosmetic Surgery: Beauty as Commodity." *Qualitative Sociology* 23 (1): 77–98.

———. 2010. "Imagining the Other in Cosmetic Surgery." *Body and Society* 16 (4): 57–76.

Good, Byron. 1994. *Medicine, Rationality, and Experience: An Anthropological Perspective.* Cambridge, UK: Cambridge University Press.

Goodman, Michael. 2011. "Female Genital Cosmetic and Plastic Surgery: A Review." *Journal of Sexual Medicine* 8 (6): 1813–25.

———. 2014. "Labiaplasty." Dr. Michael Goodman. Accessed March 6, 2014. http://www.drmichaelgoodman.com/labiaplasty-california/.

Goodman, Michael, Samantha Fashler, John Miklos, Robert Moore, and Lori Brotto. 2011. "The Sexual, Psychological, and Body Image Health of Women Undergoing Elective Vulvovaginal Plastic/Cosmetic Procedures: A Pilot Study." *The American Journal of Cosmetic Surgery* 28 (4): 219–226.

Goodman, Michael, Otto Placik, David Matlock, Alex Simopoulos, Teresa Dalton, David Veale, and Susan Hardwick-Smith. 2016. "Evaluation of Body Image and Sexual Satisfaction in Women Undergoing Female Genital Plastic/Cosmetic Surgery." *Aesthetic Surgery Journal.* Accessed June 3, 2016. doi:10.1093/asj/sjw061, 1–10.

Good Medicine. 2003. "Designer Vagina Chat Transcript." Good Medicine chat room, ninemsn, November 21. Accessed June 6, 2013. http://health.ninemsn.com.au/azindex/688918/designer-vagina-chat-transcript (site discontinued).

Grande, Elisabetta. 2004. "Hegemonic Human Rights and African Resistance: Female Circumcision in a Broader Comparative Perspective." *Global Jurist Frontiers* 4 (2). Accessed January 29, 2014. doi:10.2202/1535-1653.1145.

Green, Fiona. 2005. "From Clitoridectomies to 'Designer Vaginas': The Medical Construction of Heteronormative Female Bodies and Sexuality through Female Genital Cutting." *Sexualities, Evolution and Gender* 7 (2): 153–87.

Greer, Germaine. 2000. *The Whole Woman.* New York: Anchor Books.

———. 2006. *The Female Eunuch.* London: Harper Perennial.

Grimes, Ronald. 2000. *Deeply into the Bone: Re-inventing Rites of Passage.* Berkeley: University of California Press.

Grosz, Elizabeth. 1994. *Volatile Bodies: Toward a Corporeal Feminism.* Bloomington: Indiana University Press.

Hacking, Ian. 1996. "Normal People." In *Modes of Thought: Explorations in Culture and Cognition,* edited by David Olson and Nancy Torrance, 59–71. Cambridge, UK: Cambridge University Press.

Hald, Gert. 2006. "Gender Differences in Pornography Consumption among Young Heterosexual Danish Adults." *Archives of Sexual Behavior* 35:577–85.

Healy, David. 2006. "The New Medical Oikumene." In *Global Pharmaceuticals: Ethics, Markets, Practices*, edited by Adriana Petryna, Andrew Lakoff, and Arthur Kleinman, 61–84. Durham, NC: Duke University Press.

Herbenick, Debby, and Vanessa Schick. 2011. *Read My Lips: A Complete Guide to the Vagina and Vulva*. Lanham, MD: Rowman and Littlefield.

Herbenick, Debby, Vanessa Schick, Michael Reece, Stephanie Sanders, and James Fortenberry. 2010. "Pubic Hair Removal among Women in the United States: Prevalence, Methods, and Characteristics." *Journal of Sexual Medicine* 10:3322–30.

Heyes, Cressida. 2007a. *Self-Transformations: Foucault, Ethics and Normalised Bodies*. Oxford: Oxford University Press.

———. 2007b. "Cosmetic Surgery and the Televisual Makeover: A Foucauldian Feminist Reading." *Feminist Media Studies* 7 (1): 17–32.

———. 2007c. "Normalisation and the Psychic Life of Cosmetic Surgery." *Australian Feminist Studies* 22 (52): 55–71.

———. 2009. "Diagnosing Culture: Body Dysmorphic Disorder and Cosmetic Surgery." *Body and Society* 15:73–93.

Hodgkinson, Darryl, and Glen Hait. 1984. "Aesthetic Vaginal Labiaplasty." *Plastic and Reconstructive Surgery* 74 (3): 414–6.

Hogle, Linda. 2005. "Enhancement Technologies and the Body." *Annual Review of Anthropology* 34:695–716.

Holliday, Ruth, and Jacqueline Sanchez Taylor. 2006. "Aesthetic Surgery as False Beauty." *Feminist Theory* 7 (2): 179–95.

Honi Soit. 2013. "The Vagina Dialogues." August 21. University of Sydney Students' Representative Council, Sydney. Accessed September 1, 2013. http://www.honisoit.com/2013/08/the-vagina-dialogues/.

Horin, Adele. 2007. "One in Three Porn Viewers Are Women." *Sydney Morning Herald*, May 26. Accessed June 28, 2013. https://www.smh.com.au/articles/2007/05/25/1179601669066.html.

Horton, Richard. 1995. "Georges Canguilhem: Philosopher of Disease." *Journal of the Royal Science of Medicine* 88:316–9.

Howarth, Helena, Volker Sommer, and Fiona Jordan. 2010. "Visual Depictions of Female Genitalia Differ Depending on Source." *Journal of Medical Ethics: Medical Humanities* 36:75–9.

Hoy, David. 1999. "Critical Resistance: Foucault and Bourdieu." In *Perspectives on Embodiment: The Intersections of Nature and Culture*, edited by Gail Weiss and Honi Fern Haber, 3–22. New York: Routledge.

Huss-Ashmore, Rebecca. 2000. "'The Real Me': Therapeutic Narrative in Cosmetic Surgery." *Expedition* 42 (3): 26–38.

ISAPS. 2016. *International Study on Aesthetic/Cosmetic Procedures Performed in 2016*, International Society of Aesthetic Plastic Surgery. Accessed July 15, 2018. https://www.isaps.org/wp-content/uploads/2017/10/GlobalStatistics2016-1.pdf.

ISCG. 2008. International Society of Cosmetic Gynecology. Accessed April 17, 2012. http://www.iscgyn.com/en/aboutus.

J Sisters. 2012. "About." J Sisters. Accessed December 2, 2013. http://jsisters.com /history/ (site discontinued).

Jarrin, Alvaro. 2012. "The Right to Beauty: Cosmetic Citizenship and Medical Modernity in Brazil." Exchange, Department of Anthropology University of Chicago. Accessed May 10, 2012. http://www.academia.edu/9286492/The _Right_to_Beauty_Cosmetic_Citizenship_and_Medical_Modernity_in _Brazil.

Jemison, Micaela. 2012. "Rise in Women Seeking 'Designer Vagina.'" *Sydney Morning Herald*, November 21. Accessed September 2, 2013. https://www.smh .com.au/national/rise-in-women-seeking-designer-vagina-20121120-2903h.html.

Jenks, Chris. 2003. *Transgression*. London: Routledge.

Joe. 2013. "Is Hypertrophy of Labia Minora Normal Thing?" [Response to online forum post, updated November 25] SteadyHealth.com, London. Accessed September 2, 2013. https://www.steadyhealth.com/Is_hypertrophy_of_labia _minora_normal_thing__t53844.html#402471.

Jones, Bethany, and Camille Nurka., 2015. "Labiaplasty and Pornography: A Preliminary Investigation." *Porn Studies* 2 (1). doi:10.1080/23268743.2014 .984940.

Jones, Julie, and Jayne Raisborough. 2007. "Introduction: Situating Risk in the Everyday." In *Risk, Identities and the Everyday*, edited by Julie Jones and Jayne Raisborough, 1–18. Farnham, UK: Ashgate.

Jones, Meredith. 2008. *Skintight: An Anatomy of Cosmetic Surgery*. Oxford: Berg.

———. 2012. "The Body in Popular Culture." In *Being Cultural*, edited by Bruce Cohen, 193–209. Pearson, NZ: Auckland.

Karim, Tazin. 2012. "Medical Imaginaries and Technological Futures: Transformations of Subjectivities in Biomedicine." Somatosphere. Accessed June 8, 2012. http://somatosphere.net/2012/06/medical-imaginaries-and -technological-futures-transformations-of-subjectivities-in-biomedicine.html.

Karras, Nick. 2003. *Petals: The Journey into Self Discovery*. San Diego: Crystal River.

Kaw, Eugenia. 1993. "Medicalization of Racial Features: Asian American Women and Cosmetic Surgery." *Medical Anthropology Quarterly* 7 (1): 74–89.

Kapsalis, Terri. 1997. *Public Privates: Performing Gynecology from Both Ends of the Speculum*. Durham, NC: Duke University Press.

Kessler, Suzanne. 1998. *Lessons from the Intersexed*. New Brunswick, NJ: Rutgers University Press.

Kilbourne, Jean. 2010. *Killing Us Softly 4: Advertising's Image of Women*. Northampton, MA: Media Education Foundation.

Kipnis, Laura. 1993. *Ecstasy Unlimited: On Sex, Capital, Gender, and Aesthetics*. Minneapolis: University of Minnesota Press.

Kirtley, Chris. 1996. "Aboriginal Rock Art." *Tracce*, July 15. Footsteps of Man Archaelogical Society, Valcamonica. Accessed June 3, 2013. http://www.rupestre.net/tracce/?p=848.

Kittay, Eva. 2006. "Thoughts on the Desire for Normality." In *Surgically Shaping Children: Technology, Ethics, and the Pursuit of Normality*, edited by Erik Parens, 90–110. Baltimore, MD: Johns Hopkins University Press.

Kline, Wendy. 2010. *Bodies of Knowledge: Sexuality, Reproduction, and Women's Health in the Second Wave*. Chicago: University of Chicago Press.

Koning, Merel, Ingeborg Anne Zeijlmans, Theo Kornelis Bouman, and Berend van der Lei. 2009. "Female Attitudes Regarding Labia Minora Appearance and Reduction with Consideration of Media Influence." *Aesthetic Surgery Journal* 29 (1): 65–71.

Konrat, Georgina. 2014. "Secret Women's Business: Labiaplasty Surgery (Part 3)." Brisbane Cosmetic Clinic. Accessed April 22, 2013. https://brisbanecosmetic.com.au/secret-womens-business-labiaplasty-surgery-part-3/.

Kristeva, Julia. 1982. *Powers of Horror: An Essay on Abjection*. Translated by Leon Roudiez. New York: Columbia University Press.

Labia Library. 2017. Accessed August 20, 2017. http://www.labialibrary.org.au/.

Lakoff, George, and Mark Johnson. 1980. *Metaphors We Live By*. Chicago: University of Chicago.

Lappen, Justin, and Dana Gossett. 2010. "Changes in Episiotomy Practice: Evidence-Based Medicine in Action." *Expert Reviews Obstetrics and Gynecology* 5 (3): 301–9.

Laqueur, Thomas. 1990. *Making Sex: Body and Gender from the Greeks to Freud*. Cambridge, MA: Harvard University Press.

Lasch, Christopher. 1979. *The Culture of Narcissism: American Life in an Age of Diminishing Expectations*. New York: W. W. Norton.

Laser Vaginal Rejuvenation Institute. 2013. Laser Vaginal Rejuvenation Institute and VASER Hi Def Liposculpturing Institute of Beverley Hills. Accessed December 29, 2013. https://www.drmatlock.com/.

Lee, Marie. 2011. "Designer Vagina Surgery: Snip, Stitch, Kerching!" *The Guardian*, October 15. Accessed December 10, 2013. https://www.theguardian.com/lifeandstyle/2011/oct/14/designer-vagina-surgery.

Leonard, Lori. 2000. "Interpreting Female Genital Cutting: Moving beyond the Impasse." *Annual Review of Sex Research* 11 (1): 158–90.

Lerner, Harriet Goldhor. 1994. "And What Do Little Girls Have?" *Agenda: Empowering Women for Gender Equity*, Body Politics 23: 30–32.

Lévi-Strauss, Claude. 1969. *The Elementary Structures of Kinship*. Edited by Rodney Needham. Translated by James Bell and John von Sturmer. Boston: Beacon.

Liao, Lih-Mei, Lina Michala, and Sarah Creighton. 2010. "Labial Surgery for Well Women: A Review of the Literature." *BJOG* 117 (1): 20–25.

Liao, Lih-Mei, Neda Taghinejadi, and Sarah Creighton. 2012. "An Analysis of the Content and Clinical Implications of Online Advertisements for Female Genital Cosmetic Surgery." *BMJ Open*. Accessed January 28, 2013. doi:10.1136/bmjopen-2012-001908.

Likes, Wendy, Mario Sideri, Hope Haefner, Patricia Cunningham, and Francesca Albani. 2008. "Aesthetic Practice of Labial Reduction." *Journal of Lower Genital Tract Disease* 12 (3): 201–16.

Lloyd, Jillian, Naomi Crouch, Catherine Minto, Lih-Mei Liao, and Sarah Creighton. 2005. "Female Genital Appearance: 'Normality' Unfolds." *BJOG* 112:643–6.

Lock, Margaret, and Vinh-Kim Nguyen. 2010. *An Anthropology of Biomedicine*. Chichester, UK: Wiley-Blackwell.

Lorde, Audre. 1990. "Age, Race, Class, And Sex: Women Redefining Difference." In *Out There: Marginalization and Contemporary Cultures*, edited by Russell Ferguson, Martha Gever, Trinh Minh-ha, and Cornel West, 281–7. Cambridge, MA: MIT Press.

Mackenzie, Jean. 2017. "Vagina Surgery 'Sought by Girls as Young as Nine'." Accessed August 20, 2017. https://www.bbc.com/news/health-40410459.

Malone, Jessica. 2013. "Women and Genital Cosmetic Surgery." (Women's Health Issues Paper No. 9). Women's Health Victoria, Melbourne. Accessed February 15, 2013. https://whv.org.au/static/files/assets/ca7e9b2f/Women-and-genital-cosmetic-surgery-issues-paper.pdf.

Manderson, Lenore. 2004. "Local Rites and Body Politics: Tensions between Cultural Diversity and Human Rights." *International Feminist Journal of Politics* 6 (2): 285–307.

———. 2011. *Surface Tensions: Surgery, Bodily Boundaries, and the Social Self*. Walnut Creek, CA: Left Coast.

———. 2012. "Material Worlds, Sexy Lives: Technologies of Sexuality, Identity and Sexual Health." In *Technologies of Sexuality, Identity and Sexual Health*, edited by Lenore Manderson, 1–15. London: Routledge.

Manderson, Lenore, and Margaret Jolly. 1997. "Introduction: Sites of Desire/Economies of Pleasure in Asia and the Pacific." In *Sites of Desire/Economies of Pleasure: Sexualities in Asia and the Pacific*, edited by Lenore Manderson and Margaret Jolly, 1–26. Chicago: University of Chicago Press.

Marie Claire. 2009. "The Surgery That Saved My Sex Life." *Marie Claire*, February. Accessed June 4, 2013. https://www.paulbelt.com.au/the_surgery_that_saved_my_sex_life.

Martin, Emily. 1992. "The End of the Body?" *American Ethnologist* 19 (1): 121–40.

———. 1998. "Anthropology and the Cultural Study of Science." *Science, Technology, and Human Values* 23 (1): 24–44.

———. 2001. *The Woman in the Body: A Cultural Analysis of Reproduction*. Boston: Beacon.

Mason, Paul. 2013. *Embodiment: When Culture Becomes Anatomy* [video]. Prezi Inc. Accessed November 10, 2013. http://prezi.com/73eanzacdsoc/embodiment/.

Mass, Sylvester, and Joris Hage. Hage. 2000, "Functional and Aesthetic Labia Minora Reduction." *Plastic and Reconstructive Surgery* 105 (4): 1453–56.

Masters, William, and Virginia Johnson. 1966. *Human Sexual Response*. Toronto: Bantam Books.

Mattingly, Cheryl. 2010. *The Paradox of Hope: Journeys through a Clinical Borderland*. Berkeley: University of California Press.

McCartney, Jamie. 2014. "Changing Female Body Image through Art." The Great Wall of Vagina, UK. Accessed March 10, 2014. http://www.greatwallofvagina.co.uk/home.

McMahen, Ben. 2012. *Saving Face: Shame and Bodily Abnormality*. Master's thesis, University of Alberta. Accessed September 1, 2013. https://era.library.ualberta.ca/public/view/item/uuid:490b9209-0fd3-4780-bdce-b26f6ab621b9.

Michala, Lina, Sofia Koliantzaki, and Aris Antsaklis. 2011. "Protruding Labia Minora: Abnormal or Just Uncool?" *Journal of Psychosomatic Obstetrics and Gynecology* 32 (3): 154–6.

Moen, M., O. Storroe, A. Spydslaug, and U. Kirste. 2006. "The Normal Vulva: Morphology, Acceptance and Complaints." Paper presented to the Xth European Pediatric and Adolescent Gynaecological Congress, Budapest, May 10–13, 2006.

Mol, Annemarie. 1998. "Lived Reality and the Multiplicity of Norms: A Critical Tribute to George Canguilhem." *Economy and Society* 27 (2–3): 274–84.

———. 2002. *The Body Multiple: Ontology in Medical Practice*. Durham, NC: Duke University Press.

Moran, Claire, and Christina Lee. 2013. "Selling Genital Cosmetic Surgery to Healthy Women: A Multimodal Discourse Analysis of Australian Surgical Websites." *Critical Discourse Studies* 10 (4): 373–91.

Morgan, Kathryn. 1991. "Women and the Knife: Cosmetic Surgery and the Colonization of Women's Bodies." *Hypatia* 6 (3): 25–53.

Moynihan, Ray. 2003. "The Making of a Disease: Female Sexual Dysfunction." *BMJ* 326 (7379): 45–47.

Mulvey, Laura. 1998. *Visual and Other Pleasures*. Bloomington: Indiana University Press.

Nader, Laura. 1969. "Up the Anthropologist: Perspectives Gained from 'Studying Up.'" In *Reinventing Anthropology*, edited by Dell Hymes, 284–311. New York: Random House.

Narayan, Kirin. 1993. "How Native Is a 'Native' Anthropologist?" *American Anthropologist* 95 (3): 671–86.

Negrin, Llewellyn. 2002. "Cosmetic Surgery and the Eclipse of Identity." *Body and Society* 8 (4): 21–42.

Neill, Sallie, and Fiona Lewis, eds. 2009. *Ridley's the Vulva*, 3rd ed. Chichester, UK: Wiley-Blackwell.

Nesbitt, Shawntelle. 2001. "Venus Figurines of the Upper Paleolithic." *Totem: The University of Western Ontario Journal of Anthropology* 9 (1): 53–64.

Nguyen, Anh. 2013. "Labiaplasty." Dr. Anh Nguyen. Accessed April 12, 2013. https://www.femaleplasticsurgeon.com.au/labiaplasty.

Nurka, Camille. 2019. *Female Genital Cosmetic Surgery: Deviance, Desire and the Pursuit of Perfection*. Cham, Switzerland: Palgrave Macmillan.

Nurka, Camille, and Bethany Jones. 2013. "Labiaplasty, Race and the Colonial Imagination." *Australian Feminist Studies* 28 (78): 417–42.

O'Donnell, Jayne. 2011. "State Laws on In-Office Surgeries." *USA Today*, December 28. Accessed May 25, 2012. https://www.usatoday.com/money/perfi/basics/story/2011-12-27/state-regulations-cosmetic-plastic-surgery-offices/52247588/1.

Opening Shot. 2013. Episode: "The Vagina Diaries." ABC Television, Australia, December 1. Accessed December 4, 2013. https://www.abc.net.au/tv/programs/vagina-diaries-opening-shot-2/.

Oranges, Carlo, Andrea Sisti, and Giovanni Sisti. 2015. "Labia Minora Reduction Techniques: A Comprehensive Literature Review." *Aesthetic Surgery Journal* 35 (4): 419–31.

Orbach, Susie. 1999. "Whose Body? The Politics of the Body and the Body Politic." Keynote address at The Body Culture Conference, the annual conference of Body Image and Better Health Inc. in conjunction with VicHealth. Melbourne, Australia.

O'Regan, Kirsten. 2013. "Labiaplasty." *Guernica*, January 16. Accessed June 3, 2014. https://www.guernicamag.com/daily/kirsten-oregan-labiaplasty-part-I.

Ostrzenski, Adam. 2011. "Cosmetic Gynecology in the View of Evidence-Based Medicine and the ACOG Recommendations: A review." *Archives of Gynecology and Obstetrics* 284:617–30.

Parker, Richard. 1997. "The Carnivalization of the World." In *The Gender and Sexuality Reader*, edited by Roger Lancaster and Micaela di Leonardo, 361–77. New York: Routledge.

Parker, Rhian. 2010. *Women, Doctors and Cosmetic Surgery: Negotiating the "Normal" Body*. Basingstoke, UK: Palgrave Macmillan.

Pazmany, Els, Sophie Bergeron, Lukas van Oudenhove, Johan Verhaeghe, and Paul Enzlin. 2013. "Body Image and Genital Self-Image in Pre-menopausal Women with Dyspareunia." *Archives of Sexual Behavior* 42:999–1010.

Petryna, Adriana, and Arthur Kleinman. 2006. "The Pharmaceutical Nexus." In *Global Pharmaceuticals: Ethics, Markets, Practices*, edited by Adriana Petryna, Andrew Lakoff, and Arthur Kleinman, 1–32. Durham, NC: Duke University Press.

Phillips, Katharine. 2012. "Body Dysmorphic Disorder." In *Encyclopedia of Body Image and Human Appearance*, edited by Thomas Cash, 74–81. Cambridge, MA: Academic.

Pitts-Taylor, Victoria. 2007. *Surgery Junkies: Wellness and Pathology in Cosmetic Culture*. New Brunswick, NJ: Rutgers University Press.

Priddy, Alexa, and Jennifer Croissant. 2009. "Designer Vaginas." In *The Body in Medical Culture*, edited by Elizabeth Klaver, 173–91. Albany: State University of New York Press.

Princeton University. 2013a. "Hypertrophy." WordNet, Princeton University. Accessed August 28, 2013. http://wordnetweb.princeton.edu/perl/webwn?s= hypertrophy.

———. 2013b. "Slit." WordNet, Princeton University. Accessed April 9, 2013. http://wordnetweb.princeton.edu/perl/webwn?s=slit&sub=Search+WordNet& o2=&oo=1&o8=1&o1=1&o7=&o5=&o9=&o6=&o3=&o4=&h.

Puppo, Vincenzo. 2013. "Anatomy and Physiology of the Clitoris, Vestibular Bulbs, and Labia Minora with a Review of the Female Orgasm and the Prevention of Female Sexual Dysfunction." *Clinical Anatomy* 26:134–52.

Quill Shiv. 2011. *Labiaplasty Circa 1992* (rough draft). Accessed July 10, 2013. https://quillshiv.com/2011/06/06/labiaplasty-circa-1992/.

Rabinow, Paul. 1997. "Science as a Practice: The Higher Indifference and Mediated Curiosity." In *Cyborgs and Citadels: Anthropological Interventions in Emerging Sciences and Technologies*, edited by Gary Downey and Joseph Dumit, 193–208. Santa Fe, NM: School of American Research Press.

Radiotherapy. 2013. Radio on Demand, RRR Radio, Brunswick East, Australia, July 21. https://ondemand.rrr.org.au.

Radman, H. Melvin. 1976. "Hypertrophy of the Labia Minora." *Obstetrics and Gynecology* 48 (1 Suppl.): 78s–80s.

Ramos, Carisse. 2011. *Fun with Dick and Little Susie: The Naming of Erogenous Zones*. Bachelor's thesis, The School of the Art Institute of Chicago. Accessed June 3, 2013. http://citeseerx.ist.psu.edu/viewdoc/download?doi=10.1.1.476.1491 &rep=rep1&type=pdf.

RANZCOG. 2016. Royal Australian and New Zealand College of Obstetricians and Gynaecologists, East Melbourne, Victoria. Accessed January 29, 2016. https://www.ranzcog.edu.au.

Rees, Emma. 2013. *The Vagina: A Literary and Cultural History*. New York: Bloomsbury Academic.

Reitsma, Welmoed, Marian Mourits, Merel Koning, Astrid Pascal, and Berend van der Lei. 2011. "No (Wo)man is an Island: The Influence of Physicians' Personal Predisposition to Labia Minora Appearance on Their Clinical Decision Making: A Cross-Sectional Survey." *Journal of Sexual Medicine* 8 (8): 2377–85.

Roberts, Celia. 2007. *Messengers of Sex: Hormones, Biomedicine and Feminism*. New York: Cambridge University Press.

Robertson, Wrenna. 2011. *I'll Show You Mine*. Vancouver: Show Off Books.

Rodrigues, Sara. 2012. "From Vaginal Exception to Exceptional Vagina: The Biopolitics of Female Genital Cosmetic Surgery." *Sexualities* 15 (7): 778–94.

Rose, Nikolas. 2007. *The Politics of Life Itself: Biomedicine, Power, and Subjectivity in the Twenty-First Century*. Princeton, NJ: Princeton University Press.

Rosewarne, Lauren. 2012. "Carefree Discharges the V-bomb: But Who's Afraid of the Word 'Vagina'?" The Conversation, July 17. Accessed July 18, 2012. https:// theconversation.com/carefree-discharges-the-v-bomb-but-whos-afraid-of-the -word-vagina-8281.

Ross, Carlin. 2012. "No Hair . . . No Lips . . . Just a Slit," Betty Dodson with Carlin Ross, 15 October. Accessed June 3, 2013. http://www.drjasonwinters.com/blogs /psychology-of-sexuality/2013/01/15/carlin-ross-on-labia.

Rothman, Sheila, and David Rothman. 2003. *The Pursuit of Perfection: The Promise and Perils of Medical Enhancement*. New York: Pantheon Books.

Rouzier, Roman, Christine Louis-Sylvestre, Bernard-Jean Paniel, and Bassam Haddad. 2000. "Hypertrophy of the Labia Minora: Experience with 163 Reductions." *American Journal of Obstetrics and Gynecology* 182 (1): 35–40.

Russo, Mary. 1994. *The Female Grotesque: Risk, Excess and Modernity*. New York: Routledge.

Ryle, John. 1947. "The Meaning of Normal." *The Lancet* 249 (6436), originally published as 1 (6436): 1–5.

Sager, Dorianne. 1999. "Designer Vaginas: A Story Every Reporter Wants to Get Into." PSURG Cosmetic SurgicentreTM. Accessed June 14, 2013. http://www .psurg.com/ubc99.html.

Said, Edward. 1978. *Orientalism*. London: Routledge and Kegan Paul.

Sandel, Michael. 2004. "The Case against Perfection: What's Wrong with Designer Children, Bionic Athletes, and Genetic Engineering." *The Atlantic Monthly*, 293(3) 51–62. Accessed April 8, 2013. https://www.theatlantic.com/magazine /archive/2004/04/the-case-against-perfection/302927/.

Schechner, Richard. 1993. *The Future of Ritual: Writings on Culture and Performance*. London: Routledge.

Scheper-Hughes, Nancy, and Margaret Lock. 1987. "The Mindful Body: A Prolegomenon to Future Work in Medical Anthropology." *Medical Anthropology Quarterly* 1 (1): 6–41.

Schober, Justine, Timothy Cooney, Donald Pfaff, Lazarus Mayoglou, and Nieves Martin-Alguacil. 2010. "Innervation of the Labia Minora of Prepubertal Girls." *Journal of Pediatric Adolescent Gynecology* 23:352–57.

Sedgwick, Eve Kosofsky. 1985. *Between Men: English Literature and Male Homosocial Desire*. New York: Columbia University Press.

Sexpo. 2013. Accessed June 1, 2013. https://www.sexpo.com.au.

Shorter, Edward. 1992. *From Paralysis to Fatigue: A History of Psychosomatic Illness in the Modern Era*. New York: The Free Press.

Shweder, Richard. 2015. "Doctoring the Genitals: Towards Broadening the Meaning of Social Medicine." *The Journal of Clinical Ethics* 26 (2): 176–79.

Sinclair, Douglas. 2005. "Subspecialization in Emergency Medicine: Where Do We Go from Here?" *Canadian Journal of Emergency Medicine* 7 (5): 344–46.

Sinha-Roy, Piya. 2012. "Got White Girl Problems? Babe Walker Does, Too." Reuters, US, February 17. Accessed June 25, 2012. https://www.reuters.com /article/2012/02/17/us-whitegirlproblems-book-idUSTRE81G1XA20120217.

Somazone. 2012. Australian Drug Foundation, Melbourne. Accessed July 13, 2013. http://www.somazone.com.au/index.php?option=com_questions&task=view _detail&id=1448 (site discontinued).

Sontag, Susan. 1978. *Illness as Metaphor*. New York: Vintage.

Spitulnik, Debra. 1993. "Anthropology and the Mass Media." *Annual Review of Anthropology* 22:293–315.

Spitzack, Carole. 1988. "The Confession Mirror: Plastic Images for Surgery." *Canadian Journal of Political and Social Theory* XII (1–2): 38–50.

Spriggs, Merle, and Lynn Gillam. 2016. "Body Dysmorphic Disorder: Contradiction or Ethical Justification for Female Genital Cosmetic Surgery in Adolescents." *Bioethics* 30 (9): 706–713.

Squier, Susan. 2004. *Liminal Lives: Imagining the Human at the Frontiers of Biomedicine*. Durham, NC: Duke University Press.

Stradwick, Luke. 2009. "For Fracs Sake, Before Undergoing Cosmetic Surgery, Make Sure Your Surgeon Is Qualified." Accessed March 15, 2014. https://www .drlukestradwick.com.au/fracs-sake-undergoing-plastic-surgery-make-sure -plastic-surgeon-qualified/.

Strong, Thomas. 2007. *How to Attend a Conference in a Couple Hours*. Savage Minds: Notes and Queries in Anthropology [blog]. Accessed March 1, 2016. https://savageminds.org/2007/10/02/how-to-attend-a-conference-in-a-couple -hours.

Tanner, Claire, JaneMaree Maher, and Suzanne Fraser. 2013. *Vanity: 21st Century Selves*. Basingstoke, UK: Palgrave Macmillan.

Taussig, Michael. 2012. *Beauty and the Beast*. Chicago: University of Chicago Press.

Teens Health. 2008. "Do I Smell—And Can People Tell?" The Nemours Foundation, Jacksonville, FL. Accessed August 6, 2008. https://kidshealth.org /teen/sexual_health/girls/feminine_hygiene.html.

The Perfect Vagina. 2008. Channel 4 Television Corporation, UK, Top Documentary Films. Accessed March 7, 2009. https://topdocumentaryfilms .com/perfect-vagina/.

Tiefer, Leonore. 1996. "The Medicalization of Sexuality: Conceptual, Normative, and Professional Issues." *Annual Review of Sex Research* 7:252–82.

———. 2008. "Female Genital Cosmetic Surgery: Freakish or Inevitable? Analysis from Medical Marketing, Bioethics, and Feminist Theory." *Feminism and Psychology* 18:466–79.

Tiggemann, Marika, and Suzanna Hodgson. 2008. "The Hairlessness Norm
    Extended: Reasons for and Predictors of Women's Body Hair Removal at
    Different Body Sites." *Sex Roles* 59:889–97.
Triffin, Molly. 2010. "Warning: These Doctors May Be Dangerous to Your Vagina."
    Cosmopolitan, July: 159–161. Accessed February 19, 2014. http://i.imgur.com
    /AowC6.jpg.
Turkle, Sherry. 2008. "Always-On/Always-On-You: The Tethered Self." In
    Handbook of Mobile Communication Studies and Social Change, edited by James
    Katz, 121–37. Cambridge, MA: MIT Press.
Turner, Victor. 1967. *The Forest of Symbols: Aspects of Ndembu Ritual*. Ithaca, NY:
    Cornell University Press.
Urla, Jacqueline, and Jennifer Terry. 1995. "Introduction: Mapping Embodied
    Deviance." In *Deviant Bodies: Critical Perspectives on Difference in Science
    and Popular Culture*, edited by Jennifer Terry and Jacqueline Urla, 1–18.
    Bloomington: Indiana University Press.
Veale, David, Ertimiss Eshkevari, Nell Ellison, Ana Costa, Dudley Robinson,
    Angelica Kavouni, and Linda Cardozo. 2014. "A Comparison of Risk Factors
    for Women Seeking Labiaplasty Compared to Those Not Seeking Labiaplasty."
    Body Image 11:57–62.
Venganai, Hellen. 2016. "Negotiating Identities through the 'Cultural Practice'
    of Labia Elongation among Urban Shona Women and Men in Contemporary
    Zimbabwe." *Culture Unbound* 8 (3): 306–24.
Walby, Cathy. 2000. *The Visible Human Project: Informatic Bodies and Posthuman
    Medicine*. London: Routledge.
Walker, Babe. 2012. *White Girl Problems*. New York: Hyperion.
Wall, Shelley. 2010. "Humane Images: Visual Rhetoric in Depictions of Typical
    Genital Anatomy and Sex Differentiation." *Journal of Medical Ethics* 36:80–83.
Washabaugh, William. 2005. "The Carnival Model." In *A Life of Response: American
    Cultural Anthropology*, edited by William Washabaugh. Accessed May 3, 2012.
    https://pantherfile.uwm.edu/wash/www/102_18.htm.
Waterland, Rosie. 2013. "So I Have an Outie Vagina and I'm Meant to Feel Bad
    about It?" Mamamia, January 3. Accessed June 4, 2013. https://www.mamamia
    .com.au/social/let-it-all-hang-outie/.
Watters, Ethan. 2010. *Crazy like Us: The Globalization of the American Psyche*. New
    York: The Free Press.
Weil Davis, Simone. 2002. "Loose Lips Sink Ships." *Feminist Studies* 28 (1): 7–37.
Werner, Philip. 2013. *101 Vagina*. Melbourne: Taboo Books.
Whitcomb, Maureen. 2011. "Bodies of Flesh, Bodies of Knowledge:
    Representations of Female Genital Cutting and Female Genital Cosmetic
    Surgery." Honors thesis, State University of New York. Accessed October 10,
    2013. https://www.albany.edu/honorscollege/theses.php.

Wikimedia Commons. 2013. By Vagina039.jpg: Londoner500 Derivative Work: Lamilli (Vagina039.jpg) [Public domain]. Accessed December 29, 2013. https://commons.wikimedia.org/wiki/File:Vulva_labeled_english.jpg.

Wilding, Faith. 2001. "Vulvas with a Difference." In *Domain Errors! Cyberfeminist Practices*, edited by Maria Fernandez, Faith Wilding, and Michelle Wright. Autonomedia. Accessed August 9, 2008. https://www.obn.org/reading_room/writings/html/vulvas.html.

Williams, Simon. 1997. "Modern Medicine and the 'Uncertain Body': From Corporeality to Hyperreality?" *Social Science and Medicine* 45 (7): 1041–9.

Wolf, Naomi. 2012. *Vagina: A New Biography.* New York: HarperCollins.

Women's Health Queensland Wide Inc. 2007. "Genital Cosmetic Surgery." *Health Journey* 4:1–4.

World Health Organization. 2014. "Female Genital Mutilation." Fact Sheet No 241. Accessed November 20, 2013. https://www.who.int/mediacentre/factsheets/fs241/en/.

Wynn, Lisa, Angel Foster, and James Trussell. 2010. "Would You Say You Had Unprotected Sex If . . . ? Sexual Health Language in Emails to a Reproductive Health Website." *Culture, Health and Sexuality* 12 (5): 499–514.

Yang, Claire, Christopher Cold, Ugur Yilmaz, and Kenneth Maravilla. 2005. "Sexually Responsive Vascular Tissue of the Vulva." *BJU International* 97:766–72.

INDEX

Page numbers in *italics* refer to figures.

lesbian women, 102–3
Lévi-Strauss, Claude, 180
Liao, Lih-Mei, 19, 69–70, 211
Lim, Dr. (research participant), 70
liminality, 39–42
liposuction, 15
Lloyd, Jillian, 104, 105
Lock, Margaret, 190
Lorde, Audre, 102
Love Me (Nelson), *199*
Lumby, Catharine, 56, 60

magazines, 33–34, 47, 63, 97–99. *See also*
pornography; women's magazines
Maher, JaneMaree, 146
MakeMeHeal (message board), 131
makeover culture: the biomagical and, 68;
concept of, 21; mainstream media and, 62;
self-enhancement and self-transformation
and, 29, 123, 151–52, 159; technologies of
the self and, 146–49
male gaze, 51, 178, 179–80
male genital cosmetic surgery, 160
male genitalia, 33
Mamamia (women's website), 64–65
Manderson, Lenore, 12, 21, 22, 23, 44, 194
Mandy (woman informant): cosmetic
surgery as rite of passage and, 25; on
genital anxiety, 107; genital anxiety
and, 23; men and, xi–xvi; on pubic hair
removal, 47–48
Marcos, Dr. (medical informant), 43, 142–43,
153–54
Marie Claire (magazine), 65–66
Martin, Emily, 27, 78, 208, 209
Masters, William, 55
masturbation, 55
Matlock, David, 69, 137, 168, 185, 195
Mattingly, Cheryl, 7
McCartney, Jamie, *1*
McGaughey, Deanna, 179, 180
McKee, Alan, 56, 60
media: clean-slit aesthetic ideal and, 34,
62–67, 73–74, 203, 204–5; criticisms of
female genital cosmetic surgery in,
186–87; genital normality and, 97–103;
ideals of genital beauty and, 175;

influence of, 130–31, 133. *See also* internet;
magazines; pornography; television
Medical Board of Australia, 67
medical congresses: brotherhood and,
191–94, 196, 198; carnival and, 188–91, 198;
global reach of, 195–97; as performative,
197–99. *See also* World Congress on
Female and Male Cosmetic Genital
Surgery (Las Vegas, 2011)
medical gaze, 178–80
medical informants, gynecologists: on
age and cosmetic surgery, 90, 91–92; on
asymmetry, 106; on congresses, 195–97;
on genital aesthetics, 176; on labiaplasty,
36; on normality, 91–92; observation and
interviews with, 6, 9–10
medical informants, plastic and cosmetic
surgeons: on adolescent girls, 87–89;
advertising and, 66–67; on age and
cosmetic surgery, 17, 91, 94; on board
certification, 172; on body dysmorphic
disorder, 142; on childbirth, 92; on clean-
slit aesthetic ideal, 41; on cosmetic surgery
as fashion, 152–53; on doctor–patient
relationship, 140–41; on female genital
cutting, 134; on female sexuality, 153–54;
on feminism, 55; on genital aesthetics,
73, 175; on genital anxiety, 67–68, 109; on
hypertrophy, 105–6; on labial protrusion,
44–45, 102; on labia majora augmentation,
43; on labiaplasty, 36; on mainstream
media, 63; on normality, 103–4;
observation and interviews with, 6, 9–10;
on psychological assessments, 142–43;
on pubic hair removal, 46; on reasons for
cosmetic surgery, 19–20, 39; on reasons for
labiaplasty, 106–9
medicalization, 26–28, 211. *See also*
biomedicine
Medical Journal of Australia (journal), 172–73
medical profession: clean-slit aesthetic ideal
and, 67–73; doctor–patient relationship
and, 140–41. *See also* biomedicine;
cosmetic surgery; female genital cosmetic
surgery
medical tourism, 15
Medicare (Australia), 16, 17, 72, 106

LINDY McDOUGALL is Honorary Postdoctoral Fellow in Anthropology at Macquarie University in Sydney, Australia.

www.ingramcontent.com/pod-product-compliance
Lightning Source LLC
Chambersburg PA
CBHW020528270326
41927CB00006B/488